Dendrimers in Biomedical Applications

Dendrimers in Biomedical Applications

Edited by

Barbara Klajnert
University of Lodz, Poland

Ling Peng
Centre Interdisciplinaire de Nanoscience de Marseille, France
Email: ling.peng@univmed.fr

Valentín Ceña
Universidad de Castilla-La Mancha, Albacete, Spain

RSCPublishing

This work is a publication of the COST Action Group TD0802

ISBN: 978-1-84973-611-4

A catalogue record for this book is available from the British Library

Published by The Royal Society of Chemistry,
Thomas Graham House, Science Park, Milton Road,
Cambridge CB4 0WF, UK

Registered Charity Number 207890

Visit our website at www.rsc.org/books

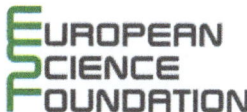

EUROPEAN
SCIENCE
FOUNDATION

ESF provides the COST Office through an EC contract

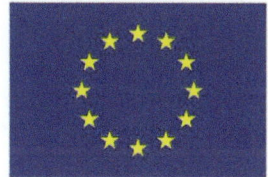

COST is supported by the EU RTD Framework programme

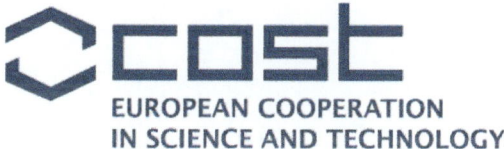

**EUROPEAN COOPERATION
IN SCIENCE AND TECHNOLOGY**

COST – the acronym for European Cooperation in Science and Technology- is the oldest and widest European intergovernmental network for cooperation in research. Established by the Ministerial Conference in November 1971, COST is presently used by the scientific communities of 36 European countries to cooperate in common research projects supported by national funds.

The funds provided by COST - less than 1% of the total value of the projects - support the COST cooperation networks (COST Actions) through which, with EUR 30 million per year, more than 30 000 European scientists are involved in research having a total value which exceeds EUR 2 billion per year. This is the financial worth of the European added value which COST achieves.

A "bottom up approach" (the initiative of launching a COST Action comes from the European scientists themselves), "à la carte participation" (only countries interested in the Action participate), "equality of access" (participation is open also to the scientific communities of countries not belonging to the European Union) and "flexible structure" (easy implementation and light management of the research initiatives) are the main characteristics of COST.

As precursor of advanced multidisciplinary research COST has a very important role for the realisation of the European Research Area (ERA) anticipating and complementing the activities of the Framework Programmes, constituting a "bridge" towards the scientific communities of emerging countries, increasing the mobility of researchers across Europe and fostering the establishment of "Networks of Excellence" in many key scientific domains such as: Biomedicine and Molecular Biosciences; Food and Agriculture; Forests, their Products and Services; Materials, Physical and Nanosciences; Chemistry and Molecular Sciences and Technologies; Earth System Science and Environmental Management; Information and Communication Technologies; Transport and Urban Development; Individuals, Societies, Cultures and Health. It covers basic and more applied research and also addresses issues of pre-normative nature or of societal importance. For more information the web address is: http://www.cost.eu

This publication is supported by COST.

PREFACE

Dendrimers are a special class of polymers with a well-defined structure and intriguing architecture bearing unique radiating branching units in the interior and numerous end groups on the surface. Unlike traditional polymers, the structures of dendrimers can be precisely controlled during their stepwise synthesis, yielding narrow polydispersity in addition to unique structural geometry and multivalent properties. Consequently, dendrimers are particularly appealing for biomedical applications. However, there is still a substantial gap in understanding how dendrimers act, and the pace of translating research from bench to bedside is far from satisfactory. It requires joint efforts from scientists with backgrounds including chemical synthesis, physical characterization, biological evaluation and clinical design. Along these lines, COST Action TD0802 "Biomedical applications of dendrimers" was established in 2008 to build a multidisciplinary European network. Its goal has been to establish a network of collaborative European research aimed at developing new medical applications based on dendrimer technology by making full use of the unique properties of dendrimers. The fruitful results of this Action have relied on its highly interdisciplinary approach in which chemists, physicists, biologists and physicians have all been involved in the collaboration. This effort has also clearly shown that it is possible to establish a successful network of cooperating research groups in a short time in Europe, which can be further continued on a long-term basis.

This book presents an overview of the-state-of-the-art in the field of dendrimer research and its biological applications. The chapters cover various aspects from the synthesis and characterization of different types of dendrimers such as polyaminoester dendrimers and multivalent dendrons (chapters 9, 12 and 13); characterization of dendrimer-based hybrid nanofibers as potential templates for 1D-objects (chapter 2); the use of different families of dendrimers for biomedical applications such as drug and genetic material delivery (chapters 3 to 6 and 10); antiamyloidogenic effects (chapter 1); anti-inflammatory actions (chapter 5) and dendrimers as sensors for drug allergy detection (chapter 7). In addition, several chapters discuss the use of molecular modeling to investigate the interaction of dendrimers with biological molecules (chapters 2, 4, 6, 8, 10 and 11).

Overall, this book can be useful for both newcomers to the field by presenting an overview of the research being performed in the field, and to the researchers working on dendrimers by presenting in-depth studies on various aspects of dendrimer synthesis and applications. We hope that more and more scientists will join the interdisciplinary research on dendrimers and make their contribution to the fast growing and fascinating world of dendrimers.

Valentin Ceña

Barbara Klajnert

Ling Peng

Contents

DENDRIMERS AS ANTIAMYLOIDOGENIC AGENTS. DENDRIMER-AMYLOID AGGREGATES MORPHOLOGY AND CELL TOXICITY

D. Appelhans[1], N. Benseny[2], O. Klementiveva[2], M. Bryszewska[3], B. Klajnert[3] and J. Cladera[2]

[1]Leibniz Institute of Polymer Research, Hohe Strasse 6, D-01069 Dresden, Germany.
[2]Biophysics Unit and Center of Studies in Biophysics, Department of Biochemistry and Molecular Biology, Universitat Autònoma de Barcelona, 08193 Bellaterra, Spain.
[3]Department of General Biophysics, Faculty of Biology and Environmental Protection, University of Lodz, Lodz, Poland.

1 SUMMARY

Dendrimers are branched polymeric structures that have been shown to have a promising antiamyloidogenic potential by interfering with the polymerization process leading to the formation of the amyloid aggregates related to conformational diseases, such as Alzheimer's and prion diseases. It has been established that there is a relationship between the morphology of the amyloid aggregates and the amyloid peptides or proteins toxicity: fibrillar structures present low or no toxicity, whereas oligomeric species and amorphous aggregates, the so called granular non-fibrillar aggregates (GNAs), are toxic to cells. When interacting with the amyloid peptide associated to the onset and development of Alzheimer's disease, dendrimers can either accelerate the formation of fibrillar structures or inhibit it. Inhibition however may mean promoting the formation of amorphous aggregates. We summarize in the present chapter the experimental evidence showing that when used in a way that favors the formation and clumping of fibrils, dendrimers (glycodendrimers in particular) can reduce amyloid toxicity. However the same glycodendrimers used under different conditions can generate toxic GNAs, an aggregated form that could represent a general morphological signature for amyloid toxicity.

2 AMYLOID AGGREGATION AND ALZHEIMER'S DISEASE.

Alzheimer's disease is one of the so called 'conformational diseases', characterized by the accumulation in the organism of a misfolded variant of a peptide or protein in the form of an amyloid deposit, usually associated to tissue regions where cell deterioration is observed. In Alzheimer's disease, a pathological condition of the Central Nervous System (CNS) which evolution implies the degeneration of cognitive functions, amyloid plaques are typically observed in histological preparations from the affected brains[1,2]. Such plaques, observed under the electron microscope are made of very thin (approximately 10 nm in diameter) and long (micrometers) amyloid fibrils (Fig. 1A). The main component of amyloid fibrils is the amyloid peptide, a 40-42 residues long peptide (Fig. 1 B) which is the proteolytic product of the Amyloid Precursor Protein (APP). APP is a membrane protein

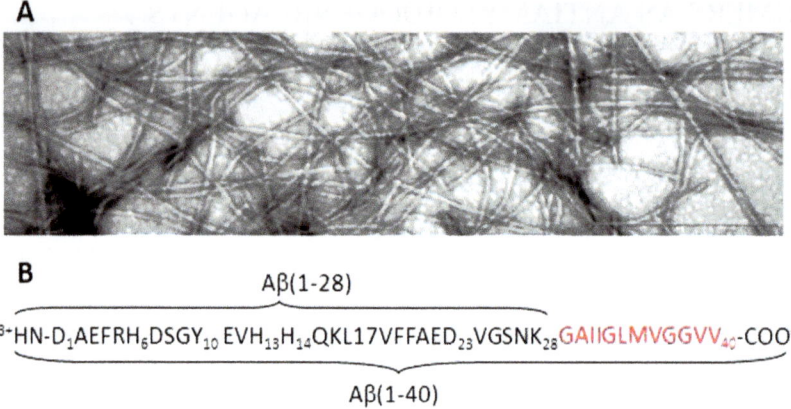

Figure 1 *(A) Electron micrograph of the typical amyloid fibrils detected in the amyloid plaques that form in brains affected by Alzheimer's disease. (B) Aminoacidic sequence Aβ(1-40); in red, the hydrophobic residues, from the intramenbrane part of APP (the amyloid precursor protein). Aβ(1-28) corresponds to the hydrophyllic portion of the peptide and it has been as well used as an amyloid peptide because it can aggregate forming fibrillar structures equivalent to those formed by the whole peptide.*

which function in the CNS is yet not well established and that can be processed by three different secretases: when cleaved by the α and β secretases a non-amyloidogenic peptide is generated; however when processed by the β and γ secreatases, a mixture of 40 and 42 residues long amyloid peptides, with a high tendency to aggregate is produced into the extracellular space of the CNS.

2.1 Amyloid Peptide Aggregation and Cell Toxicity.

The formation of amyloid fibrils has been thoroughly studied in vitro[3]. The amyloid peptide is structured in the fibril in the form of a cross β-sheet and fibril formation follows a nucleation-dependent polymerization mechanism (Fig. 2). During the lag phase of the typically sigmoid-shaped kinetics different forms of non-fibrillar, low and high molecular weight intermediates are formed. There is a mounting amount of evidence pointing to some of these non-fibrillar species that form during the nucleation phase as the amyloid species that may cause cytotoxicity, whereas mature fibrils would have very low toxicity[4].

In the search for compounds that would inhibit cell deterioration in Alzheimer's disease, there is a marked interest in finding compounds which are able to inhibit the formation of amyloid deposits either by promoting the removal of the amyloid peptide from the CNS or by inhibiting the formation of the toxic amyloid species or blocking their action. Given the non-toxic character of amyloid fibrils it has to be considered that one way of avoiding the amyloid peptide toxicity could be via its rapid association into fibrils.

Many studies can be found in the literature dedicated to study the effects of a very diverse number of compounds on the amyloid peptide aggregation kinetics[5]. In many cases, it is considered that the power of a compound to inhibit fibril formation represents the possibility that such a compound could be useful to inhibit the peptide's cell toxicity. However, when evaluating the results of such studies, one has to consider the possibility

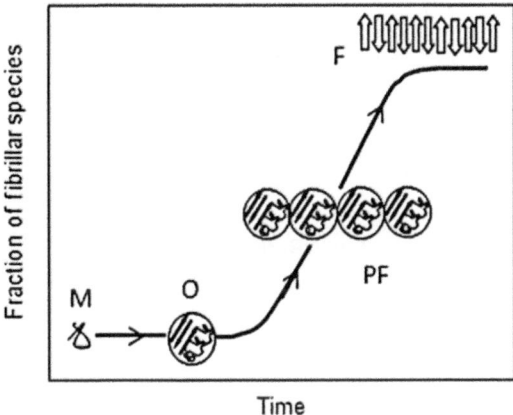

Figure 2 *Amyloid fibril formation kinetics schematic illustration (nucleation-dependent polymerization process). Monomeric peptides or proteins (M) combine during a lag phase into oligomeric nuclei (O). The transition between monomers and nuclei during this so called nucleation phase may take place through the formation of different oligomeric intermediates (dimers, trimers, etc.). The nucleation phase is followed by an elongation phase during which protofibrillar structures (PF) form by combination of nuclei. Finally protofibrils convert into amyloid fibrils (F).*

that the fact of inhibiting the formation of fibrils, may implicate the accumulation of non-fibrillar toxic species, high and low molecular weight intermediates, or the accumulation of the so-called (toxic) 'Granular Non-fibrillar Aggregates' (GNAs).

2.2 Granular Non-Fibrillar Aggregates (GNAs).

When we consider a protein folding energy landscape diagram[6] like the one depicted in Fig. 3, it can be seen that amyloid fibrils represent a misfolded form of a peptide or protein which can arise sometimes, given the right conditions, from some of the many intermediate (high energy) forms present at the beginning of the process, between which the structure of the peptide or protein fluctuates. The misfolded, fibrillar form, represents a minimum of energy which is even lower than that of the native form. However, fibrils are not the only misfolded, stable form. Peptides and proteins can aggregate as well in the form of amorphous, non-fibrillar aggregates.

It has been mentioned above that it is believed nowadays that the toxic forms of the amyloid peptide, have to be looked for, in Alzheimer's disease, among those species formed during the nucleation phase of the fibril formation process. In a recent work carried out by the group of Josep Cladera in Barcelona (Spain) in collaboration with Jan Maly's group in Usti nad Labem (Czech Republic) we have described, in the case of Alzheimer's disease, the formation of a kind of amorphous, non-fibrillar aggregates, which have been named 'Granular Non-fibrillar Aggregates' (GNAs)[7] (Fig. 4), that could have an important role in cell toxicity. GNAs have been proposed as an off-pathway mechanism in amyloid aggregation. Its formation is related to relevant physiological parameters in Alzheimer's disease, such as an acid medium (pH between 5 and 6.5) or the interaction of the peptide with negatively charged biological membranes. Formation of amorphous toxic aggregates has been as well described as a consequence of the interaction of the amyloid peptide with Cu^{2+}, another significant factor related to the development of the pathology.

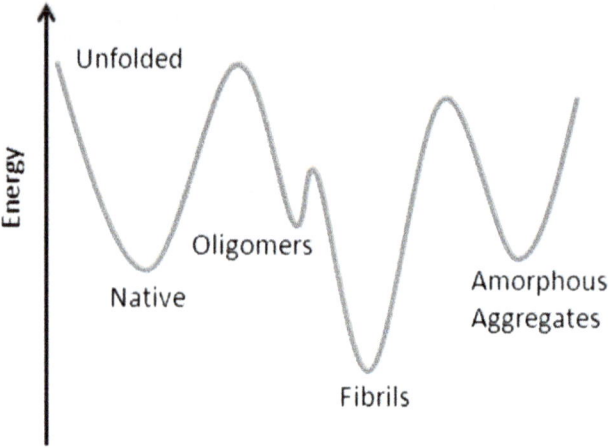

Figure 3 *Protein folding energy landscape under physiological and misfolding conditions. The shape of the graph shows the energy of the protein conformations moving toward its native or misfolded condition through multiple inter- and intramolecular contact arrangements. Under certain environmental conditions, fluctuating intermediate species can follow the path that leads to the formation of misfolded structures: amorphous aggregates and fibrils[6,23].*

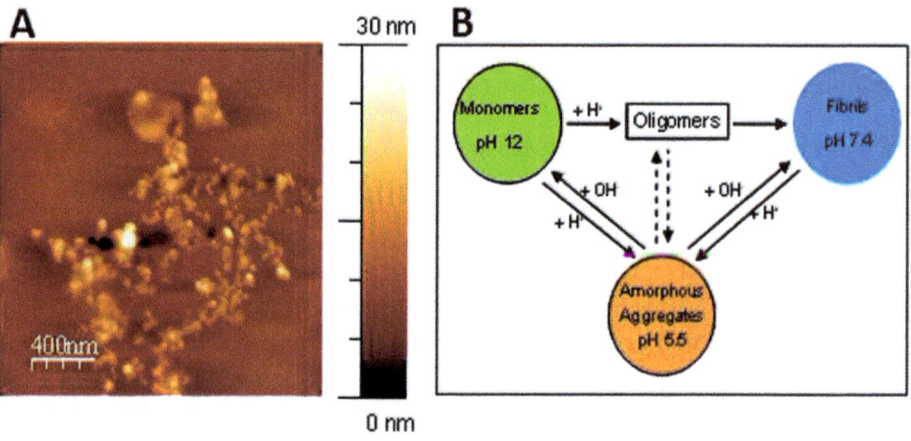

Figure 4 *(A) AFM image of amorphous aggregates (GNAs) formed by the peptide Aβ(1-40) at pH 5.5. The color scale refers to the height of the granular aggregates detected on the mica surface on which the sample was deposited. (B) Aβ(1-40) aggregation diagram: by lowering the pH from 12 (the pH at which the peptide is kept unaggregated in vitro in the stock solution) to 7.4, the typical nucleation-dependent polymerization process is triggered; lowering the pH implies the formation of granular non-fibrilar aggregates (described at pH 5.5). Fibrils can form from non-fibrilar aggregates by increasing the pH at 7.4 and vice-versa. The unaggregated state of the peptide can be reverted to from the non-fibrilar state by increasing the pH at 12. (Adapted with permission from Curr Alzheimer Res. 2012; 9(8):962-71).*

3 INTERACTION OF DENDRIMERS WITH ALZHEIMER'S AMYLOID PEPTIDES. AGGREGATE MORPHOLOGY AND TOXICITY.

In the past seven years, in a series of collaborations between the labs of Maria Bryszewska and Barbara Klajnert in Lodz (Poland), Jean Pierre Majoral in Toulouse (France), Francesca Ottaviani in Urbino (Italy), Dietmar Appelhans in Dresden (Germany) and Josep Cladera in Barcelona (Spain)[8-13,18,24], dendrimers have been shown to be capable of interfering *in vitro* with the formation of the amyloid aggregated structures typically related to the onset and development of Alzheimer's disease and prion diseases. This makes dendrimers potentially useful as compounds that could prevent or inhibit the action of the cytotoxic amyloid species. Such a possibility has come out in the first place from observations showing that dendrimers (PAMAM and phosphorus dendrimers) could interfere with the aggregation kinetics of two amyloid model peptides: the hydrophilic Aβ(1-28) (28 residues long) bit of the 40-42 residues long amyloid peptide (Fig. 1) found in Alzheimer's plaques and a segment of the human prion protein (the Prp185-206 peptide). In summary it has been found that PAMAM and phosphorus dendrimers can interfere with amyloid fibril formation by either accelerating fibril formation or by slowing down and/or inhibiting its formation.

3.1 Interaction of PAMAM Dendrimers with the Aβ(1-40) Amyloid Peptide.

Fig. 5, shows the influence of PAMAM dendrimers on the aggregation process of the Alzheimer's whole amyloid Aβ(1-40) peptide. Amyloid fibril formation can be easily monitored using the fluorescence dye Thioflavin T (ThT). The dye becomes only fluorescent when interacting with the well-ordered β-sheet structures present in amyloid fibrils, so it is a good method to detect the appearance of fibrils. Fig. 5 reveals the sygmoid-shaped curve corresponding to the fibril formation kinetics of Aβ(1-40), where the typical lag (nucleation) phase followed by the elongation phase are clearly observed. Similarly to what had been observed for Aβ(1-28), PAMAM dendrimers may, in the case of Aβ(1-40), either accelerate fibril formation (this happens at low dendrimer/peptide ratios) or inhibit it (at higher dendrimer/peptide ratios). According to the ThT fluorescent measurements, when the peptide interacts with PAMAM dendrimers at a low dendrimer/ peptide ratio there is a clear shortening of the nucleation phase, the presence of the dendrimer accelerates nuclei formation, but, as in the case of the amyloid peptide alone, ThT fluorescence increases until its value reaches a plateau. This is already indicative of the fact that under such conditions the peptide will still form fibrils at the end of the process. However, what is the morphology of the peptide-dendrimer aggregates at the end of the process when they interact at high dendrimer/peptide ratios and no ThT fluorescence increase is observed? This can be checked using electron microscopy. Three electron micrographs, corresponding to the end of three of the kinetics shown in Fig. 5, are shown in Fig. 6. As expected, Aβ(1-40) forms the typical amyloid fibrils when let to aggregate alone or in the presence of PAMAM dendrimers at low dendrimer/peptide ratios. However, when the dendrimer is present at high dendrimer/peptide ratios, no fibrillar structures are present in the electron micrograph. Only amorphous aggregates, similar in shape to those (toxic ones) described for the peptide at low pH or in the presence of Cu^{2+} ions to which we have referred above (GNAs), can be observed. In the case of the dendrimer/Aβ(1-40) complexes though, are these structures toxic to cells? When using PAMAM dendrimers, their intrinsic cell toxicity makes it impossible to answer the question. In order to measure cell toxicity, the use of biocompatible dendrimers having similar effects to those of

PAMAM on amyloid aggregation is necessary. This, as we shall see in the next section, can be achieved using maltose-decorated dendrimers.

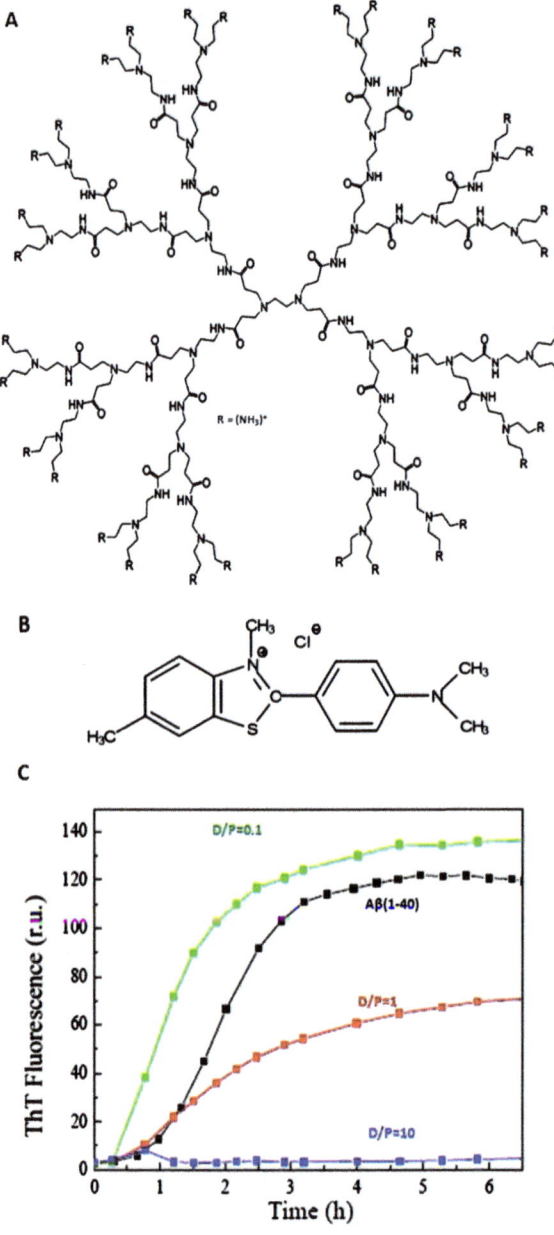

Figure 5. *(A) Molecular structure of a Generation 3 (G3) PAMAM dendrimer. (B) Molecular structure of Thioflavin T (ThT) the dye that becomes fluorescent when intercalates into the amyloid fibrils and is used to monitor fibril formation kinetics. (C) Effect of G3 PAMAM dendrimers on the fibrils formation kinetics of Aβ(1-40) at different dendrimer/peptide (D/P) ratios. Peptide concentration was always 25 μM, pH 7.4, 37°C ThT 35 μM.*

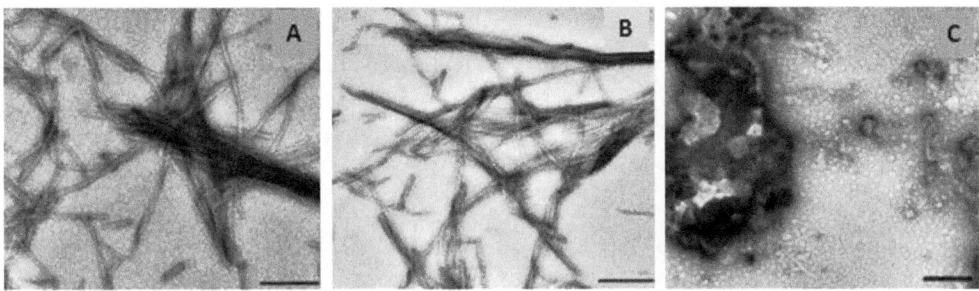

Figure 6. *Electron micrographs corresponding to the end of three of the Aβ(1-40) kinetics shown in Fig. 5. (A) end of the aggregation process of Aβ(1-40) alone; (B) end of the aggregation process of Aβ(1-40) in the presence of G3 PAMAM at D/P=0.1; (C) end of the aggregation process of Aβ(1-40) in the presence of G3 PAMAM at D/P=10. Bar: 200 nm.*

3.2 Interaction of Glycodendrimers with the Aβ(1-40) Amyloid Peptide.

The intrinsic cell toxicity of PAMAM dendrimers, with high superficial electrical charge density, is thought to be related to their capacity of establishing very strong interactions of electrostatic nature with biological structures. Glycodendrimers, dendrimers in which the surface is decorated with polysaccharides, have been recently shown in different works to be useful compounds to overcome cell toxicity[14,15]. In the case of glycodendrimers, the interaction with biological macromolecules would proceed via the establishment of hydrogen bonds. Glycodendrimers have already been shown to have remarkably low or zero toxicity towards different cell lines and experiments on their properties when interacting with biological systems (hemolytic power, interaction with HSA and PrP185–208) have been reported[14,15]. Fig. 7 illustrates how PPI-maltose glycodendrimers, generations 4 and 5, are not toxic to PC12 and SH-SY5Y cells up to 50 μM dendrimer concentration and have a low toxic effect between 50 and 100 μM. These two cell lines have been routinely used as neuronal models to test cell toxicity[16,17].

As shown in a recent work by the labs of Josep Cladera in Barcelona (Spain) and Dietmar Appelhans in Dresden (Germany)[18] the interference capacity of glycodendrimers on the nucleation-dependent aggregation of Aβ(1–40), as illustrated for PPI-maltose generation 4 in Fig. 8, turns out to be very similar to the effect of PAMAM dendrimers (shown in Fig. 5): at low dendrimer–peptide ratios there is a slight acceleration of fibril formation; as the dendrimer/peptide ratio is increased the rate and the amount of fibrils at the end of the process decrease. In the case of PPI-maltose generation 5 glycodendrimers, a complete inhibitory effect of the ThT fluorescence increase (fibril formation) has been observed at any dendrimer/peptide ratio. When considering the similar effect of PAMAM and gycodendrimers on amyloid aggregation we have to consider the fact that in both cases the observed effect depends on the dendrimer-peptide ratio. At low ratios, dendrimers are not able to hamper fibril formation, that is, they cannot inhibit the elongation phase that takes place by combination of amyloid nuclei. And as a matter of fact, at low dendrimer-peptide ratios dendrimers become (although the molecular mechanism is unknown) as amyloid nucleation accelerators, shortening the nucleation phase and accelerating the formation of fibrils. It is reasonable to think that in the case of PAMAM dendrimers this nucleation effect could take place mainly through the establishment of electrostatic interactions

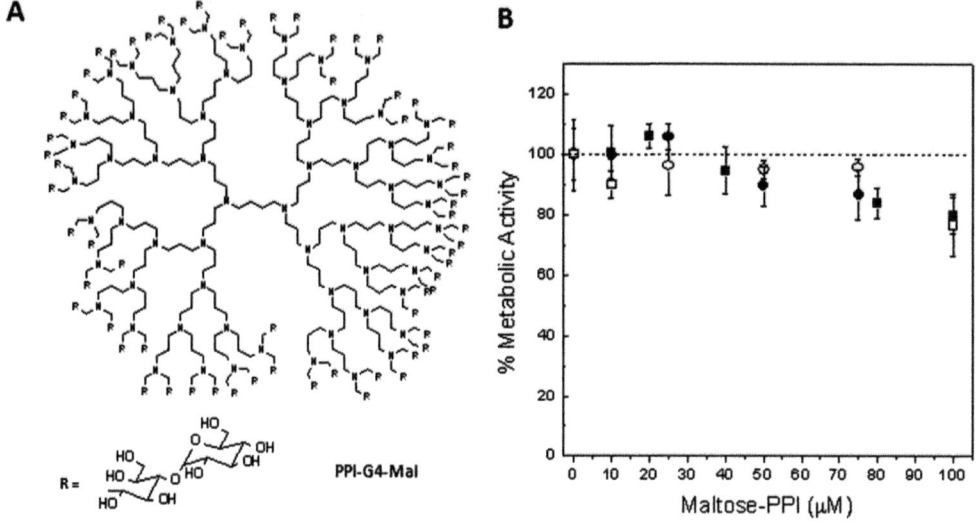

Figure 7 *(A) Molecular structure of a generation 4 PPI-maltose glycondendrimer. (B) Effect of PPI-maltose dendrimer concentration on cell metabolic activity: PC12 (circles) and SH-SY5Y (squares) cells; PPI-G4-Mal (full symbols) and PPI-G5-Mal (empty symbols); Statistics: no significant difference exists between any of the experimental points shown and the control (ANOVA analysis, $p < 0.05$, n=3). (Adapted with permission from Biomacromolecules. 2011; 12(11):3903-9. Copyright 2011 American Chemical Society).*

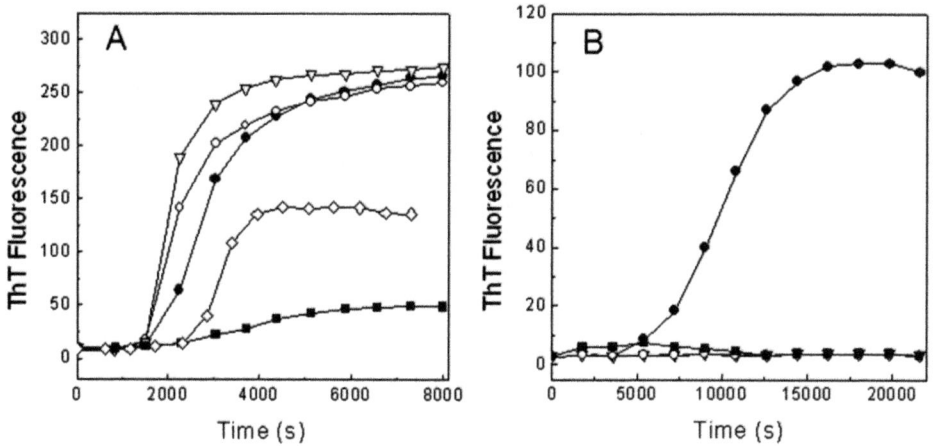

Figure 8 Effect of PPI-maltose dendrimers on the aggregation kinetics of Aβ(1-40).
(A) Effect of PPI-G4-Mal on Aβ(1-40) fibril formation; (B) Effect of PPI-G5-Mal on Aβ(1-40) fibril formation. (-•-) Aβ(1-40) 25 μM (control); (-∇-) Aβ(1-40) + dendrimer at dendrimer/peptide ratio = 0.1; (-o-) Aβ(1-40) + dendrimer at dendrimer/peptide ratio = 1: (-◇-) Aβ(1-40) + dendrimer at dendrimer/peptide ratio = 5; (-■-) Aβ(1-40) + dendrimer at dendrimer/peptide ratio = 10. Temperature was 37°C and pH 7.4. Peptide concentration was in all cases 25 μM, pH 7.4, 37°C, ThT 35 μM. (Adapted with permission from Biomacromolecules. 2011; 12(11):3903-9. Copyright 2011 American Chemical Society).

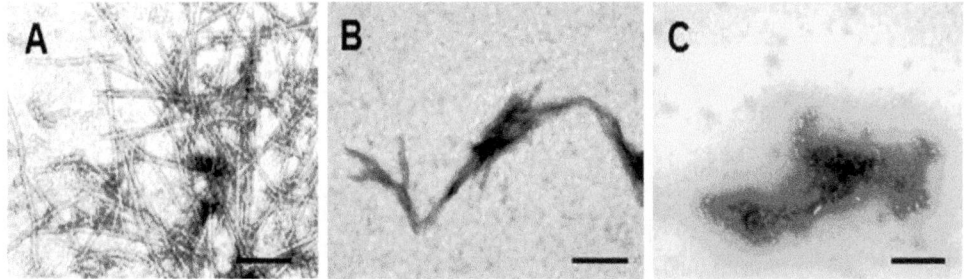

Figure 9 *Morphology of Aβ(1-40) and dendrimer-Aβ(1-40) amyloid aggregates. Electron microscopy micrographs of: Aβ(1-40) incubated at pH 7.4 (coexistence of fibrils and globular oligomers) (A); Aβ(1-40) incubated at pH 7.4 in the presence of PPI-G4-Mal (detection of clumped fibrils (B); Aβ(1-40) incubated at pH 7.4 in the presence of PPI-G5-Mal (detection of granular non-fibrilar, amorphous aggregates) (C). Bar: 200 nm. (Adapted with permission from Biomacromolecules. 2011; 12(11):3903-9. Copyright 2011 American Chemical Society).*

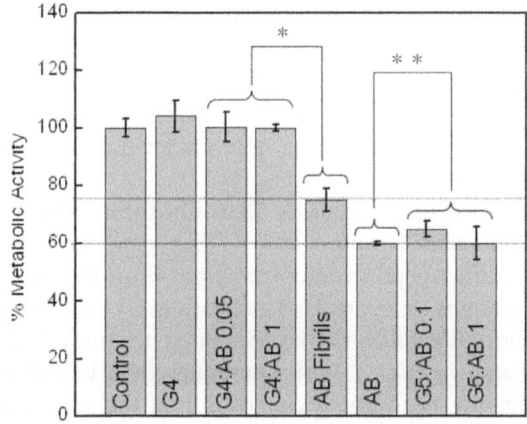

Figure 10 *Effect of PPI-Mal dendrimers-Aβ(1-40) complexes on cell toxicity: (control) PC12 cells in the absence of dendrimers and/or Aβ(1-40); (G4) effect of PPI-G4-Mal 2.5μM in the absence of peptide; (G4:AB 0.05) effect of a mixture of PPI-G4-Mal-Aβ(1-40) at dendrimer/peptide ratio of 0.05, incubated for 12 hours at pH 7.4 previous addition to the cell culture; (G4:AB 0.1) effect of a mixture of PPI-G4-Mal-Aβ(1-40) at dendrimer/peptide ratio of 0.1 incubated for 12 hours at pH 7.4 previous addition to the cell culture; (AB Fibrils) Aβ(1-40) incubated for 12 hours at pH 7.4 previous addition to the cell culture; (AB) Aβ(1-40) added into the cell culture without incubation; (G5:AB 0.1) effect of a mixture of PPI-G5-Mal-Aβ(1-40) at dendrimer/peptide ratio of 0.1 incubated for 12 hours at pH 7.4 previous addition to the cell culture; (G5:AB 1) effect of a mixture of PPI-G5-Mal-Aβ(1-40) at dendrimer/peptide ratio of 1, incubated for 12 hours at pH 7.4 previous addition to the cell culture. Peptide concentration was in all cases 25 μM. Statistics: *: Significantly different; * *: no significantly different (ANOVA analysis, p < 0.05, n=3). (Adapted with permission from Biomacromolecules. 2011; 12(11):3903-9. Copyright 2011 American Chemical Society).*

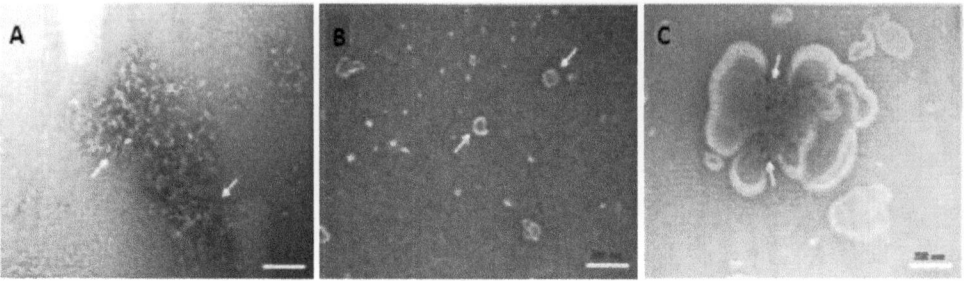

Figure 11 *Electron micrographs of a 23 residues long fusion peptide form the HIV protein gp41 after being added into aqueous buffer (formation of amorphous aggregates) (A); electron micrograph of unilamelar, 100 nm in diameter liposomes (B); fused liposomes after addition of the aggregated peptides into the liposome suspension. Bar: 200 nm.*

between the amyloid oligomers that constitute the nuclei and the dendrimer, whereas in the case of glycodendrimers the effect would come through the formation of hydrogen bonds between the amyloid dendrimers and the surface of the dendrimers. At high dendrimer-peptide ratios, the dendrimer concentration would be enough to hamper the combination of the amyloid nuclei that results in the formation of fibrils. Again the interaction between PAMAM dendrimers and amyloid nuclei would be of electrostatic nature and the interaction between glycodendrimers and the nuclei would take place through the formation of hydrogen bonds.

The electron microscope (Fig. 9) reveals that fibril formation inhibition causes the formation of globular non-fibrillar aggregates (GNAs, generated by incubating dendrimer and peptide at high dendrimer/peptide ratios), whereas fibril formation enhancement favors fibril clumping (fibril clumps generated by incubating G4 maltose glycodendrimers with Ab(1–40) at low dendrimer/peptide ratios, compared to normal fibrils). As it has been hypothesized by Klementieva et al.[18] fibril clumping could be due to the fact that at low dendrimer-peptide ratio, the dendrimers cannot inhibit the formation of fibrils, whereas once formed the same dendrimers may act as a 'glue', bringing the fibrils together in the form of clumps, through the establishment of hydrogen bonds.

It seems therefore that the effect of dendrimers on amyloid aggregation would be greatly due to the properties of the dendrimer surface. Klementieva et al.[18] have estimated that the differential effect of G4 and G5 glycondendrimers is most likely due to the difference in the maltose surface density. An effect due to the electric charge density in model lipid membranes has been as well described by Benseny-Cases et al.[7] Beyond dendrimers and lipid vesicles, they may be other globular polymeric structures with surfaces able to interact with amyloids, that could have similar effects and that may be worth investigating.

The intrinsic biocompatibility of glycodendrimers permits to evaluate the toxic capacity of both fibrillar (clumped fibrils) and amorphous glycodendrimer/Aβ(1-40) complexes. When PC12 cell viability is assessed it can be observed that fibril clumping, achieved by using G4 at low dendrimer peptide ratios (G4:AB 0.05 and G4:AB 1 in Fig. 10), renders amyloid fibrils non-toxic. However, fibril formation inhibition, using G5 at any dendrimer/peptide ratio (G5:AB 0.1 and G5:AB 1 in Fig. 10) or G4 at high dendrimer/peptide ratios (G4:AB 10, not sown in fig. 10), generates toxic GNAs (Fig. 10).

3.3 Generalization of Amorphous GNAs as a Toxic Peptide Aggregated Form.

We have already mentioned that, besides the amorphous aggregates detected when dendrimers interact with the amyloid peptide, GNAs form as well under different conditions (pH, Cu^{2+}, negatively charged membranes)[7]. The destabilizing power of GNAs, can be extended to other amyloid peptides, since its toxic power has been as well described for poly-glutamine peptides related to Huntington's disease and for the SH3 domain of PI3, a model amyloid peptide[19-21]. In these works, the authors point to amorphous aggregation as a possible general structural amyloid organization related to toxicity. Outside the amyloid world, it has been described in Josep Cladera's lab[22] that the membrane destabilizing effects of the so called fusion peptides from HIV's gp41 protein that induce membrane fusion, depend on this peptide adopting the form of an amorphous β-sheet aggregate. Such fusion peptide aggregates, are morphologically very similar to the amyloid GNAs as it can be seen in Fig. 11.

4 CONCLUSION

In this chapter, we have analyzed the interference of dendrimers with the aggregation process of the Alzheimer's amyloid peptide Aβ(1-40), paying special attention to the relevance that the resulting dendrimer-peptide aggregated complexes morphology could have in relation to the peptide cytotoxicity. Dendrimers can interfere with amyloid fibril formation either by accelerating the formation of amyloid fibrils or by inhibiting it. From a morphological point of view, the end products are different: when dendrimers (either PAMAM or glycodendrimers) favor fibril formation, amyloid fibrils are detected at the end of the polymerization reaction. In the case of glycodendrimers these fibrils are clearly clumped. However, when dendrimers inhibit fibril formation, the resulting product has the form of a β-sheet amorphous, granular aggregate, which resembles the amorphous, granular, toxic aggregates formed by Aβ(1-40) under different experimental conditions. Such dendrimer-amyloid amorphous complexes turn out to be as well toxic to cells, as it can be proved when using biocompatible glycodendrimers. Interestingly however, when dendrimers are used in a way that promotes the formation of crumpled fibrils, a clear decrease in the cytotoxicity of the amyloid peptide is observed. The relationship between morphology and toxicity is schematically summarized in Fig. 12 for the interaction of dendrimers and Aβ(1-40). In general, these observations, coming out of the studies on the interaction of dendrimers with amyloid peptides carried out *in vitro*, point towards a possible use of dendrimers (in particular glycodendrimers) as antiamyloidogenic agents in Alzheimer's disease. That is, when used in a way that promote fibril formation. But there is also a warning, in the sense that conditions must be controlled, when translating the use of dendrimers into *in vivo* conditions, in order to avoid the formation of toxic amorphous aggregates.

Finally, it is important to point out that in the present chapter we have addressed, mainly from a morphological point of view, two characteristic dendrimer-aggregate complexes: amorphous aggregates (toxic) and fibrils (non-toxic). However, it has been shown that dendrimers can act sometimes upon an amyloidogenic cellular infection, without enhancing fibril formation or fibril's clumping, but rather by clearing up the presence of amyloid aggregated forms form the cellular system. This has been shown for example for glycodendrimers acting on cell infected by the prion protein in a work by Fisher et al.[15].

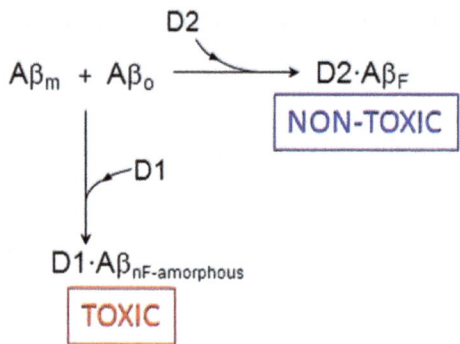

Figure 12. *Schematic proposal of a molecular mechanism explaining the formation of the different PPI-maltose dendrimers-Aβ(1-40). Dendrimers (D1: PAMAM dendrimers at high dendrimer/peptide ratio; G5 PPI-Mal at any dendrimer/peptide ratio; G4 PPI-Mal at high dendrimer/peptide ratio) can interact with Aβ(1-40) generating toxic amorphous, granulated aggregates (GNAs); However, dendrimers (D2: PAMAM dendrimers at low dendrimer/peptide ratio; G4 PPI-Mal at low dendrimer/peptide ratio) can interact with Aβ(1-40) enhancing fibril formation, and reducing, in the case of glycodendrimers, the peptide toxicity.*

References

1   C. Haass and D. J. Selkoe, *Nat Rev Mol Cell Biol*, 2007, **8**, 101-112.
2   S. B. Prusiner, *Dev Biol Stand*, 1991, **75**, 55-74.
3   N. Benseny-Cases, M. Cocera and J. Cladera, *Biochem Biophys Res Commun*, 2007, **361**, 916-921.
4   K. N. Dahlgren, A. M. Manelli, W. B. Stine, Jr., L. K. Baker, G. A. Krafft and M. J. ç LaDu, *J Biol Chem*, 2002, **277**, 32046-32053.
5   C. W. Cairo, A. Strzelec, R. M. Murphy and L. L. Kiessling, *Biochemistry*, 2002, **41**, 8620-8629.
6   T. R. Jahn and S. E. Radford, *FEBS J*, 2005, **272**, 5962-5970.
7   N. Benseny-Cases, O. Klementieva, J. Malý and J. Cladera, *Curr. Alzheimer Res.*, 2012, **9**, Epub ahead of print.
8   B. Klajnert, M. Cortijo-Arellano, M. Bryszewska and J. Cladera, *Biochem Biophys Res Commun*, 2006, **339**, 577-582.
9   B. Klajnert, J. Cladera and M. Bryszewska, *Biomacromolecules*, 2006, **7**, 2186-2191.
10 B. Klajnert, M. Cortijo-Arellano, J. Cladera, J. P. Majoral, A. M. Caminade and M. Bryszewska, *Biochem Biophys Res Commun*, 2007, **364**, 20-25.
11 B. Klajnert, M. Cangiotti, S. Calici, J. P. Majoral, A. M. Caminade, J. Cladera, M. Bryszewska and M. F. Ottaviani, *Macromol Biosci*, 2007, **7**, 1065-1074.
12 B. Klajnert, M. Cortijo-Arellano, J. Cladera and M. Bryszewska, *Biochem Biophys Res Commun*, 2006, **345**, 21-28.
13 B. Klajnert, Cangiotti, M., Calici, S., Ionov, M., Majoral, J.P., Caminade, A.M., Cladera, J., Bryszewska, M., Ottaviani, M.F., *New J Chem*, 2009, **33**, 1087-1093.
14 B. Klajnert, D. Appelhans, H. Komber, N. Morgner, S. Schwarz, S. Richter, B. Brutschy, M. Ionov, A. K. Tonkikh, M. Bryszewska and B. Voit, *Chemistry*, 2008, **14**,

7030-7041.

15 M. Fischer, D. Appelhans, S. Schwarz, B. Klajnert, M. Bryszewska, B. Voit and M. Rogers, *Biomacromolecules*, 2010, **11**, 1314-1325.

16 J. Bieschke, S. J. Siegel, Y. Fu and J. W. Kelly, *Biochemistry*, 2008, **47**, 50-59.

17 O. Simakova and N. J. Arispe, *J Neurosci*, 2007, **27**, 13719-13729.

18 O. Klementieva, N. Benseny-Cases, A. Gella, D. Appelhans, B. Voit and J. Cladera, *Biomacromolecules*, 2011, **12**, 3903-3909.

19 H. Mukai, T. Isagawa, E. Goyama, S. Tanaka, N. F. Bence, A. Tamura, Y. Ono and R. R. Kopito, *Proc Natl Acad Sci USA*, 2005, **33**, W148-153.

20 M. Bucciantini, S. Rigacci, A. Berti, L. Pieri, C. Cecchi, D. Nosi, L. Formigli, F. Chiti and M. Stefani, *FASEB J*, 2005, **19**, 437-439.

21 M. Bucciantini, E. Giannoni, F. Chiti, F. Baroni, L. Formigli, J. Zurdo, N. Taddei, G. Ramponi, C. M. Dobson and M. Stefani, *Nature*, 2002, **416**, 507-511.

22 V. Buzón, E. Padrós and J. Cladera, *Biochemistry*, 2005, **44**, 13354-13364.

23 E. Herczenic and F.B.G. Gebbink, *FASEB J*, 2008, **22**, 2115-2133.

24 T. Wasiak, M. Ionov, K. Nieznanski, H. Nieznanska, O. Klementieva, M. Granell, J. Cladera, J.P. Majoral, A.M. Caminade and B. Klajnert, *Mol Pharm*, 2012, **9**, 458-469.

DENDRIMER-BASED HYBRID FIBERS AS POTENTIAL PLATFORM FOR 1D-OBJECTS IN NANOTECHNOLOGY

A. Fahmi,[1] D. Appelhans,[2] A. Danani,[4] G.M. Pavan[4] and B. Voit[2,3]

[1]Faculty Technology and Bionics, Rhine-Waal University of Applied Sciences, D-47533 Kleve, Germany
[2]Leibniz Institute of Polymer Research, D-01069 Dresden, Germany
[3]Organic Chemistry of Polymers, Technische Universität Dresden, 01062 Dresden, Germany
[4]Laboratory of Applied Mathematics and Physics (LaMFI), University of Applied Sciences of Southern Switzerland (SUPSI), Centro Galleria 2, Manno, 6928, Switzerland

1 INTRODUCTION

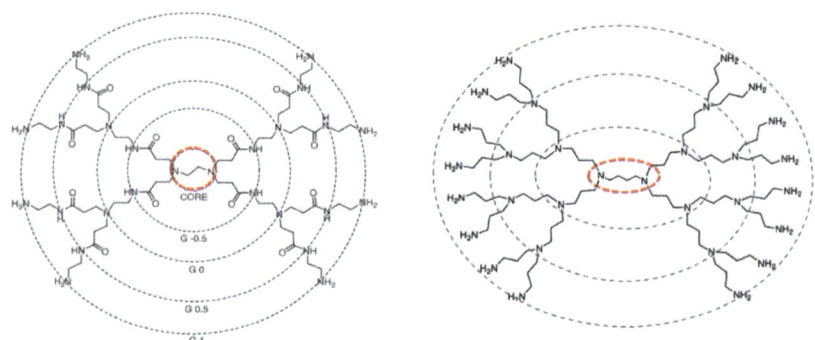

Figure 1 *The structures of a polyamidoamine (G1-PAMAM) and poly(propylene imine) (G2-PPI) dendrimer*[Footnote I]

Nanofabrication via directed self-assembly has emerged as a promising approach for novel functional materials with unique optical, magnetic, and electronic properties.[1-4] This book chapter reviews recent progress in research on dendrimer-based hybrid fibers as potential template for 1D-Objects in nanotechnology.[5-7] Emphasis has been given to the controlled self-assembly of organic-inorganic hybrid nanomaterials, which are all based on amino terminated poly(propylene imine) (PPI) dendrimers in combination with inorganic components. Herein, we give a brief overview of dendritic architectures as encapsulating, stabilizing and directing agents, followed by the presentation of a simple approach towards

---

[Footnote I] Following suggestion from D.A. Tomalia and M. Rookmaker for "Poly(propyleneimine) Dendrimers" in *Polymer Data Handbook* [Second edition, (James E. Mark, editor) Oxford University Press, New York, 979-982 (2009)], the nomenclature for Tomalia-type PAMAM dendrimers can be adopted also for PPI dendrimers. This means that we, then, discuss the hybrid nanofiber formation of 1st up to 4th generation only instead of 2nd – 5th generation PPI dendrimers in our previous papers. Explicitly, we present the results from the 3rd generation PPI dendrimer which was described as 4th generation PPI dendrimers in our previous papers. We motivate all to use the right nomenclature for PPI dendrimers in their future papers.

μm-lengths dendrimer-based hybrid fibers, which can be further used as potential template for 1D-Objects in nanotechnology.

The remarkable properties of dendritic polymers are their structural diversity leading to a wide range of potential applications in materials science, catalysis, and biomedical research.[8-18] Dendrimers with various architectures and functionalities have attracted particular attention because their regular, compartmentalized, and well-defined architecture allows chemical modification at either the core or the shell. Thus far, only two types of dendritic scaffolds, namely polyamidoamine (PAMAM) and poly(propylene imine) (PPI), have been commercialized, because the synthesis of dendrimers is generally very tedious and time-consuming and requires repeating purification steps and exact characterization. Figure 1 shows the typical structure of PAMAM and PPI dendrimers.

Two fundamental approaches can be adopted to design dendritic frameworks.[10,11,19] One approach is to initially attach branching monomer units to a reactive core molecule. The obtained periphery is then activated for the reaction with more monomer units, where upon subsequent iterations result in higher generation dendrimers. Since the two steps can be repeated, the so-called divergent approach is better suited for the preparation of larger quantities of dendrimers. The divergent growth method was first reported by Vögtle et al. (1978)[20] where an iterative sequence of Michael reactions and hydrogenation steps was used for the synthesis of cascade-like oligoamines. PPI dendrimers are prepared via the same synthetic protocol. Similar to the oligoamines, PPI scaffolds are highly-branched polyalkylamines bearing primary amines as terminal end-groups. The dendrimer interior bears internal voids and consists of tertiary trispropylene amine units. In the early 1980s Tomalia et al.[21] first synthesized a broad variety of PAMAM dendrimers starting from ammonia or ethylenediamine as a core. PAMAM dendrimers can be prepared bearing surface primary amino groups (full generations) or terminal carboxylic acid groups (half-generations) (Figure 1).

Dendritic polymers are attracting considerable interest for the construction of dendritic nanocarriers for drug solubilization and delivery.[13,15-18] Both, the interior branches and surface functional groups can be modified. Hydrophobic dyes and drugs can be selectively solubilized by the dendritic scaffolds, due to the cavities generated by the complete molecular structure of dendrimer.[22,23] The encapsulation of guest molecules is generally driven by supramolcular, non-covalent weak binding interactions such as hydrophobic and van der Waals interactions. Therefore, dendrimers are considered as unimolecular polymeric micelles.[24] The utility of polymeric micelles for solubilization of lipophilic guest molecules is well known and results from their particular core-shell architecture with a well-defined hydrophobic interior and hydrophilic shell. Being nanosized macromolecules, dendrimers respond to external stimuli. Like proteins, dendritic polymers adapt a tight-packed (native) or an extended (denatured) conformation, depending on solvent, pH, and ionic strength.[24-27]

Nanotechnology aims to design materials possessing new fundamental properties and functions on the molecular, supramolecular, and macromolecular size scale.[1-4,28-34] As nanotechnology becomes increasingly important in daily life, a wide range of fabrication techniques have been developed in order to produce highly ordered nanostructures and functional devices. The formation of well-ordered structures by the process of controlled self-assembly has been a unique opportunity for the engineering of functional hierarchical materials. Many types of self-assembled nanostructures have been described, as for example, surfactant and polymeric micelles,[35,36] lipid vesicles,[37] dendrimers,[8-11,13,14,16] microemulsions,[38] gels,[39] and liquid crystals.[40] Another interesting application of dendrimers is to generate hybrid organic-inorganic nanostructures.[41] In combination with inorganic components dendrimer-based hybrid materials present a valuable functional system for nanostructuring.[41-44] For example, the directed self-assembly of PPI dendrimers via complexation with inorganic cations is a simple concept for fabricating micrometer long nanofibers.[5,6] Selective decoration of the hybrid fibers with, for example, metallic gold (Au) nanoparticles leads to multifunctional 1D nanostructures, which exhibit interesting physical properties. In this way, a variety of well-defined, more complex nanostructures can be obtained. With regard to their potential for nanotechnological applications, multifunctional 1D nanostructures (nanofibers) enable applications in optics,[3,45] sensors,[46] and nanoelectronics[47,48] as well as bioscience and life sciences.[49-51]

2 METHOD AND RESULTS

2.1 Fabrication of nanofibers via self-assembly of PPI dendrimers in the presence of Cd (II) ions

We employed the directed self-assembly of PPI dendrimers via complexation with cadmium (II) ions as a simple approach for fabricating micrometer long nanofibers.[5,6] The resulting hybrid nanofibers can be used as platform for additionally selective decoration of them with metallic nanoparticles. This may lead to multifunctional 1D nanostructures with interesting physical properties in nanotechnology. Herein, we present a simple approach towards 1D nanostructures and show that the dendrimer-based fibers can be used as a template to guide the nucleation and growth of gold (Au) nanoparticles along the hybrid nanofibers' surface.

Cd(II)-complexed PPI nanofibers are formed as a stable dispersion in aqueous solution. The simple and fast preparation is based on the formation of multiple coordination bonds between the dendrimers and the ions.[5] In the presence of PPI dendrimers the cations coordinate under the experimental conditions employed to the peripheral primary amines. Hence, cadmium ions can act as a linker and promote the unidirectional self-assembly of the dendritic scaffolds in aqueous solution. For example, when cadmium acetate $(Cd(CH_3COO)_2)$ is added to an aqueous solution of 3rd generation PPI dendrimer (PPI-G3) (0.3 mM, 10:1 ratio), one observes the formation of tens of micrometer long fibers (Figure 2). As the aqueous dendrimer solution is treated with the cadmium salt, the pH decreases to 8.3. Thus the ionic strength increases as a result of a higher total ion concentration. Cadmium acetate is water soluble. As a result, the salt completely dissociates into its component ions. Due to its partially empty d orbitals, cadmium ions preferentially form complexes with ammonia, amines, halide ions, and cyanide. This indicates interaction similarities with most of the transition metals series ions.[52] As shown in Figure 2, Cd(II) ions are partially bound to the dendrimer surface. Due to pH decrease induced by the addition of salt (increased ionic strength), the dendrimers are partially protonated. Figure 2 illustrates the cation-induced self-assembly of PPI dendrimers into nanofibers.[5]

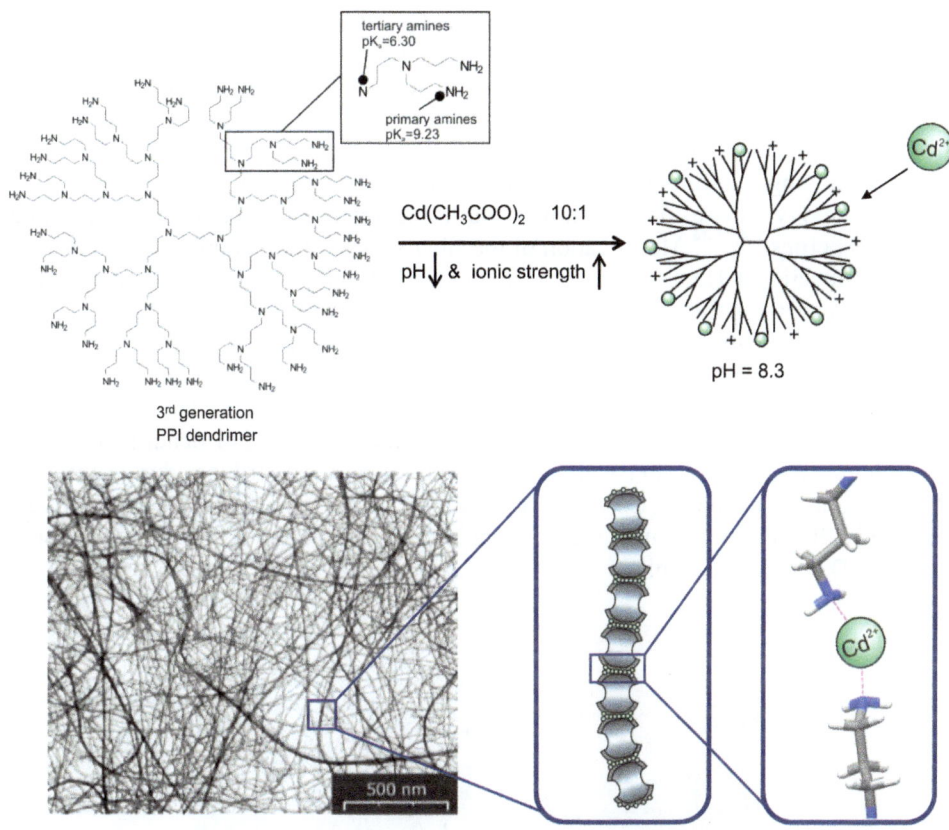

Figure 2 *Cation-induced self-assembly of poly(propylene imine) (PPI) dendrimers into organic-inorganic hybrid nanofibers. The fibers are formed as a stable dispersion in water. Cd(CH₃COO)₂ is added to aqueous dendrimer solution in a molar ratio of 10:1. The cations coordinate to the peripheral primary amines, thus leading to the formation of micrometer long fibers. Reproduced from reference 5 with permission.*

In order to complement the self-assembling process by direct structural data, atomic force microscopy (AFM) and transmission electron microscopy (TEM) was performed for aqueous sample solutions of PPI-based nanofibers. As can be seen from Figure 3a, nanofibers with homogeneous diameters of 4-6 nm are formed. A first indication of the fiber formation is that the dendrimer solutions turn slightly turbid upon the addition of the cadmium salt. However, dynamic light scattering experiments confirmed the increase in hydrodynamic radius from 2.1 nm for the unmodified PPI dendrimer to > 500 nm for Cd(II)-complexed dendrimer fibers. These results clearly indicate that the nanofibers are formed already in aqueous solutions and not during film deposition. TEM images in Figure 3b,c reveal that the micrometer-long fibers are randomly distributed on the substrate and only a few bundles with larger diameters can be observed.

This is most likely due to a repulsive charge interaction between the dendritic architectures. As mentioned above, the PPI dendrimers are partially decorated with Cd(II) ions and possess partially protonated primary amino groups. Due to the remaining positive surface charge, nanofiber growth perpendicular to the fiber axis as well as aggregation of the fibers into bundles is less favored. From the TEM image in Figure 3d it can be seen that within the bundles, the nanofibers are aligned parallel. Upon exposure to the electron beam Cd(II) is reduced to Cd(0). Therefore, cadmium appears as dark spots in the TEM image. Most striking, a regular distribution of small Cd clusters along the dendrimer nanofibers is observed, which supports our hypothesis of the growth mechanism described above. Semiconductor nanofibers with special optical and electronic properties can be prepared by adding a sulfur/selenium precursor under ambient conditions.

Nanotechnology aims to develop novel, multifunctional 1D nanostructures with unique physical properties.[1-4,28-34] Modification of the fiber surface, for example, by metallization, yields multifunctional 1D nanostructures that extend the range of accessible applications.[5] A simple concept for the decoration of dendrimer/Cd(II) nanofibers with, for example, metallic gold nanoparticles is shown in Figure 4. A gold precursor (chloroauric acid, $HAuCl_4$) is added to dilute aqueous solutions of the nanofibers (PPI-G3-Cd(CH$_3$COO)$_2$) in a certain molar ratio, for example, PPI-G3:HAuCl$_4$ = 1:1 or 1:3. The gold precursor coordinates selectively to the peripheral primary amines of the PPI dendrimers, and Au nanoparticles are obtained after wet-chemical reduction. Most striking, during the course of the reaction the nanoparticles follow the contour of the nanofibers. Hence, the Cd(II)-complexed PPI nanofibers can be used to template Au nanoparticles and direct their spatial order into 1D particle assemblies.

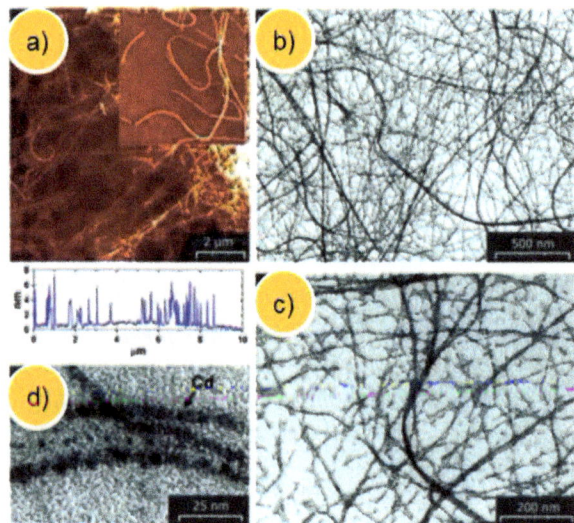

Figure 3 *Atomic force microscopy (AFM) and transmission electron microscopy (TEM) images of self-assembled nanofibers derived from 3rd generation poly(propylene imine) dendrimers in the presence of cadmium acetate. The inset in (a) shows a magnified view of an ensemble of fibers with monodisperse diameters (image size 2 μm). The TEM image in (d) is a magnified view showing the enrichment of Cd(0) clusters in the nanofibers. Reproduced from reference 5 with permission.*

Gold nanoparticles are generally produced through the reduction of chloroauric acid. Different methods (Turkevich, Burst, and Perrault) have been adopted to synthesize Au nanoparticles.[53] Most commonly, sodium citrate, sodium borohydride, and hydrochinone are being used. Both, the Turkevich and Perrault protocol allow for the preparation of Au nanoparticles in aqueous solution. Cd(II)-complexed PPI nanofibers were prepared by using sodium citrate as reducing agent.

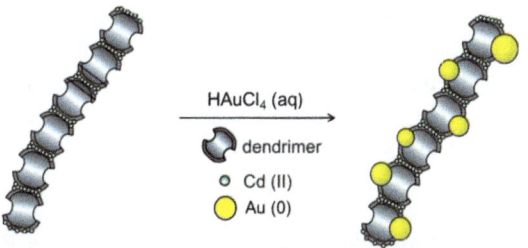

Figure 4 *Metallisation of Cd(II)-complexed poly(propylene imine) (PPI) nanofibers with gold. HAuCl₄ coordinates selectively to the peripheral primary amines of the PPI dendrimers. Au nanoparticles are obtained after wet-chemical reduction. Reproduced from reference 5 with permission.*

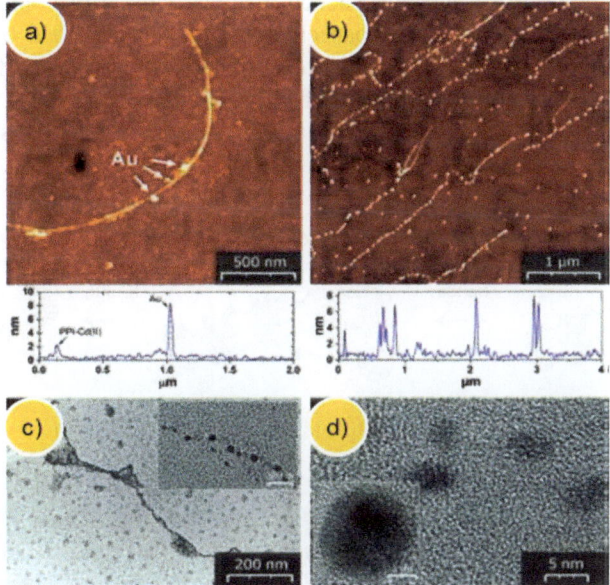

Figure 5 *AFM images of gold metallized nanofibers of PPI-G3–Cd(II). The fibers are decorated with gold nanoparticles; the molar ratio of PPI-G3:Au is a) 1:1, b) 1:3. The c) TEM and d) high-resolution (HR) TEM images show a regular distribution of Au nanoparticles along the fiber contour. The insets in the TEM images are magnified views of individual Au nanoparticles. Reproduced from reference 5 with permission.*

The AFM images in Figure 5a,b show gold-metallized nanofibers of PPI-G3–Cd(II), where necklace-like structures of Au nanoparticles are obtained which preferably mimic the contour of the nanofibers. The nucleation and growth of the Au particles are governed by the kinetics of both the coordination of HAuCl₄ to the primary amines of PPI-G3 and the reduction of the gold precursor to metallic gold. Moreover, the degree of metallization can be adjusted through the molar ratio of PPI-G3:HAuCl₄; a higher density of Au particles decorating the nanofibers is achieved at higher concentrations of gold precursor. For example, only a few Au nanoparticles are formed at molar ratios of PPI-G3:HAuCl₄ = 1:1 (Figure 5a), while regular necklace structures of nanofibers decorated with Au particles can be obtained at PPI-G3:HAuCl₄ = 1:3 (Figure 5b). Markedly, the spacing of the Au nanoparticles appears to be relatively constant along the nanofibers and the Au particles show a narrow size distribution, especially under the consideration that no additional stabilizer was employed during their preparation. The average particle size, as determined from TEM measurements (Figure 5c), is 5.4 nm with a standard deviation of 0.9 nm. Moreover, the presence of fringes in the HRTEM image (Figure 5d) suggests that the particles are crystalline.

2.2 Hybrid nanoalloys – Fabrication of CdSe nanoparticles-PPI dendrimer hybrid nanofibers decorated with Au nanoparticles along nanofibers contour

Our previous studies on Cd(II)-complexed PPI aggregates[5] stimulated us to do further investigations in order to fabricate novel, functional nanofibers with unique physical properties. For example, the preparation of highly anisotropic one dimensional nanostructures composed of closely packed nanoparticle arrays and their associated collective vectorial properties are of particular interest in the field of nanoelectronics, optoelectronics, biosensor, and nanodevice technology.[6] The purpose of this paragraph is to demonstrate the fabrication of well-defined nanostructures based on various non-covalent interactions among densely ordered CdSe nanoparticles within self-assembled PPI dendrimers.

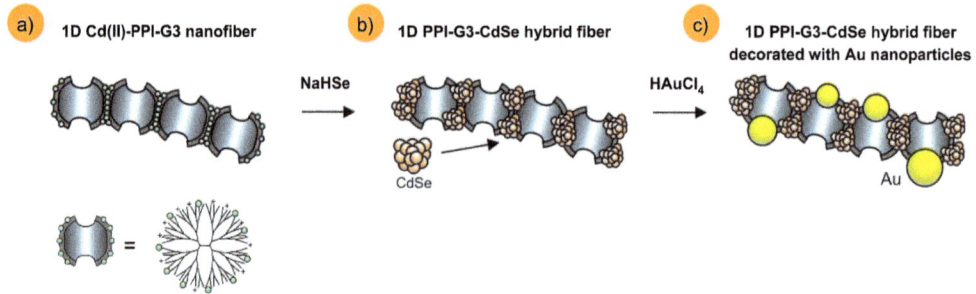

Figure 6 *Schematic illustration of various hybrid fibers. (a) Unidirectional self-assembly of 3rd generation poly(propylene imine) (PPI-G3) dendrimers in the presence of of Cd(II). (b) Cd(II)-PPI dendrimer nanofibers templating CdSe particles into hybrid nanofibers. (c) Metallisation of PPI-G3-CdSe nanofibers with gold nanoparticles. Reproduced from reference 6 with permission.*

A particular feature of this fabrication method is that the CdSe nanoparticles are prepared *in-situ* within the PPI matrices at a moderate pH and room temperature. Dendrimer-CdSe nanofibers are first prepared by a wet chemical method in aqueous solution. The hybrid nanofibers, however, can then be used as scaffolds to assemble spatially discrete Au nanoparticles along the PPI dendrimer-CdSe nanofibers. In this way, functional hybrid nanoalloys are obtained with interesting optical properties. Figure 6 gives a schematic illustration of the preparation of the hybrid nanoalloys.[6]

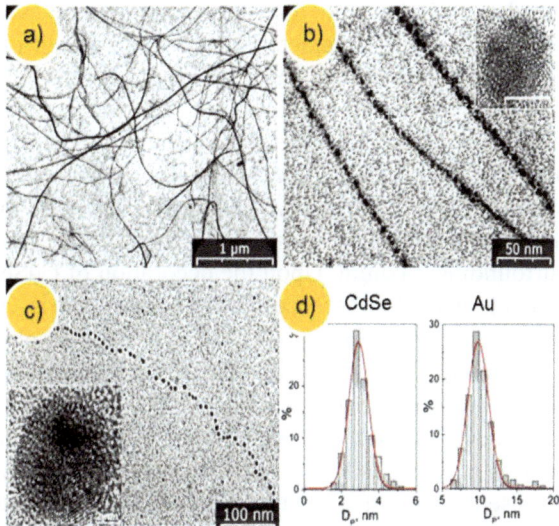

Figure 7 *TEM micrographs of self-assembled nanofibers based on dendrimer-stabilised CdSe nanoparticles (a, b). The insets in (b and c) are high resolution TEM micrographs with scale bar of 2 nm. TEM micrographs are showing crystalline CdSe nanoparticles within the fibers using 3rd generation poly(propylene imine) dendrimer. The nanofibers are metallized leading to form necklace-like structures of Au nanoparticles along the nanofiber's contour (c). The inset in (c) is a high resolution TEM micrograph showing a crystalline Au nanoparticle. Histograms of the particle size distribution are shown in (d) for both the CdSe and the Au nanoparticles. Reproduced from reference 6 with permission.*

In a typical experiment, the PPI dendrimer-CdSe hybrid nanofibers were prepared by mixing aqueous solutions (0.3 mM) of the 3rd generation PPI dendrimer (PPI-G3) and a solution (0.3 M) of cadmium acetate (Cd(CH$_3$COO)$_2$) in a specific molar ratio to form Cd(II)-PPI-G3 nanofibers (Figure 6a). A freshly prepared solution of NaSeH (0.05 M) was then injected into a solution of 10 mL of Cd(II)-PPI complex under inert (N$_2$ or Ar) atmosphere. The solution turned bright yellow immediately upon the addition of NaSeH, thus indicating the formation of small CdSe nanocrystals (Figure 6b). In the last step, a gold precursor (HAuCl$_4$) was added to dilute aqueous solutions of the PPI-G3-CdSe fibers in a certain molar ratio, e.g. PPI-G3-CdSe:HAuCl$_4$ = 1:1 or 1:3. From Figure 6c it can be seen that the gold precursor coordinates selectively to the available peripheral primary amines of the CdSe hybridfibers to form discrete alignment of the Au nanoparticles along the fibers. Various techniques were finally applied to characterize the thus obtained fibers. AFM and TEM were used to study the morphology of the nanoalloys, whereas optical properties were investigated by means of UV-Vis spectroscopy and photoluminescence. Figure 7 shows the TEM micrographs of the hybrid nanofibers based on self-assembled CdSe particles stabilized with PPI-G3 dendrimers. The dendrimer is mainly used to template CdSe nanoparticles *in-situ* followed by the assembly into hybrid nanofibers. The fibers have an average diameter of 6.4 nm and a length of up to 10 μm. Each nanofiber preferably adapts the diameter of the PPI-G3 dendrimer. Noteworthy, the PPI-G3 scaffold does not only template the CdSe nanoparticles and drive the formation of nanofibers in aqueous solution, but also confines the growth of the particles leading to a low polydispersity. Thus, analysis of the TEM micrographs yields a mean CdSe nanoparticle diameter of 2.9 nm with a standard deviation of 0.6 nm (Figure 7d).

Decorating the hybrid nanofibers with discrete Au nanoparticles change significantly their optical properties.[6] The optical characteristics of both the PPI-G3-CdSe nanofibers and the Au decorated assemblies were evaluated by using UV-Vis and photoluminescence (PL) spectroscopy. We have found that adsorption of Au nanoparticles onto the surface of the PPI dendrimer-CdSe nanofibers has a significant effect on their optical properties. For example, hybrid nanofibers of PPI-G3-CdSe exhibit a strong fluorescence emission band at λ_{max} = 570 nm (Figure 8a). It is well known that the position of the emission band of semiconductor quantum dots (QDs) depends on the particle size, the density within the nanofibers and the surrounding medium. Upon the decoration of CdSe nanofibers with Au nanoparticles, the characteristic fluorescence of the CdSe QDs is completely quenched (Figure 8b). Thus, only a very weak emission at λ_{max} = 553 nm is observed. Additionally, the presence of Au nanoparticles in the solution is indicated by the appearance of the typical surface plasmon resonance band at λ_{SPR} = 530 nm in the UV-Vis absorption spectra. These results indicate that self-assembled nanofibers containing fluorescent CdSe QDs in aqueous solutions may not only be used as labels or markers in biotechnological applications, but also as sensors for the detection of other (metallic) species in solution.

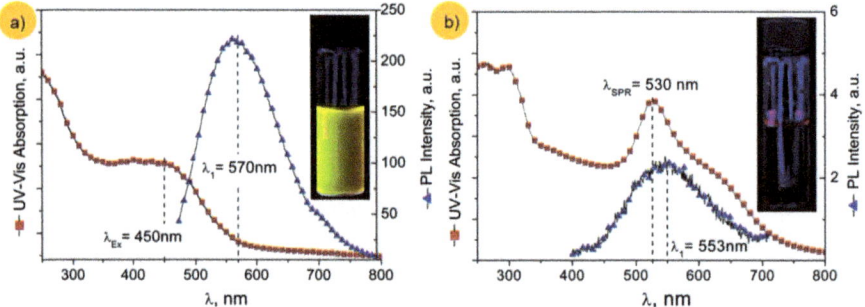

Figure 8 *UV-Vis and photoluminescence (PL) spectra of (a) nanofibers of dendrimer-stabilised CdSe quantum dots and (b) the same nanofibers after metallization with Au. The insets are optical photographs of aqueous solutions of nanofibers taken under UV-illumination. Reproduced from reference 6 with permission.*

2.3 Controlling the self-assembly and disassembly of dendrimer-based nanofibers in aqueous solution

The hybrid nanofibers described herein have been demonstrated to possess interesting functionalities and properties, because these materials can be functionalized in different ways to obtain hybrid conductor or semiconductor devices.[5,6] The purpose of this paragraph is to present the main factors that control the unidirectional dendrimer aggregation in aqueous solution. Controlling the self-assembly of dendrimer-based nanofibers is crucial. Apart from solution conditions (pH and ionic strength) possible parameters that control the self-assembly and disassembly are for example, dendrimer size (generation), types of ion sources (salt), and PPI:cation ratio.

Precise control over the fiber length could not be achieved by simply varying the dendrimer generation, PPI:Cd(II) ratio, and solution pH.[5] A crucial factor for the growth of 1D dendrimer fibers in water is the presence of a charge and shape asymmetry in the Cd(II)-complexed polymers, because a shape and charge asymmetry (or anisotropy) occurs more likely in dendrimers with a sufficiently flexible scaffold. In fact, micrometer-long nanofibers could only be obtained with 3rd generation and 4th generation dendrimers as a result of the higher flexibility of the dendritic scaffold.[5] For lower generations, however, fewer and considerably shorter fibers were found. Amino terminated PPI dendrimers are structurally defined, monodispersed polymers.[10,11]

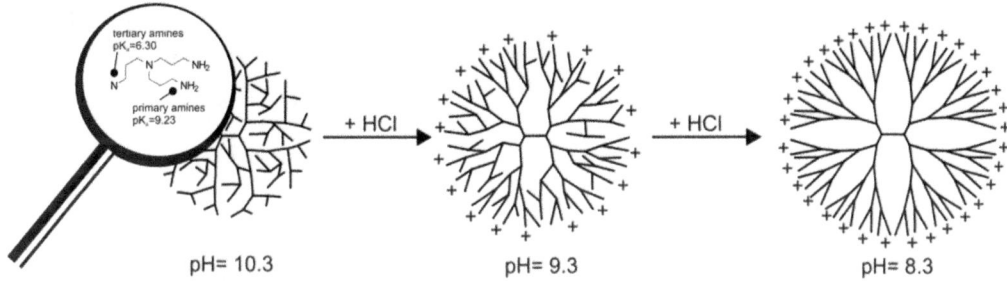

Figure 9 *Change of dendrimer conformation in aqueous solution as a function of pH. The surface charge gradually increases as the pH is lowered to 8.3.*

As shown in Figure 9, a 3rd generation amino-terminated PPI dendrimer consists of an interior based on 30 tertiary amine groups and a periphery of 32 primary amines. The primary amino groups at the dendrimer's surface are more alkaline (pK_a = 9.23) than the interior tertiary amino groups (pK_a = 6.30). This particular property is due to an environmental effect that allows for selective protonation of the dendrimer's surface at moderate pH, while the interior amino groups remain uncharged.[52] Amines closer to the core are generally expected to have a lower pK_a relative to identical functional groups located at the surface of the dendrimer. As a result of selective protonation, the conformation of amino-terminated PPI dendrimer changes, because the globular shape of the PPI dendrimer strongly depends on external factors, such as the type of surrounding medium (polarity), its acidity and ionic strength. Figure 9 shows, schematically, the expected conformational change of 3rd generation amino-terminated PPI dendrimers (PPI-G3) at different pH conditions. At high pH and ionic strength the PPI dendrimers tend to adopt a compact, globular shape, while the opposite conditions lead to an extended conformation. At high pH almost all surface functional groups are deprotonated, thus giving rise to a noncharged surface. Backfolding therefore results in an increased molecular density in the interior of the dendrimer. Acidification, however, causes a partial protonation of the terminal amine groups, where upon a gradual increase in surface charge towards positive is observed. As a result, an asymmetric shape and charge distribution is observed. The complete protonation of the peripheral amine groups does not allow backfolding of the terminal groups and yields an overall globular shape. Considering a pK_a of 9.23 and by using the Henderson–Hasselbach equation the extent of ionization of amino groups can be estimated.[25] Thus, at pH 8.3 almost all terminal amino groups of PPI-G3 are protonated.

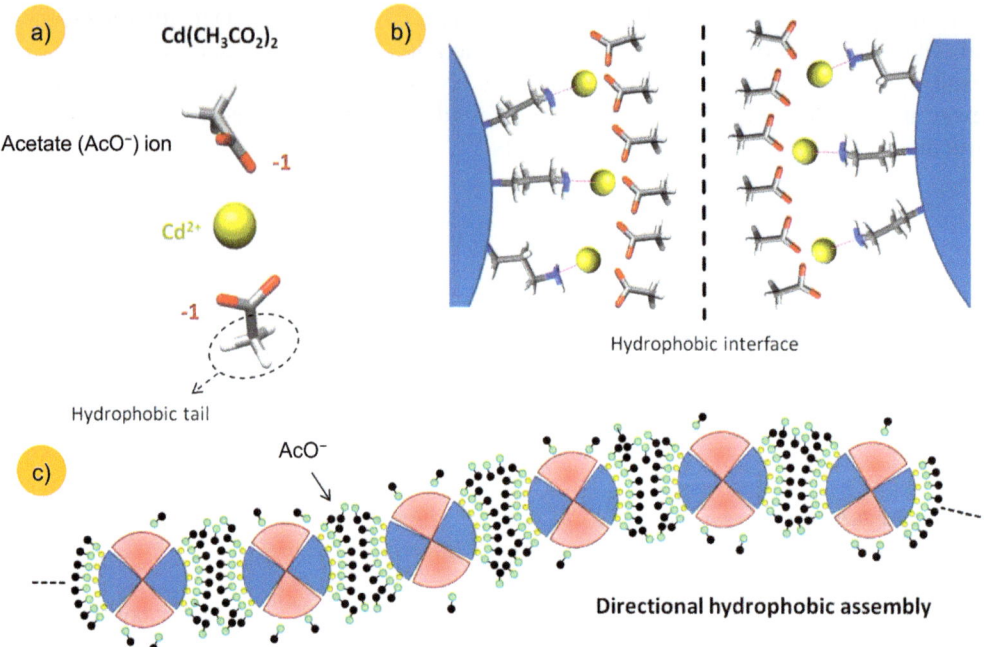

Figure 10 *Ionic-selective mechanism of dendrimer-fibers formation. (a) The entire mechanism is controlled by acetate ions. (b) The particular features of AcO⁻ generate a self-assembly controlled by hydrophobic forces – the tail-tail coupling of AcO⁻ ions recalls the mechanism of formation of lipid bilayers. (c) Dendrimers aggregation along preferential directionality is due to hydrophobic anisotropy at D's surface which drives to aggregation of blue hydrophobic domains. Reproduced from reference 5 with permission.*

It is well known that cations or anions strongly interact with the charged surface of a dendritic molecule.[55-59] Therefore, the influence of the type of ion on fiber formation has been explored in depth by using molecular dynamics (MD) simulations.[7] Results for Cd(CH₃COOH)₂ were discussed in terms of ion association to the charged dendrimer surface and compared with cadmium derivatives like CdCl₂ and CdSO₄. First, we created a model for PPI-G3 dendrimer (D) in aqueous solution. For this purpose, the cadmium ions (10 Cd(II)) were coordinated uniformly and randomly to 10 of the total 32 amino surface groups of the unfolded PPI dendrimer. Due to the solution pH of 8.3, the remaining surface groups were mainly addressed to be protonated (22 NH₃⁺). A single unfolded dendrimer was finally equilibrated in a periodic box containing water and the respective ions. MD simulations demonstrate some very interesting results. Although the cadmium ions are partially bound to the dendrimer surface, acetate ions (AcO⁻) seem to play the major role in controlling the monodimensional dendrimer assembly in aqueous solution. As shown in Figure 10, negatively charged AcO⁻ ions are strongly attracted by the surface cadmium ions, because the positive charge of each Cd(II) decorated NH₂–Cd²⁺ segment is double that present on the NH₃⁺ group. Hence, acetate ions preferably coordinate to the NH₂–Cd²⁺ segment groups of the dendritic scaffold (Figure 10). As a result, very tight and stable primary dendrimer-Cd(II)-acetate (D-AcO⁻) complexes are formed.

The strong attraction and stable coordination between surface Cd(II) and the negatively charged acetate ions have an important impact on the aggregation phenomena studied here.

As illustrated in Figure 10b, the NH$_2$-Cd(II) surface groups of D are surrounded by AcO$^-$ tails (highly hydrophobic CH$_3$ groups) which intuitively transforms the symmetrical and spherical shaped dendrimers into asymmetric building blocks. As a general consequence, however, this phenomenon subdivides the surface of D into hydrophilic (red) and hydrophobic (blue) domains where the latter ones tend to aggregate as represented conceptually by the schemes of Figure 10b,c. Within the D−AcO$^-$ primary complexes, hydrophobicity is entirely focused onto the blue domains. The directional assembly of PPI dendrimers can therefore be attributed to the hydrophobic anisotropy at D's surface. In this context it is of interest to note that solvation energy (G$_{sol}$) analysis indeed demonstrated that when acetate ions stabilize over D's surface, the resulting dendrimer-ion primary complex D−AcO$^-$ is greater than ten times more hydrophobic than the native dendrimer D.

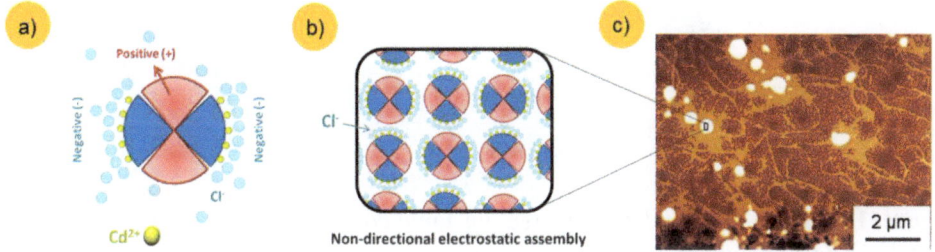

Figure 11 *CdCl$_2$ (3 mM) does not generate nanofibers of poly(propylene imine) dendrimers (D) (0.3 mM) in water. The non-directional aggregation of D-Cl$^-$ complexes is generated by the electrostatic attraction between the oppositely charged red and blue surface domains which induce the formation of multiple globular super-assemblies in solution with ~0.5-1 µm of size. Reproduced from reference 7 with permission.*

Noteworthy, while red domains (NH$_3^+$ groups) are in general hydrophilic and positively charged, the characteristics of the blue ones (NH$_2$−Cd(II)) depend on the coordinated anions. Contrary to AcO$^-$, chloride ions (Cl$^-$) induce an overall negative surface charge on the blue domains, whereas the red ones remain positively charged (Figure 11a). As a result of electrostatic attraction between the oppositely charged red (NH$_3^+$) and blue (NH$_2$−Cd(II)−Cl$^-$) domains, a nondirectional aggregation of many D−Cl$^-$ primary complexes is observed (Figure 11b). Thus, atomic force microscopic (AFM) studies showed that in a solution of 3 mM CdCl$_2$, no formation of fibers occurs for the same PPI-G3 dendrimers (0.3 mM PPI) under the same conditions. This clearly demonstrates the absence of any assembly directionality. As can be seen from Figure 11c, spherical aggregates with a diameter of around 0.5 to 1 µm are formed.

The lack of directionality in the assembly generated by CdCl$_2$ is due to the symmetry of Cl$^-$ ions, and was also verified for other transition-metal based salts with symmetric anions (i.e., CdSO$_4$). The peculiar partition of D's surface into different red and blue surface domains is intrinsically dependent upon the concentration of the respective ions owing to the partial Cd^{2+} coordination of the dendrimers surface. Thus, AFM measurements showed that already at 1:20 dendrimer−Cd(CH$_3$COO)$_2$ molar ratio, the assembly loses directionality and the fibers are almost entirely replaced by supramolecular assemblies with globular shape.

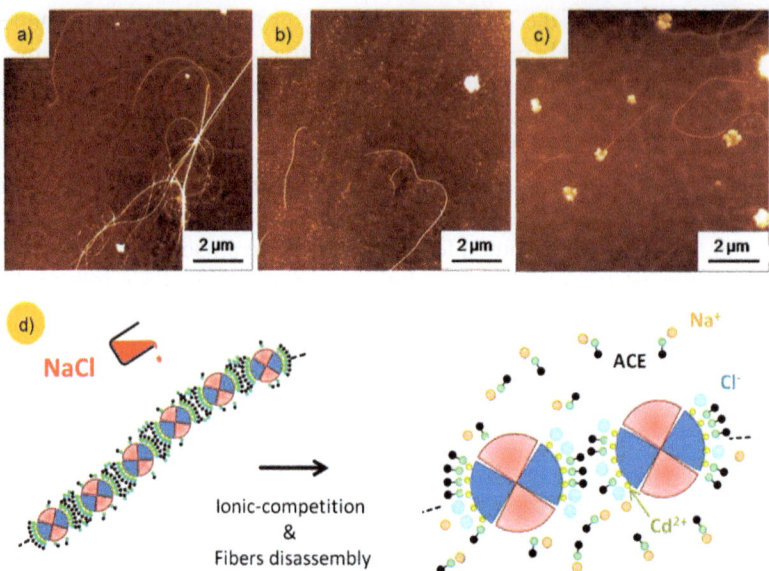

Figure 12 *Fibers-disassembly triggered by ionic-competition. (a) AFM image of PPI-Cd(CH₃COO)₂ nanofibers on silicon substrate. Fibers are formed dissolving 0.3 mM PPI G3 dendrimer in distilled water solution with 3 mM Cd(CH₃COO)₂ (a molecular ratio with the dendrimers of 10:1). (b) After the addition of only 0.3 mM NaCl in solution (1:1 molar ratio with the dendrimer) most of the dendrimer fibers start do disassemble and to disappear from the solution substituted by a general dispersity. (c) When the NaCl salt concentration is increased to 3 mM (the same concentration in solution of Cadmium acetate) the fibers start to be replaced by particles as was evidenced in CdCl₂ solution. (d) Fibers disassembly is induced by ionic-competition; at D's surface Cl⁻ (cyan) replace AcO⁻ ions (green and black) due to a higher affinity for Cd (II) (yellow). Reproduced from reference 7 with permission.*

Self assembly and aggregation directionality are both governed exclusively by ions, making the mechanism of nanofiber formation a real "ion-selective" process.[7] This in turn suggests that it is also possible to use other ions to trigger disassembly, as for example by using simple NaCl salt. Figure 12 demonstrates the efficacy of this principle. As soon as 0.3 mM of NaCl is introduced into the hybrid system (Figure 12a) the nanofibers start to disassemble rapidly (Figure 12b). Moreover, when the NaCl concentration is increased to 3 mM (Figure 12c) the fibers start to be substituted by globular aggregates with again 0.5–1 µm of size. This disassembly process, however, is due to ion-competition; Cl⁻ replaces AcO⁻ ions at dendrimer's surface. As a result, AcO⁻ anions diffuse in solution (Figure 12d). It is evident that the presence of Cl⁻ at D's surface eliminates the hydrophobic surface anisotropy which controls the unidirectional assembly.

3 CONCLUSION

The fabrication of nanostructures via directed self-assembly has emerged as a promising approach for novel functional materials with unique optical, magnetic, and electronic properties.   The aim of this book chapter has been to present recent approaches to dendrimer-based hybrid fibers as potential template for 1D-Objects in nanotechnology. We first presented a simple and fast method to fabricate bimetallic nanofibers via self-assembly of PPI dendrimers in the presence of cadmium acetate. Dendrimers-aggregation and assembly-directionality are both controlled by acetate anions and molecular dynamics simulation demonstrated that acetate ions from dissociated $Cd(CH_3COO)_2$ generate selectively cationic PPI-dendrimers fibers through hydrophobic-modification. Noteworthy, this well-defined directional assembly of cationic dendrimers is absent for other cadmium derivatives, i.e. $CdCl_2$ or $CdSO_4$. However, self-assembly and aggregation directionality are both governed exclusively by ions, making the mechanism of nanofiber formation a real "ion-selective" process supported by necessary hydrophobic-hydrophobic interactions. Since fibers-disassembly can be triggered by using NaCl salt, the fabrication methods described herein represents a simple and cost effective tool to control actively such self-assembled functional nanomaterials.

The preparation of highly anisotropic one dimensional nanostructures composed of closely packed nanoparticle arrays and their associated collective vectorial properties are of particular interest in the field of nanoelectronics, optoelectronics, biosensor, and nanodevice technology. Interestingly, the obtained hybrid organic-inorganic nanofibers can be used as a scaffold to guide the nucleation and growth of Au-nanoparticles along the hybrid nanofibers surface. We demonstrated the fabrication of well-defined nanostructures based on complexation interactions among densely ordered CdSe nanoparticles within self-assembled PPI dendrimers. A particular feature of this fabrication method is that the CdSe nanoparticles are prepared in-situ within the PPI matrices at a moderate pH and room temperature. The directed self-assembly of PPI dendrimers mediating the in-situ confinement of CdSe nanoparticles is a versatile tool for preparing dendrimer-CdSe hybrid nanofibers. These nanofabrication approach via directed self-assembly opens a new avenue for the generation of novel and well-defined hybrid 1D-Objects possess unique optical, magnetic, and electronic properties, those functional materials will have a bright future in many applications. However, more translational research is necessary to evaluate their potential applications in bio- and nanotechnology.

Acknowledgement

The authors acknowledge the COST action TD0802, 'Dendrimers in Biomedical Applications', in favoring this collaborative research program. Dr. Anderas Mohr and Dr. Marek Maly are thankfully acknowledged for the useful discussions.

References

1   A.P. Alivisatos, *Science*, 1996, **271**, 933.
2   S.A. Empedocles and M.G. Bawendi, *Science*, 1997, **278**, 2114.
3   W.U. Huynh, J.J. Dittmer and A.P. Alivisatos, *Science*, 2002, **295**, 2425.
4   G. Yu and C.M. Lieber, *Pure Appl. Chem.*, 2010, **82**, 2295.
5   T. Pietsch, N. Cheval, D. Appelhans, N. Gindy, B. Voit and A. Fahmi, *Small*, 2011, **7**, 221.
6   A. Fahmi, D. Appelhans, N. Cheval, T. Pietsch, C. Bellmann, N. Gindy and B. Voit, *Adv. Mater.*, 2011, **23**, 3289.
7   M. Garzoni, N. Cheval, A. Fahmi, A. Danani and G.M. Pavan, *J. Am. Chem. Soc.*, 2012, **134**, 3349.
8   F. Zeng and S.C. Zimmerman, *Chem. Rev.*, 1997, **97**, 1681.
9   A.W. Bosman, H.M. Janssen and E.W. Meijer, *Chem. Rev.*, 1999, **99**, 1665.

10 G.R. Newkome, C.N. Moorefield, and F. Vögtle, *Dendrimers and Dendrons: Concepts, Syntheses, Applications*, Wiley-VCH, Weinheim, 2001.

11 J.M.J. Frechet and D.A. Tomalia, *Dendrimers and Other Dendritic Polymers*, John Wiley & Sons, Ltd, Chichester, UK, 2001.

12 R. van Heerbeek, P.C.J. Kamer, P.W.N.M. van Leeuwen and J.N.H. Reek, *Chem. Rev.*, 2002, **102**, 3717.

13 S.H. Medina and M.E.H. El-Sayed, *Chem. Rev.*, 2009, **109**, 3141.

14 D. Astruc, E. Boisselier and C. Ornelas, *Chem. Rev.*, 2010, **110**, 1857.

15 L. M. Bronstein and Z.B. Shifrina, *Chem. Rev.*, 2011, **111**, 5301.

16 A. Mohr and R. Haag, in *Applications of Supramolecular Chemistry*, CRC Press, Boca Raton, US, 2012.

17 *Dendrimers, Dendrons and Dendritic Polymers: Discovery, Applications, the Future,"* D.A. Tomalia, J.B. Christensen and U. Boas, Cambridge University Press, NY (2012).

18 A.R. Menjoge, R.M. Kannan and D.A. Tomalia, *Drug Discovery Today*, 2010, **15** (5/6), 171.

19 S.M. Grayson and J.M.J. Fréchet, *Chem. Rev.*, 2001, **101**, 3819.

20 E. Buhleiner, W. Wehner and F. Vögtle, *Synthesis*, 1978, 155.

21 D.A. Tomalia, H. Baker, J. Dewald, M. Hall, G. Kallos, S. Martin, J. Roeck, J. Ryder and P. Smith, *Polym. J.*, 1985, **17**, 117.

22 M. Shema-Mizrachi, G.M. Pavan, E. Levin, A. Danani and N.G. Lemcoff, *J. Am. Chem. Soc.*, 2011, **133**, 14359.

23 J. Lim, G.M. Pavan, O. Annunziata and E.E. Simanek, *J. Am. Chem. Soc.*, 2012, **134**, 1942.

24 W. Chen, D.A. Tomalia, and J.L. Thomas, *Macromolecules*, 2000, **33**, 9169.

25 I. Lee, B.D. Athey, A.W. Wetzel, W. Meixner and J.R. Baker, *Macromolecules*, 2002, **35**, 4510.

26 Y. Liu, V.S. Bryantsev, M.S. Diallo and W.A. Goddard III, *J. Am. Chem. Soc.*, 2009, **131**, 2798.

27 J. Khandare, A. Mohr, M. Calderón, P. Welker, K. Licha and R. Haag, *Biomaterials*, 2010, **31**, 4268.

28 J.J. Storhoff and C.A. Mirkin, *Chem. Rev.*, 1999, **99**, 1849.

29 Z. Tang, N.A. Kotov and M. Giersig, *Science*, 2002, **297**, 237.

30 E. Katz and I. Willner, *Angew. Chem. Int. Ed.*, 2004, **43**, 6042.

31 R.A. Sperling, P.R. Gil, F. Zhang, M. Zanella and W.J. Parak, *Chem. Soc. Rev.*, 2008, **37**, 1896.

32 H. Zhang and D. Wang, *Angew. Chem.*, 2008, **120**, 4048.

33 B.A. Grzybowski, C.E. Wilmer, J. Kim, K.P. Browne and K.J.M. Bishop, *Soft Matter*, 2009, **5**, 1110.

34 X. Qi, C. Xue, X. Huang, Y. Huang, X. Zhou, H.Li, D. Liu, F. Boey, Q. Yan, W. Huang, S. De Feyter, K. Müllen and H. Zhang, *Adv. Funct. Mater.*, 2010, **20**, 43.

35 M.J. Rosen and J.T. Kunjappu, *Surfactants and Interfacial Phenomena*, John Wiley & Sons, Ltd, Hoboken, US, 4th edn., 2012.

36 K. Holmberg, B. Jönsson, B. Kronberg and B. Lindman, *Surfactants and Polymers in Aqueous Solution*, John Wiley & Sons, Ltd, 2nd edn., 2002.

37 A.-K. Awizio, *From Lipid Bilayers to Synaptic Vesicles: Atomic Force Microscopy on Lipid-based Systems*, VDM Verlag, 2008.

38 P. Kumar and K.L. Mittal, *Handbook of Microemulsion Science and Technology*, Marcel Dekker Inc, 1999.

39 Y. Osada and A.R. Khokhlov, *Polymer Gels and Networks*, Marcel Dekker Inc, 2001.

40 S. Chandrasekhar, *Liquid Crystals*, Cambridge University press, 2nd edn., 1992.
41 Q. Wang, J.L. Mynar, M. Yoshida, E. Lee, M. Lee, K. Okuro, K. Kinbara and T. Aida, *Nature*, 2010, **463**, 339.
42 J.G. Worden, Q. Dai and Q. Huo, *Chem. Commun.*, 2006, 1536.
43 R.W.J. Scott, H. Ye, R.R. Henriquez and R.M. Crooks, *Chem. Mater.*, 2003, **15**, 3873.
44 A. Fahmi, T. Pietsch, D. Appelhans, N. Gindy and B. Voit, *New J. Chem.*, 2009, **33**, 703.
45 V.I. Klimov, A.A. Mikhailovsky, S. Xu, A. Malko, J.A. Hollingsworth, C.A. Leatherdale, H.-J. Eisler and M.G. Bawendi, *Science*, 2000, **290**, 314.
46 J. Kong, N.R. Franklin, C. Zhou, M.G. Chapline, S. Peng, K. Cho and H. Dai, *Science*, 2000, **287**, 622.
47 X. Duan, Y. Huang, Y. Cui, J. Wang and C.M. Lieber, *Nature*, 2001, **409**, 66.
48 M.S. Gudiksen, L.J. Lauhon, J. Wang, D.C. Smith and C.M. Lieber, *Nature*, 2002, **415**, 617.
49 W.C.W. Chan and S. Nie, *Science*, 1998, **281**, 2016.
50 M. Bruchez, M. Moronne, P. Gin, S. Weiss and A.P. Alivisatos, *Science*, 1998, **281**, 2013.
51 T.A. Taton, C.A. Mirkin and R.L. Letsinger, *Science*, 2000, **289**, 1757.
52 S.A. Hasan, Q. Fariduddin, B. Ali, S. Hayat and A. Ahmad, *J. Environ. Biol.*, 2009, **30**, 165.
53 P.E. Chow, *Gold Nanoparticles: Properties, Characterization and Fabrication*, Nova Science Publishers, Inc., 2010.
54 R.W.J. Scott, O.M. Wilson and R.M. Crooks, *J. Phys. Chem. B*, 2004, **109**, 692.
55 M.S. Diallo, S. Christie, P. Swaminathan, L. Balogh, X. Shi, W. Um, C. Papelis, W.A. Goddard III and J.H. Johnson, *Langmuir*, 2004, **20**, 2640.
56 M.S. Diallo, S. Christie, P. Swaminathan, J.H. Johnson and W.A. Goddard III, *Environ.Sci. Technol.*, 2005, **39**, 1366.
57 M.S. Diallo, K. Falconer, J.H. Johnson and W.A. Goddard III, *Environ. Sci. Technol.*, 2007, **41**, 6521.
58 M.S. Diallo, W. Arasho, J.H. Johnson and W.A. Goddard III, *Environ. Sci. Technol.*, 2008, **42**, 1572.
59 K.A. Marvin, J.A. Johnson, S.E. Rodenbusch, L. Gong, D.A. Vanden Bout and K.J. Stevenson, *Anal. Chem.*, 2012, **84**, 5154.

NATURAL AND SYNTHETIC BIOMATERIALS AS COMPOSITES OF ADVANCED DRUG DELIVERY NANO SYSTEMS (ADDNSS). BIOMEDICAL APPLICATIONS

K. Gardikis [1], E. A. Mourelatou [1], M. Ionov [2], A. Aserin [3], D. Libster [3], B. Klajnert[2], M. Bryszewska[2], N. Garti [3], J.-P. Majoral [4], K. Dimas [5] and C. Demetzos [1,*]

[1] Faculty of Pharmacy, Department of Pharmaceutical Technology, Panepistimiopolis Zografou 15771, University of Athens, Greece
[2] Department of General Biophysics, Faculty of Biology and Environmental Protection, University of Lodz, Poland
[3] Casali Institute of Applied Chemistry, The Institute of Chemistry, The Hebrew University of Jerusalem, Edmond J. Safra Campus, Givat Ram, Jerusalem 91904, Israel
[4] Laboratoire de Chimie de Coordination CNRS, Toulouse, France
[5] Department of Pharmacology, Faculty of Medicine, University of Thessaly, Biopolis, Larisa.

1 INTRODUCTION

The most common problems/challenges concerning bioactive molecules are their **A**bsorption, bio**D**istribution, **M**etabolism and **E**xcretion, referred to as the ADME profile of the drug. Excipients, an essential part of the drug formulation have been traditionally used in order to ameliorate the ADME profile of the bioactive substance. Since the late 1960s and especially during the last decade, excipients –named drug delivery systems- have evolved to the extent that they represent a very important component of the drug compound playing a key role in the final formulation almost as important as the bioactive ingredient[1] a role that has begun to take new dimensions with the arrival of nanotechnology. Nanotechnology is the multi-disciplinary scientific field that is changing the philosophy and the modalities of almost every contemporary scientific application. Drug delivery is one of the scientific fields that benefits to a large extent from this technologic breakthrough by the formation of Drug Delivery nanoSystems (DDnSs). The new nano-scale drug carriers offer the possibility of increasing the Therapeutic Index (TI) of known or new drug molecules by increasing their effectiveness, diminishing their toxicity against physiological tissues and achieving controlled and sustained therapeutic levels of the drug for prolonged time. The proper choice of a drug delivery agent can alter the solubility and ameliorate the stability of candidate drugs, improving their overall ADME profile[2].

Sustained release systems provide beneficial behavior because of their ability to maintain therapeutic blood levels of the administered drug for an extended period of time. The above systems do not release drugs in a zero order kinetics, but provide a slow first order released profile. Controlled release systems can be effective if the release of the drug can be modulated by the biomaterials from which the system has been produced[3]. The design of a Modulatory Controlled Release System in nano scale level (MCRnS) needs biomaterials which can modulate the release of the encapsulated drug. Parenteral administration which is used to administer potent drugs with an 'immediate' effect but with serious adverse effects is a challenging field for the design and development of DDnSs. Furthermore achieving a controlled release profile through modulating the drug release with appropriate biomaterials (natural or synthetic) is an additional challenge. The most widely used vesicles composed of natural biomaterials in DDnSs are liposomes. They are able to encapsulate either lipophilic or hydrophilic drugs in their lipidic bilayers or aqueous interior respectively. It has been proved that they are able to ameliorate the pharmacokinetic and pharmacological profile of many drugs [4-6] giving way to the appearance of several liposomal formulations in the market. The application of liposomes is limited because of their thermodynamic instability, giving rise to phenomena such as aggregation, fusion or drug leakage upon storage. However these problems have been significantly tackled with freeze drying [7-8]. As far as synthetic DDnSs are concerned, polymers are the most widely used. Dendrimers and hyperbranched polymers (HBPs) seem to be very promising categories of polymers.

Dendrimers, a so-called 4th new architectural class of polymers, represent a relatively new category of drug delivery vehicles[9-11]. The dendritic macromolecular structure is well-defined and consists of a central core, branching units and terminal functional groups which can be further chemically modified. Due to their precise architecture, dendrimers are monodisperse, which gives them a significant advantage over other generally polydisperse nanoparticles and allows for greater control over their pharmacodynamic profile. Furthermore, as drug delivery vehicles, they can be used either for encapsulation of bioactive compounds in their core or covalent or non-covalent attachment of bioactive compounds at their periphery. They also offer other potential advantages such as prolongation of drug circulation time, protection of a drug from its surroundings, increase of drug stability (and possibly effectiveness) and the ability to target diseased tissue[12-15].

HBPs are a relatively young class of dendritic polymers that has lately attracted much attention in the research field and their effectiveness in replacing dendrimers as drug carriers is under study. HBPs are characterized by a high degree of branching, a three dimensional architecture and multiple terminal functional units[16]. Compared to dendrimers, they are polydisperse, due to their random branching and the existence of linear units in their structure. However they are obtained via one-step reactions, through the statistical polymerization of ABx (x being the number of repeating units)- type monomers by means of condensation or addition procedures, which makes them low-cost, easily produced high functional products. Although current advances in research of polymers with highly branched architecture have created opportunities for the development of new drug delivery systems, the research of HBPs as drug carriers is still in its infancy. Several approaches have been performed including the entrapment or the non-covalent attachment of drug molecules to HBPs (drug complexes or unimolecular micelles), the covalent conjugation of drug molecules to the terminal groups of HBPs and the drug loading in multimolecular micelle cores [17]. The combination of two nanocarriers of different nature, liposomes and polymers, in one nanoparticle took place for the first time in the beginning of last decade [18-19] and gained such attention ever since [20-24]. This new mixed system was categorized as an efficient class of Modulatory Liposomal Controlled Release Systems (MLCRS) [25] that belong to the MCRnSs. The MCRnSs have been classified into conventional DDnSs (cDDnSs) and advanced DDnSs (aDDnSs). Polymeric or lipidic nanosystems belong to cDDnSs. The aDDnSs can be characterized as mixed nanosystems due to the combination of different in nature biomaterials, for example a synthetic with a natural biomaterial. The nature of the biomaterials (same or different) used is a crucial.

In the first case the system should be defined as **hy**bridic (**hy**-), for example liposomes in liposomes [26] while in the second case as **chi**meric (**chi**-) [21, 27], from the ancient Greek mythology, for example dendrimers in liposomes. The attention of the scientific community **chi**-aDDnSs has been attracted due to two significant advantages over conventional nanocarriers and especially liposomes: a) the increase of the drug load up taken by the system and b) the modification of the drug release from the **chi**-aDDnS compared to that of the conventional liposomal formulation leading to higher TI [18, 21, 25].

This article is a review of the attempts for the creation of aDDnSs comprised of liposomes and polymers focusing on the interactions of the structural components and their biomedical applications.

2 aDDnSs CONSISTING OF LIPOSOMES AND DENDRIMERS

2.1 aDDnSs containing PAMAM Dendrimers

The first attempt for the creation of a single nanocarrier consisting of liposomes and dendrimers was the work performed by Khopade et al. [18]. In that study, cationic polyamidoamine (PAMAM) dendrimers were incorporated in the aqueous interior of liposomes in order to increase the encapsulation efficiency of the acidic anticancer drug methotrexate. The loading of the drug was indeed increased proportionally to dendrimer generation while the leakage of the drug from the system decreased. The results from this work were impressive, though limited data on the physicochemical interactions between the components were provided. A further study of such systems was made by Papagiannaros, Demetzos et al. [23] in which a PAMAM G4-doxorubicin complex was formed prior to encapsulation in liposomes. From the results obtained this system seems to be quite promising in terms of drug release and cytotoxic activity against cancer cell lines. The above studies demonstrated the superiority of PAMAM dendrimers containing aDDnSs compared to conventional liposomal carriers but did not provide adequate information in order to explain the physicochemical processes responsible for this amelioration. It is worth mentioning that a number of studies have focused on the physicochemical interactions between PAMAM dendrimers and non-liposomal or liposomal lipidic membranes. The immobilization of anionic liposomes with PAMAM G4 has been explored using FT-IR, X-ray diffraction and Surface Plasmon Resonance (SPR) [22] and the results revealed that PAMAM G4 dendrimers may be used to fabricate porous carrier films on the liposome surface through which ions or small molecules can be diffused and subsequently released from liposomes. Another study by ^{31}P NMR and AFM, using neutral liposomes and lipid bilayers interacting with PAMAM G7 dendrimers gave similar results which were attributed to the formation of lipid-dendrimer aggregates [28-29]. A very important method for studying physicochemical interactions in complex systems such as aDDnSs is Differential Scanning Calorimetry (DSC). Recently our groups have published several reports of thermal analysis data for the interaction of dendrimers with model lipid membranes or liposomes[30-34].

The first serious attempt for the investigation of the physicochemical interactions between liposomes and dendrimers in a single aDDnS was performed by Gardikis, Demetzos et al.[24]. In that study anionic PAMAM (G3,5) dendrimers were incorporated into liposomes consisted of dipalmitoyl phosphatidyl choline (DPPC) and dipalmitoyl phosphatidyl glycerol (DPPG) and the anticancer drug Doxorubicin (Dox) was loaded into the aDDnSs. PAMAM G3,5 was chosen because of the high probability of the creation of electrostatic complexes with the positively charged Dox in the pH of the interior of the liposome. The loading of Dox was significantly increased in the case of the aDDnS compared to the conventional liposome (dendrimer free DPPC/DPPG), as expected. The physicochemical interactions between the components of the empty or loaded systems were studied with thermal analysis (micro DSC) and the results were in line with a picture of phase separation between DPPC/DPPG lipids and PAMAM dendrimer that promotes the stability of the liposome membrane and the cooperativity of the relevant gel-to-liquid crystalline transition, which is enhanced in the simultaneous presence of the dendrimer and the drug. This process implies a practically complete displacement of the dendrimer and the drug into the aqueous core of the liposome, the membrane of which behaves like a simple multilamellar (non liposomal) lipid membrane (MLB). As a result, the inner core of the liposome contained large amounts of PAMAM-Dox complex was protected by a very stable membrane. The interactions between PAMAM and the lipid membrane were found to be entropy driven, indicating absence or minor direct molecular interactions. These results were generally validated through respective investigations on hydroxyl-terminated dendrimers of lower generations, indicating that the crucial factor for the creation of a stable and effective (in terms of drug loading and controlled release of the drug) aDDnS is rather the induction of phase separation on the lipid membrane than the nature or branching degree of the polymer used. The data from the above work were applied for the design of a study investigating the pharmacological effect of PAMAM containing aDDnSs[2]. In that study, PAMAM G3,5 was incorporated in liposomes consisted of dioleyl phosphatidyl choline (DOPC) and dipalmitoyl phosphatidyl glycerol (DPPG) for the formation of a new aDDnS. In this aDDnSs, Dox was encapsulated and the final product was subjected to lyophilization. The physicochemical properties of the system, in terms of drug loading efficiency, *in vitro* release profile, thermotropic behavior, fluorescent spectroscopic behavior and *in vitro* pharmacological toxicity were assessed versus the respective conventional liposomal system (DOPC/DPPG). It has been shown that PAMAM dendrimers interact with both hydrophilic and lipophilic part of the liposomal membrane while upon Dox loading, the electrostatic complex probably migrates in the interior of the liposomal cavity, verifying the findings from the previous work in a very different lipidic system. The results revealed the superiority of the aDDnS as far as encapsulation efficiency; drug release profile and pharmacological profile are concerned. Furthermore, the Dox-aDDnS system was easily lyophilized retaining its physicochemical characteristics upon reconstitution, thus overcoming the well-known stability disadvantages of conventional liposomal vesicles.

2.2 aDDnSs containing Polyether-Polyester Dendrimers

The lipidic system DOPC/DPPG was also used for the creation of an aDDnS containing newly synthesized hydroxyl terminated polyether-polyester (PEPE) dendrimers of first and second generation, namely PG1 and PG2 **(Figure 1)**.

It has to be noticed that polyether-polyester dendrimers have demonstrated the capability to penetrate the Blood Brain Barrier (BBB). In a study published by Dhanikula et al. [35] it was reported that glycosylated PEPE may efficiently deliver methotrexate (MTX) in avascular human glioma tumor spheroids. In this study authors demonstrated that MTX-loaded PEPE dendrimers were more potent than free MTX as well as effective against MTX-resistant glioma cells. Thus, authors concluded that these dendrimers could deliver MTX across BBB in high amounts and can penetrate into the central necrotic regions of a vascular tumor spheroids suggesting that glucosylated PEPE dendrimers can serve as potential delivery system for the treatment of gliomas. Dox was also used as a model drug and the physicochemical characteristics of the drug delivery system were assessed using DSC and fluorescence spectroscopy.

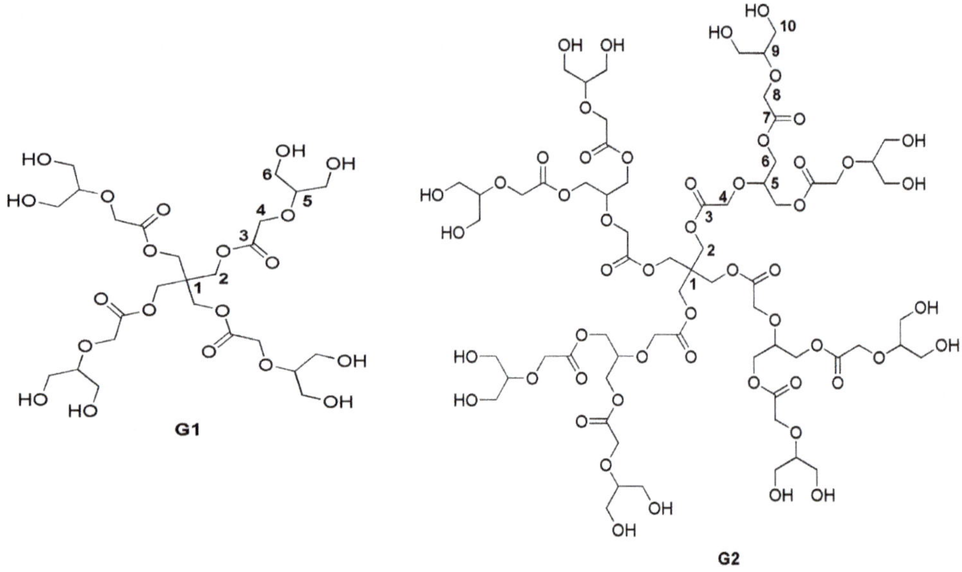

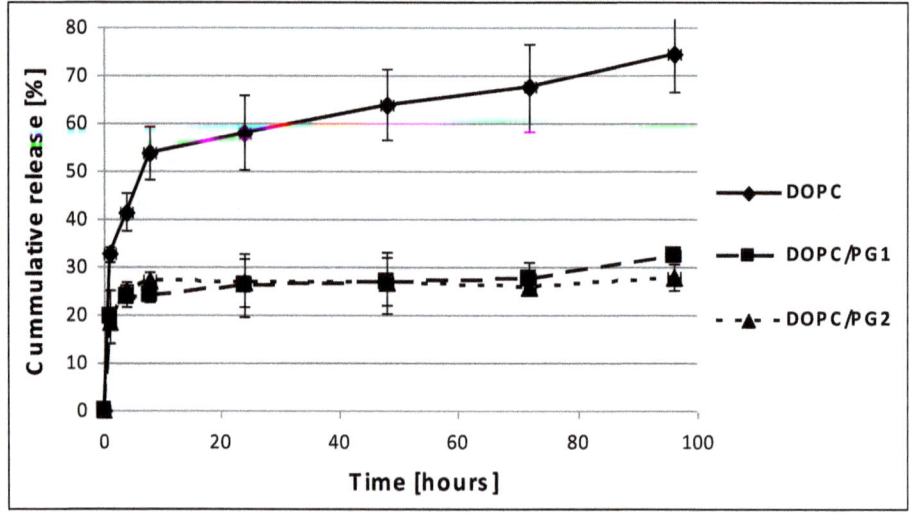

Figure 1 *Generation 1 and 2 (**G1&G2**) PG dendrimers.*

Figure 2 *In vitro release of Dox-loaded pure liposomes (DOPC) or **chi**-aDDnSs (DOPC/PG1, DOPC/PG2) in RPMI 5%* [27]

The aDDnS which has been produced exhibited high drug loads and slower *in vitro* release rate compared to the respective conventional liposomes (**Figure 2**). The physicochemical studies revealed a strong, concentration dependent, interaction between the lipidic chains of DOPC and PG1 or PG2 dendrimers. On the other hand, the interaction of the polar head groups of the lipids with both dendrimers was found to be not significant. Furthermore the interaction between lipids and dendrimers was found to be of entropic nature, as expected, leading to the conclusion that probably no bond formation between lipids and dendrimers took place but the interactions were of steric nature and were favored in the interior of the acyl chains. The larger PG2 dendrimer at high incorporated concentrations induced a clear phase separation of the lipid bilayer due to its size, leading to higher encapsulation percentage into the more thermodynamically favorable aqueous interior of a unilamellar liposomal vesicle.

In a recently published article by our group[27], PG1 dendrimer was incorporated into aDDnS liposomes which composed of DOPC/CHOL/PG1 and Dox was encapsulated, while the liposomal system composed of DOPC/CHOL without PG1 was also studied. EPC/CHOL liposomes were also produced for the same purpose (commercial product 'Myocet' replica). The DOPC/CHOL/PG1 liposomal system did not denmostrate any significant changes to the release rate of Dox compared to that of the conventional system (i.e. DOPC/CHOL). On the contrary, the aDDnSs composed of EPC/CHOL/PG1 presented significant retardation of Dox release compared to the conventional liposomes composed of EPC/CHOL.

This fact could be attributed to the PG1/Dox molar ratio that was found to be 0,32 for DOPC/CHOL aDDnSs, while it was 0,50 for EPC/CHOL aDDnSs. Probably the increased relative concentration of dendrimer in the case of EPC is responsible for the retardation of the leakage of Dox. The *in vitro* activity studies revealed that both liposomal and **chi**-aDDnSs preparations were able to retain the growth inhibiting activity of the free anthracycline while they reduced drug's toxicity (i.e. exhibited much higher LC_{50}s) against the two cell lines tested. Thus, all systems under consideration increased the Therapeutic Index (TI) of Dox.

As a conclusion, it was shown that EPC/CHOL as aDDnS can encapsulate Dox more effectively and release it slower than the respective liposomes ('Myocet' replica). In other words, without any further production step, a final lyophilized product ready for the shelf, exhibiting more interesting kinetic properties while retaining the TI of the commercial product can be prepared – a fact that gives hope to such systems for further *in vivo* investigations.

2.3 aDDnSs consisting of Liposomes and HBPs

Recently other polymeric materials with dendritic architecture known as hyperbranched polymers (HBPs) have been used for the preparation of aDDnSs [36,37]. HBPs low cost and ease of production have rendered them quite attractive for use in the field of drug delivery. Their properties mainly depend on the nature of their terminal units. However their imperfect structure (existence of dendritic and linear terminal units) and subsequent increased polydispersity, often leads to more complex behaviors compared to the perfectly branched dendrimers. However, in comparison to the well established linear biodegradable polyesters, such as poly(lactic acid) (PLA), poly(glycolic acid) (PGA), and poly(lactic-co-glycolic acid) (PLG), HBPs might offer the advantage of adjustable polymer degradation and erosion. This may be of particular interest for drug delivery systems designed for parenteral use, as a carefully adjusted drug release and polymer degradation rate is a prerequisite [38]. In a study done by Suttiruengwong and his colleagues [38] the authors studied the microencaspulation and release kinetics of commercially available HBPs. In this study the authors concluded that commercially available HBPs such as the Boltorn H3200 and the Hybrane 1500 could be candidates for controlled-release applications depending though on the delivery strategies (types of release, encapsulation, and degradability). They also notice that these HBPs can offer another emerging application such as in a polymer blend system to increase the hydrophilic characteristic of the drug excipients, concluding that they potentially can be used in biomedical applications assuming though that significant issues such as their toxicity and biocompatibility could be overcome in the future.

For the development of a new **chi**-aDDnS composed of liposomes and dendritic materials, HBPs belonging to the class of aliphatic polyesters were incorporated in liposomes of two different lipid compositions: a) distearoyl phosphatidyl choline (DSPC) and dipalmitoyl phosphatidyl glycerol (DPPG) and b) distearoyl phosphatidyl choline (DSPC) and cholesterol (CHOL). The exact positioning of the HBPs in the liposomal vesicle, as well as the interactions between the two basic components (lipidic and polymeric) were elucidated by means of Attenuated Total Reflectance – Fourier Transform Infrared Spectroscopy (ATR-FTIR), Pulse Generated Spin Echo – Nuclear Magnetic Resonance (PGSE-NMR), ^{31}P-NMR [35] and micro-DSC. The HBPs used were prepared from 2,2-dimethylol propionic acid (bis-MPA) as monomer and a polyol (epoxylated pentaerythritol) as a core, resulting in multiple hydroxyl groups as terminal units. An important feature of aliphatic polyester HBPs is the existence of an extensive network of *inter-* and *intra-* molecular hydrogen bonds, which results in the polymers having a rather compact structure [39,40]. HBPs of different pseudo-generation number (G2, G3 and G4 with 16, 32 and 64 terminal hydroxyl groups respectively) were used in order to examine its dependence on liposome-HBP interaction. PGSE-NMR measurements demonstrated that the incorporation of HBPs in liposomes is successful since the diffusion coefficients of liposomes and incorporated HBPs have values of the same order, suggesting that polymers and liposomes diffuse as one complex. For a better understanding of HBPs-liposomes interactions ATR-FTIR studies were performed to these new aDDnSs, from where it was revealed that HBPs, in DSPC/DPPG liposomes, are incorporated in the head group region of the liposomes lipid bilayer. This positioning takes place after competing with water molecules bonded in this area (hydration shell), thus resulting in the modification of the head groups degree of hydration. Moreover ^{31}P-NMR studies demonstrated that HBPs incorporation also affects the mobility of the phospholipids polar head group, which is inversely proportional to HBPs pseudo-generation number. This insertion is significantly affected by the lipid bilayer composition, since it has been found that in cholesterol containing liposomes, HBPs intercalation is being restricted. Finally the interactions between HBPs and DSCP/DPPG liposomes do not present a linear trend with HBPs pseudo-generation number, since stronger interactions are noticed with G2 and G4 HBPs compared to G3 HBP. Additionally Dox has been encapsulated in these aDDnSs, in order to assess their drug encapsulation efficiency. In this case, similar results with previous studies performed on aDDnSs composed of liposomes and dendrimers have been obtained; incorporation of HBPs significantly increased the encapsulation of Dox. Moreover thermal analysis of these systems (micro-DSC) revealed the induction of phase separation when HBPs were incorporated, which demonstrates the entropic nature of interaction between the lipidic and dendritic materials. Upon drug encapsulation this phase separation is being abolished, indicating that similar mechanism, as mentioned for aDDnSs containing dendrimers, takes place. Overall it can be established that for **chi**-aDDnSs containing HBPs, three parameters are of vital importance for the development of an effective drug carrier: **1**. Liposome composition, **2**. Number of functional hydroxyl groups and **3**. Compactness of structure as defined by the *inter-* and *intra-* hydrogen bond network formed in the HBPs molecules. The thorough study of aDDnSs composed of liposomes and HBPs is ongoing and aims at investigating the underlying mechanisms involved in drug loading, release and pharmacological behavior of the final system.

3 CONCLUSION

It has been shown that aDDnSs represent a breakthrough category of drug delivery systems, especially as far as highly toxic molecules with low T.I. (such as anticancer agents) are concerned. aDDnSs have been shown to significantly: a) increase the load of the bioactive substance into the system, which is very important both for manufacturing-economic reasons and for toxicity reasons (as less quantity of carrier is used for the same amount of drug), b) lower the release rate of the encapsulate drug, a fact that could create a more controlled and/or sustained release profile of the drug in the bloodstream, leading to lower toxicity and higher effectiveness c) advanced pharmacological toxicity compared to the free drug and at least equal toxicity compared to the respective conventional liposomal formulation. A plethora of physicochemical data has begun to shed light to the interactions of the components of these complicate systems that seem to be responsible for the advantages presented by the aDDnSs. It has been demonstrated that, differently to what Khopade et al. had suggested in the first article concerning aDDnSs, pH and solubility gradient is presumably not the basis of the drug release modulation. The amelioration of the release profile is not caused, mainly, by the forces developed between dendrimer and drug but by the induction of a more "stable" and, probably, less permeable lipid membrane due to the existence of the dendrimer-drug complex in the interior of the vesicle. It has been shown that the cumulative release of Dox from aDDnSs of exactly same lipid composition incorporating dendrimers of totally different size and chemistry follows exactly the same pattern, independently of the nature of the interactions between dendrimer and Dox. The thermotropic behavior of empty aDDnSs was found to be different, depending on the size and chemistry of the incorporated dendrimer. Very interestingly, when Dox was loaded to three **chi** aDDnSs partly composed of PG1, PG2, PAMAM and HBPs, the thermotropic behavior of the lipid membrane was extremely alike. The results revealed that the incorporation of Dox promoted the stability of the liposome membrane and the cooperativity of the relevant lipid gel-to-liquid crystal transition. Combining this result with the exact similarity of the release profile of Dox from the PAMAM, PG1 and PG2 containing aDDnSs it is concluded that the choice or the design of the dendrimer should be influenced by its ability to induce phase separation to the lipid membrane, at least as far as Dox is concerned. Upon Dox loading, thermal analysis has demonstrated that the dendrimer, Dox, as well as their complex probably migrate in the interior cavity of the liposome without interfering significantly with the physicochemical properties of the membrane while leading to structural and energetic changes of the lipid bilayer. The next step concerning aDDnS investigation is a deeper understanding of the physicochemical mechanisms and interactions of the components of such systems, the testing of various bioactive substances and different dendrimers or HPBs and, most important of all, the biological evaluation of aDDnSs through extensive *in vivo* investigations.

Acknowledgements
This work was supported by the COST Action TD0802 .

References

1. G. Pifferi and P. Restani, *Il Farmaco,* 2003, **58**, 541
2. K. Gardikis and D. S. Fessas, Marco; Dimas, Konstantinos; Tsimplouli, Chrisiida; Ionov, Maksim; Demetzos, Costas, *Journal of Nanoscience and Nanotechnology,* 2011, **11**, 3764
3. N. Garti, G. Hoshen and A. Aserin, *Colloids and Surfaces B: Biointerfaces,*
4. S. A. Abraham, D. N. Waterhouse, L. D. Mayer, P. R. Cullis, T. D. Madden and M. B. Bally, *Methods in Enzymology,* 2005, **Volume 391**, 71
5. U. Massing and S. Fuxius, *Drug Resistance Updates,* 2000, **3**, 171
6. R. M. Schiffelers and G. Storm, *International Journal of Pharmaceutics,* 2008, **364**, 258
7. S. Hatziantoniou, K. Dimas, A. Georgopoulos, N. Sotiriadou and C. Demetzos, *Pharmacological Research,* 2006, **53**, 80
8. K. Miyajima, *Advanced Drug Delivery Reviews,* 1997, **24**, 151
9. E. Buhleier, W. Wehner and F. Vogtle, *Synthesis-Stuttgart,* 1978, 155
10. D. A. Tomalia, A. M. Naylor and W. A. Goddard, *Angewandte Chemie-International Edition in English,* 1990, **29**, 138
11. D. A. Tomalia and J. M. J. Fréchet, *Journal of Polymer Science Part A: Polymer Chemistry,* 2002, **40**, 2719
12. R. Esfand and D. A. Tomalia, *Drug Discovery Today,* 2001, **6**, 427
13. E. R. Gillies and J. M. J. Frechet, *Journal of the American Chemical Society,* 2002, **124**, 14137
14. E. R. Gillies and J. M. J. Frechet, *Drug Discovery Today,* 2005, **10**, 35
15. S. Svenson and D. A. Tomalia, *Advanced Drug Delivery Reviews,* 2005, **57**, 2106
16. A. Hult, M. Johansson and E. Malmström, *Branched Polymers II,* 1999, 1
17. Y. Zhou, W. Huang, J. Liu, X. Zhu and D. Yan, *Advanced Materials,* 2010, **22**, 4567
18. A. J. Khopade, F. Caruso, P. Tripathi, S. Nagaich and N. K. Jain, *International Journal of Pharmaceutics,* 2002, **232**, 157
19. G. Purohit, T. Sakthivel and A. T. Florence, *International Journal of Pharmaceutics,* 2001, **214**, 71
20. S. Ballut, A. Makky, B. Loock, J. P. Michel, P. Maillard and V. Rosilio, *Chemical Communications,* 2009, 224
21. K. Gardikis, S. Hatziantoniou, M. Bucos, D. Fessas, M. Signorelli, T. Felekis, M. Zervou, C. G. Screttas, B. R. Steele, M. Ionov, M. Micha-Screttas, B. Klajnert, M. Bryszewska and C. Demetzos, *Journal of Pharmaceutical Sciences,* 2010, **99**, 3561
22. M. L. Moraes, M. S. Baptista, R. Itri, V. Zucolotto and O. N. Oliveira Jr, *Materials Science and Engineering: C,* 2008, **28**, 467
23. A. Papagiannaros, K. Dimas, G. T. Papaioannou and C. Demetzos, *International Journal of Pharmaceutics,* 2005, **302**, 29
24. K. Gardikis, S. Hatziantoniou, M. Signorelli, M. Pusceddu, M. Micha-Screttas, A. Schiraldi, C. Demetzos and D. Fessas, *Colloids and Surfaces B: Biointerfaces,* 2010, **81**, 11
25. R. K. Tekade, P. V. Kumar and N. K. Jain, *Chemical Reviews,* 2009, **109**, 49

26.   V. Saroglou, S. Hatziantoniou, M. Smyrniotakis, I. Kyrikou, T. Mavromoustakos, A. Zompra, V. Magafa, P. Cordopatis and C. Demetzos, *Journal of Peptide Science,* 2006, **12**, 43

27.   K. Gardikis, C. Tsimplouli, K. Dimas, M. Micha-Screttas and C. Demetzos, *International Journal of Pharmaceutics,* **402**, 231

28.   A. Mecke, S. Uppuluri, T. M. Sassanella, D.-K. Lee, A. Ramamoorthy, J. J. R. Baker, B. G. Orr and M. M. Banaszak Holl, *Chemistry and Physics of Lipids,* 2004, **132**, 3

29.   S. Hong, J. A. Hessler, M. M. Banaszak Holl, P. Leroueil, A. Mecke and B. G. Orr, *Journal of Chemical Health and Safety,* 2006, **13**, 16

30.   D. Wrobel, M. Ionov, K. Gardikis, C. Demetzos, J. P. Majoral, B. Palecz, B. Klajnert and M. Bryszewska, *Biochimica Et Biophysica Acta-Molecular and Cell Biology of Lipids,* 2011, **1811**, 221

31.   M. Ionov, K. Gardikis, D. Wrobel, S. Hatziantoniou, H. Mourelatou, J. P. Majoral, B. Klajnert, M. Bryszewska and C. Demetzos, *Colloids and Surfaces B-Biointerfaces,* 2011, **82**, 8

32.   K. Gardikis, S. Hatziantoniou, K. Viras, M. Wagner and C. Demetzos, *International Journal of Pharmaceutics,* 2006, **318**, 118

33.   B. Klajnert and R. M. Epand, *International Journal of Pharmaceutics,* 2005, **305**, 154

34.   B. Klajnert, J. Janiszewska, Z. Urbanczyk-Lipkowska, M. Bryszewska and R. M. Epand, *International Journal of Pharmaceutics,* 2006, **327**, 145

35.   R.S. Dhanikula, A. Argaw, J.F. Bouchard and P. Hildgen, *Molecular Pharmaceutics,* 2007, **5**, 105

36.   E.A. Mourelatou, D. Libster, I. Nir, S. Hatziantoniou, A. Aserin, N. Garti and C. Demetzos, *The Journal of Physical Chemistry B*, 2011, **115**, 3400

37.   A. Breitenbach, Y.X. Li andT.T. Kissel, *Journal of Controlled Release*, 2000, **4**, 167

38.   S. Suttiruengwong, J. Rolker, I. Smirnova and W. Arlt, *Pharmaceutical Development and Technology,* 2006,**11**, 55

39.   E.Žagar and J. Grdadolnik , *Journal of Molecular Structure*, 2003, **658**, 143

40.   I. Tanis, D. Tragoudaras, K. Karatasos and S.H. Anastasiadis, *The Journal of Physical Chemistry B*, 2009, **112**, 5356

CATIONIC CARBOSILANE DENDRIMERS AS NON-VIRAL VECTORS OF NUCLEIC ACIDS (OLIGONUCLEOTIDE OR siRNA) FOR GENE THERAPY PURPOSES

R. Gómez,[1,5] F. J. de la Mata,[1,5] J. L. Jiménez-Fuentes[2], P. Ortega,[1,5] B. Klajnert,[3] E. Pedziwiatr-Werbicka,[3] D. Shcharbin,[3,6] M. Bryszewska[3] M. Maly,[4,7] J. Maly,[4] M.J. Serramía,[2,5] R. Lorente[2,5] and M. A. Muñoz-Fernández[2,5]

[1] Departamento de Química Inorgánica, Universidad de Alcalá, Campus Universitario, E-28871 Alcalá de Henares (Spain).
[2] Laboratorio Inmuno Biología Molecular. Hospital General Universitario Gregorio Marañón. Madrid (Spain).
[3] Department of General Biophysics, University of Lodz, Pomorska str. 141/143, Lodz 91-236, Poland
[4] J. E. Purkinje University, Ceske mladeze 8, 400 96 Usti nad Labem (Czech Republic)
[5] Networking Research Center on Bioengineering, Biomaterials and Nanomedicine (CIBER-BBN), Spain.
[6] Institute of Biophysics and Cell Engineering of NASB, 27 Akademicheskaja St., Minsk, 220072, Belarus.
[7] University of Applied Science of Southern Switzerland, Lab Appl Math & Phys LAMFI, CH-6928 Manno (Switzerland)

1 INTRODUCTION

In the last few years many anti-viral drugs have been developed to fight against HIV-1 infection and have been proved to control infection. Highly active antiretroviral therapy (HAART) has made an immense impact on fighting the HIV/AIDS pandemic, however, it still possesses major drawbacks such as the need of keeping greater than 95% adherence to be effective and it is a life-long therapy. The additional problems of availability and drug cost, side effects of the treatment, the emergence of drug resistance, the wide array of viral isolates, high mutability of the virus, and coinfections with other diseases such as tuberculosis or hepatitis, among many other issues, demand the research into addressing HIV infection to be continued and further expanded with the objective of making new discoveries and improving current therapies.

Intensification of successful antiretroviral therapy has been proposed as a strategy that could control residual replication, diminish the HIV latent reservoirs, and be useful for eradication purposes.[1] However, recently reported studies have failed to show any significant impact of treatment intensification on residual HIV viremia in patients with chronic infection treated with HAART.[2] As a consequence, intensification is close to be rejected for eradication purposes.

Therefore, the HIV/AIDS pandemic will not be eradicated without substantial new developments and innovation. A new approach should focus on improving the efficacy and safety of short nucleic acids (oligonucleotides and/or RNA interference (RNAi)-based antiviral drugs) and how this technology is being developed as a new therapeutic tool to fight against HIV infection. The mechanism of RNAi involves short double-stranded segments of RNA termed short interfering RNA (siRNA). The introduction of these oligonucleotides into the cytoplasm of the cell results in degradation of mRNA complementary to the sequence contained in the siRNA.[3] RNAi is a technique that has been used to successfully target HIV replication.[4] However, there still exist some problems that need to be addressed such as obstacles in delivery, target cell transfection, stability/degradation, transient activity, secondary effects, toxicity caused by delivery vector, and resistance all hinder the path of carrying out *in vivo* experiments with RNAi and further developing RNAi as a new therapy for clinical use. Furthermore, new advances of these issues can be addressed by using the correct delivery vector. Therefore, a great deal of research is being put into finding a suitable partner and chauffeur for these valuable small nucleic acid (SNA) molecules. The ideal delivery agent should protect the oligonucleotide (ODN) from binding unspecifically to serum proteins and should protect the siRNA from degradation. Also, it should transport ODN or siRNA to the target cells or tissues and facilitate their transfection into the cytoplasm of the cells. The ideal delivery should remain fairly innocuous all the time and should cause little or no adverse effects.

To overcome these drawbacks and to make gene therapy (GT) a real alternative, non-viral vehicles such as cationic liposomes, conventional polymers, or dendrimers, have been developed. Once in contact with negatively charged DNA [oligodeoxynucleotides (ODNs) or siRNA], cationic systems form electrostatic complexes with the nucleic acids, namely lipoplexes, polyplexes, or dendriplexes respectively. The use of liposomes for transfection purposes was first described in 1987.[5] Cationic lipids prepared for this purpose are commercially available (i.e. Cytofectin™ or Lipofectin™). However, they have side-effects such us lung inflammatory reactions,[6] and a possible failure of transfection in the presence of serum. The main drawback of the use of conventional degradable polymers as delivery agents is their thermodynamic instability, that results in a short *in vivo* life-time of the active species, besides their polydispersity.[7]

Dendrimers represent an alternative approach for the transfection of SNAs in a wide range of cells. Dendrimers are nanoscopic monodisperse polymers with highly branched three dimensional structures that have shown a wide potential for biological applications.[8] The major advantage of dendrimers over the rest of the vehicles is based on their uniform structure and versatile modification of their skeletons and surfaces, which gives the basis for a precise characterization of the complex [vector/nucleic acid or vector/drug] and a more accurate and systematic research of the delivery process. These systems have shown stability and non-immunogenic properties for their potential use in a high variety of therapeutic applications and have been successfully used as carriers for delivery of nucleic acids and drugs.[9]

The first report using dendritic macromolecules for transfection was presented in 1993 using poly(amidoamine) (PAMAM) dendrimers,[10] and since then, extensive studies have been performed.[11] Good results are typically achieved with sixth or seventh generation dendrimers. However, the transfection efficiency can be increased two- to three-fold when the PAMAM is activated by heat treatment (*e.g.* Superfect™) or in the case of flexible PAMAM structures designed.[11d]

Another class of potential transfecting agents are the phosphorus-containing dendrimers,[12] which can be synthesized up to the twelfth generation. The dendritic surface has been grafted with protonated or methylated terminal tertiary amines and examined as transfecting agents for the luciferase gene in 3T3 cells. The efficiency increased as a function of the dendrimer generation, although a constant value was reached between generation three and five. Furthermore, these dendrimers exhibit improved transfection efficiency when serum is present.

Other kinds of dendritic macromolecules, such as polypropylenimine (PPI),[13] and poly(lysine)[14] dendrimers, have also been studied as potential DNA or ODN carriers. For instance, low generation PPI dendrimers have also shown gene transfection ability *in vitro* with low cytotoxicity, although at higher generations toxicity increases and prohibits their use.

With regards to the use of carbosilane dendrimers in GT our research groups have recently noted that carbosilane dendrimers have shown promising biocompatibility, protection against serum proteins or nucleases and transfection profiles.[15-21] Here, in this chapter, we provide an overview of the use of carbosilane dendrimers as a new approach in the treatment of HIV infection.

2 METHODS AND RESULTS

2.1 Synthesis of Dendrimers

2.1.1 Amine-Terminated Carbosilane Dendrimers

We have studied the synthesis of new carbosilane dendrimers containing amine groups at their periphery as precursors for cationic dendrimers. For this purpose, two general strategies have been developed: (i) the alcoholysis of the well-known chlorosilane-terminated dendrimers, $nG\text{-}(SiCl_y)_x$, using alcohol-amine systems, and (ii) hydrosilylation of allyl amines with Si-H terminated dendrimers, $nG\text{-}(SiH_y)_x$.

Dendrimers formed by alcoholysis of dendritic Si-Cl bonds: chlorosilane-terminated dendrimers of type $nG\text{-}(SiCl)_x$ ($n = 1$, 2 and 3; $x = 4$, 8 and 16) were synthesized as reported previously[22] and formed the starting materials for the preparation of new dendrimers via alcoholysis reactions. Different amino-alcohols were used, like [3,5-$(NMe_2CH_2CH_2O)_2](C_6H_3)CH_2OH$ (**I**) , $Me_2NCH_2CH_2N(Me)CH_2CH_2OH$ (**II**) and *N,N*-dimethylethanolamine (**III**). Chlorosilane-terminated dendrimers were treated with stoichiometric amounts of the amine-alcohols **I-III** in diethylether and in the presence of an excess of NEt_3, to afford the corresponding amine-terminated dendrimers nG-$[Si\{OCH_2(C_6H_3)\text{-}3,5\text{-}(OCH_2CH_2NMe_2)_2\}]_x$ ($n = 1$, $x = 4$ (**1**); $n = 2$, $x = 8$ (**2**); $n = 3$, $x = 16$ (**3**)); nG-$[Si\{O(CH_2)_2N(Me)(CH_2)_2NMe_2\}]_x$ ($n = 1$, $x = 4$ (**4**); $n = 2$, $x = 8$ (**5**); $n = 3$, $x = 16$ (**6**)) ; nG-$[Si\{O(CH_2)_2NMe_2\}]_x$ ($n = 1$, $x = 4$ (**7**); $n = 2$, $x = 8$ (**8**); $n = 3$, $x = 16$ (**9**)) in high yields as colorless or yellow oils (see Scheme 1). All these derivatives are soluble in all common organic solvents, but insoluble in water.

Dendrimers formed by hydrosilylation with dendritic Si-H bonds: Si-H terminated carbosilane dendrimers of type $nG\text{-}(SiH)_x$ ($n = 1$ and 2; $x = 4$ and 8) were synthesized as reported previously[22d,e] and used in the hydrosilylation of allylamine to afford the corresponding dendrimers nG-$[Si(CH_2)_3NH_2]_x$ ($n = 1$, $x = 4$ (**10**); $n = 2$, $x = 8$ (**11**)) in high yields as colorless oils (see Scheme 2).

2.1.2 Ammonium-Terminated Carbosilane Dendrimers

The formation of the ammonium-terminated dendrimers was performed adding MeI to the parent dendrimers **1-9** in diethylether (see Scheme 1) to afford the corresponding quaternized systems nG-[Si{OCH$_2$(C$_6$H$_3$)-3,5-(OCH$_2$CH$_2$NMe$_3^+$I$^-$)$_2$}]$_x$ (n = 1, x = 4 (**12**); n = 2, x = 8 (**13**); n = 3, x = 16 (**14**)); nG-[Si{O(CH$_2$)$_2$N$^+$(Me$_2$)(CH$_2$)$_2$NMe$_3^+$}2I$^-$]$_x$ (n = 1, x = 4 (**15**); n = 2, x = 8 (**16**); n = 3, x = 16 (**17**)) or nG-[Si{O(CH$_2$)$_2$NMe$_3^+$}I$^-$]$_x$ (n = 1, x = 4 (**18**); n = 2, x = 8 (**19**); n = 3, x = 16 (**20**)) as white solids.

For dendrimers **10** and **11**, the protonation was achieved by adding stoichiometric amounts or an excess of HCl to produce nG-[Si(CH$_2$)$_3$NH$_3^+$Cl$^-$]$_x$ (n = 1, x = 4 (**21**); n = 2, x = 8 (**22**)) as white solids (see Scheme 2).

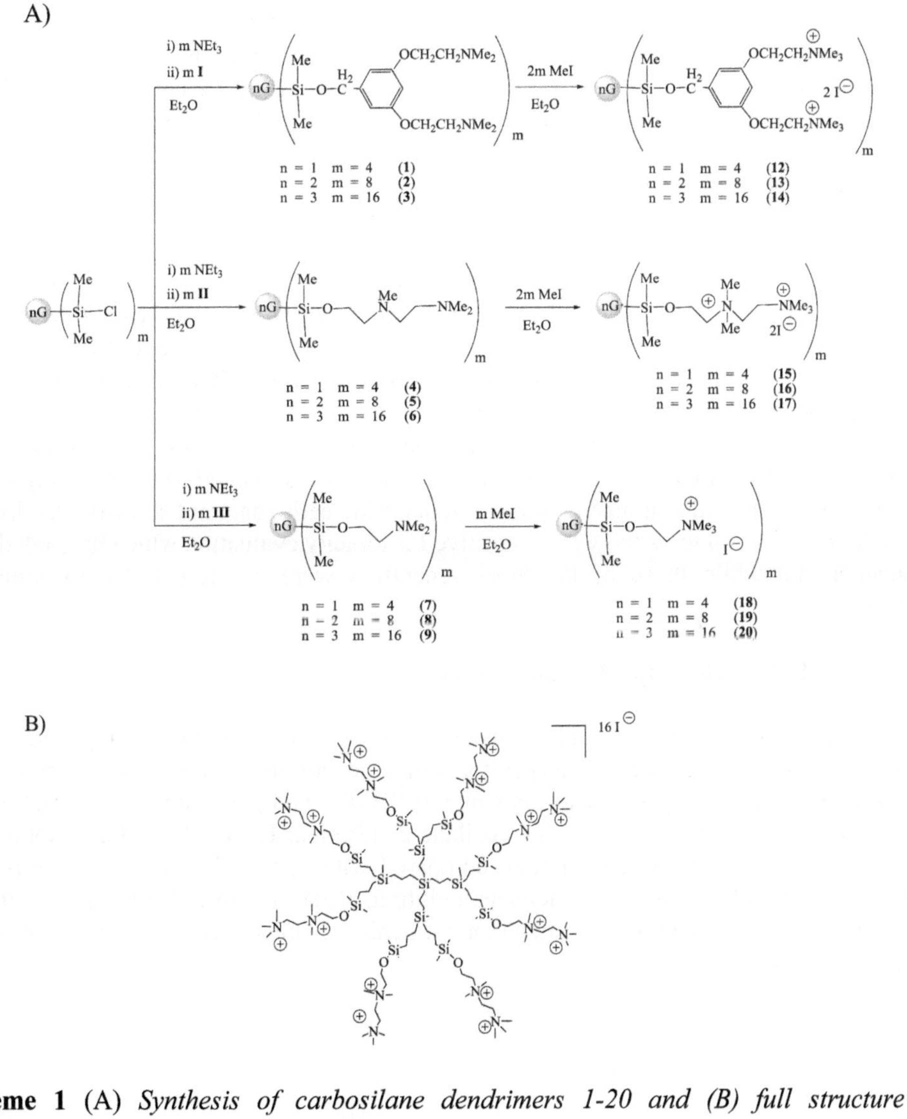

A)

B)

Scheme 1 (A) *Synthesis of carbosilane dendrimers 1-20 and (B) full structure of dendrimer **16**, also denoted as 2G-NN16.*

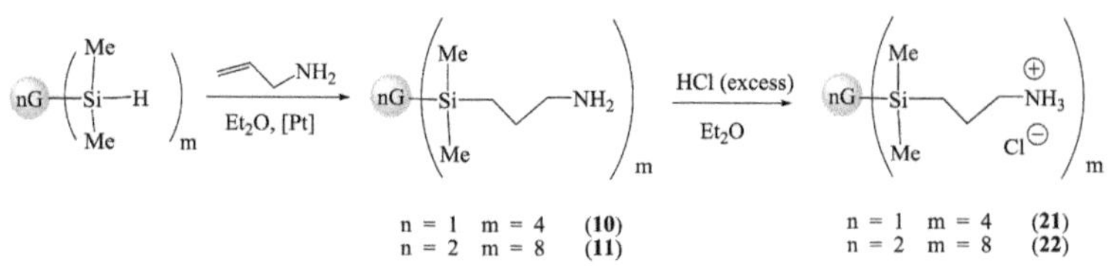

$$n = 1 \quad m = 4 \quad \textbf{(10)}$$
$$n = 2 \quad m = 8 \quad \textbf{(11)}$$

$$n = 1 \quad m = 4 \quad \textbf{(21)}$$
$$n = 2 \quad m = 8 \quad \textbf{(22)}$$

Scheme 2 *Synthesis of water stable carbosilane dendrimers*

All compounds **12-22** are water-soluble, although solubility decreases on increasing the generation. The dendrimers based on the presence of Si-O bonds decomposed slowly via hydrolysis of those bonds. However, the hydrolysis rates of the dendrimers **12-14** containing quaternized groups derived from amino-alcohol **I**, are considerably attenuated respecting to those dendrimers having the fragment **II** and **III**. Opposite to this, dendrimers **21** and **22** based on Si-C bonds are completely stable towards hydrolysis.

The NMR spectroscopic and analytical data of derivatives **12–22** are consistent with their proposed structures (Scheme 1-2) and corroborated by molecular modeling.[23]

2.2 Toxicity Evaluation of Dendrimers

The toxicities of quaternized second generation carbosilane dendrimers **13**, **16**, **19** and **22** were evaluated in a wide range of immune cell types, including primary cultures of peripheral blood mononuclear cells (PBMCs) and purified CD4 T lymphocytes using different methods: (i) visual exam under phase-contrast light microscope, (ii) MTT assay (Figure 1A-B), (iii) Flow cytometry (Figure 1C), or (iv) Trypan Blue (Figure 1D) uptake, showing good toxicity profiles in the range of 1-5 μM. From these studies, the most compatible dendrimer resulted to be the second generation dendrimer 2G-[Si{O(CH$_2$)$_2$N$^+$(Me$_2$)(CH$_2$)$_2$NMe$_3$$^+$}2I$^-$]$_8$ (**16**), which is also called 2G-NN16 (Figure 1). We had the same results in macrophages and dendritic cells (data not shown). Dendrimers of the first generation were too water-sensitive for toxicity evaluation which precluded data rationalization, while those of the third generation were not tested due to solubility problems.

2.3 Antigenicity, Lymphoproliferative Assay

When a new macromolecule is under consideration for a potential biologic application, it is important not to constitute an unspecific antigenic stimulus (unless it is needed for development of immunogens). The challenge of PBMCs and purified CD4 T-lymphocytes with different concentrations of the carbosilane dendrimers **13**, **16**, **19** and **22**, looking for induction/not induction of proliferation, compared with that achieved with an unspecific mithogenic stimuli such as phytohaemagglutinin (PHA) showed that none of the carbosilane dendrimers used constituted an antigenic stimulus at the tested concentrations (2 and 5 μM) (Figure 2).

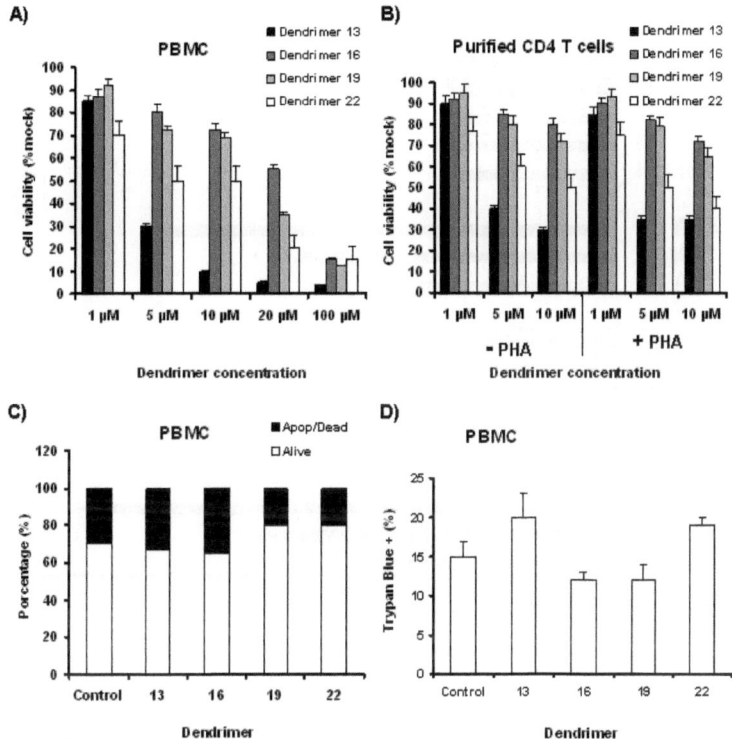

Figure 1. *A-B) Quantification of mitochondrial activity (MA) of PBMCs by MTT after 48 h of incubation with a curve of different dendrimer concentrations in PBMCs and purified CD4 T cells. MA is expressed as percentage with respect to the MA of the untreated cells (control). C) Evaluation of the percentage of live cells against the percentage of cells corresponding to dead/apoptotic cells by flow cytometry in PBMCs after 72 h of incubation with different dendrimers. D) Percentage of cells positive for Trypan Blue after 72 h of incubation with dendrimers. Data show three independent experiments.*

2.4 Toxicity Evaluation of Dendriplexes

Dendriplex formation in different conditions were previously studied by a multi-disciplinary approach using electrophoresis, fluorescence methods, laser Doppler electrophoresis, dynamic light scattering (DLS), atomic force microscopy (AFM), transmission electron microscopy (TEM) and molecular modeling.[23] Electrophoresis with ODN or siRNA, using the quaternized second generation dendrimers **13**, **16**, **19** and **22**, showed dendriplex formation at very low electrostatic charge ratio (+)/(−) of 2/1.[16,19]

Therefore, toxicity profiles of dendriplexes formed by all carbosilane dendrimers were studied by the same methods and conditions as above including primary cultures of PBMCs and purified CD4 T lymphocytes: (i) visual exam under phase-contrast light microscopy, (ii) MTT assay (Figure 3A-B), or (iii) LDH assay (Figure 3C-D). The dendriplexes showed good toxicity profiles in the range tested of 1-10 μM. As an example, Figure 3 shows the results obtained with the dendrimer **16** (also called 2G-NN16). Our results clearly show that dendrimer alone is slightly more toxic than when complexed with ODN or siRNA.

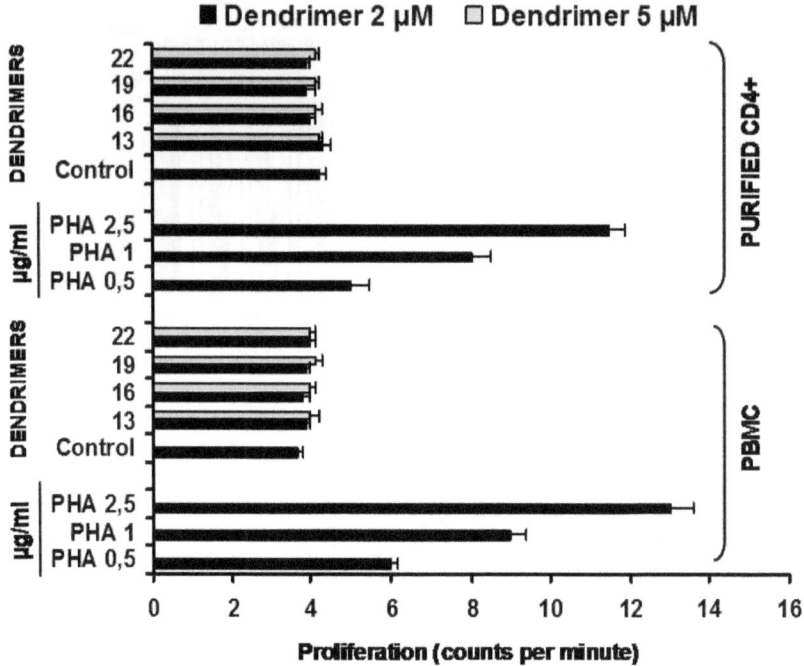

Figure 2. *Lymphoproliferative assay: antigenicity of the carbosilane dendrimers in proliferation of PBMCs or CD4 T cells exposed to two different concentrations of each dendrimer (2 and 5 μM) and compared with that achieved with the mitogen phytohemagglutinin (PHA) to different doses. Data show three independent experiments.*

2.5 Protection from Serum Proteins and RNases

Treatment of dendriplexes with the anionic detergent sodium dodecyl sulfate disrupted the complexes indicating that the nature of the union in such dendriplexes is merely electrostatic (data not shown). However, dendriplexes were not dissociated by serum proteins like bovine and human serum albumins tested by gel electrophoresis and fluorescence experiments. As follows from Figure 4 B in the presence of BSA the fluorescence polarization of ODN/dendrimer complexes did not change. This means that BSA does not affect ODN/dendrimer complexes. On the other hand, dendrimer interactions with BSA were tested by quenching of BSA fluorescence upon addition of dendrimers in different concentrations.

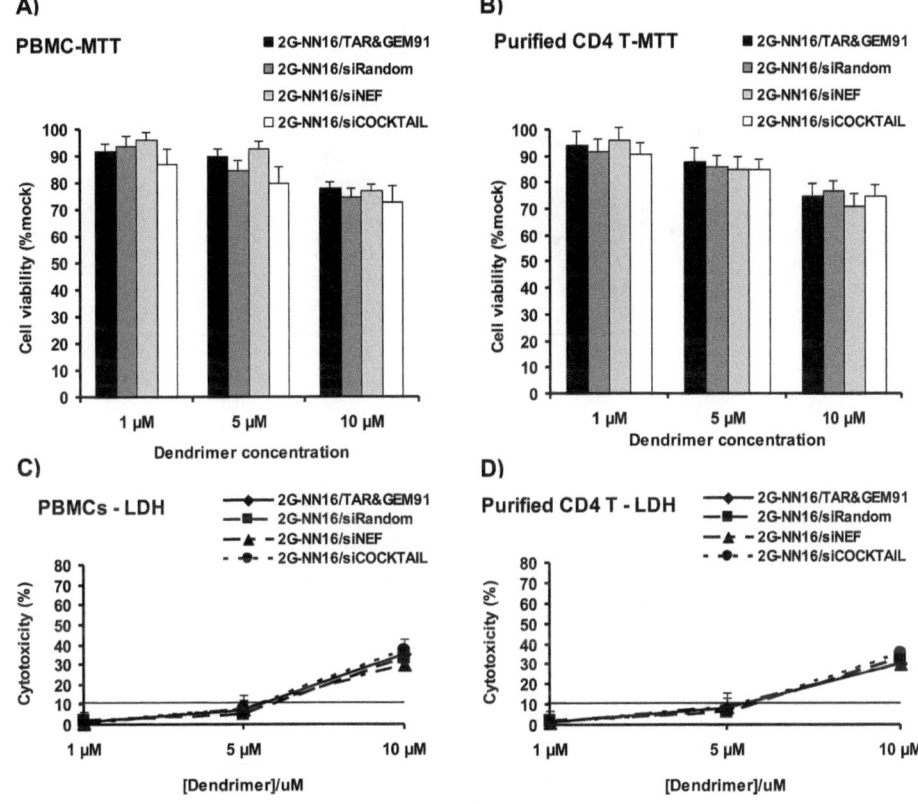

Figure 3. *Effect of dendriplexes on PBMCs and purified CD4 T cells viability. MTT assay of PBMCs (A) or purified CD4 T cells (B) 20 h after being treated with dendriplex. A toxicity limit was set at 80% for metabolic activity. Membrane rupture was detected by quantifying lactate dehydrogenase (LDH) concentration in supernatants from dendriplexes treated PBMCs (C) and purified CD4 T cells (D) after 24 hours. A toxicity limit was set at 10% LDH release. Cells were submitted to treatment with dendriplexes (2G-NN16/ODN or 2G-NN16/siRNAs). All points were performed in triplicate. Dendrimer 2G.NN16 is also named as* **16**.

As follows from Figure 4C, dendrimer did not affect the quenching of internal and external Trps of BSA. In contrast, the results on the interaction between AF attached to BSA surface and dendrimer show that the dendrimer can quench AF fluorescence. This means that the interactions between carbosilane dendrimers and BSA are weak and occur preferentially at protein surface.

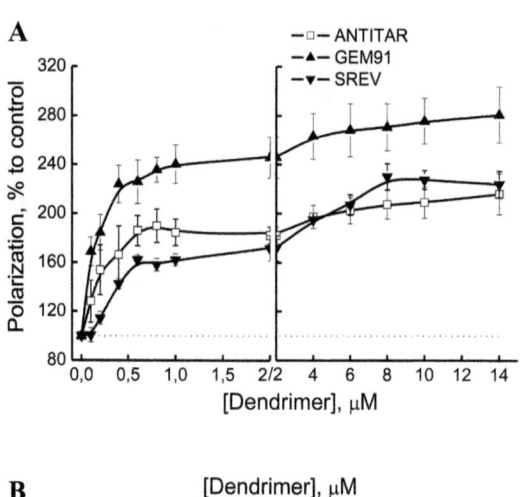

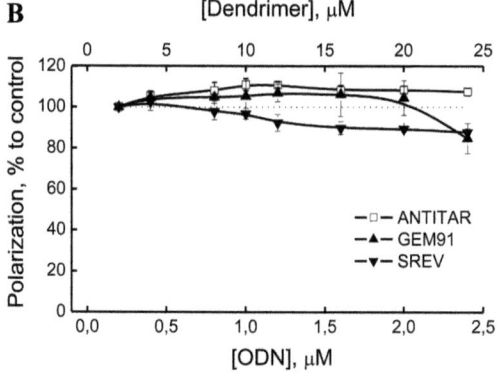

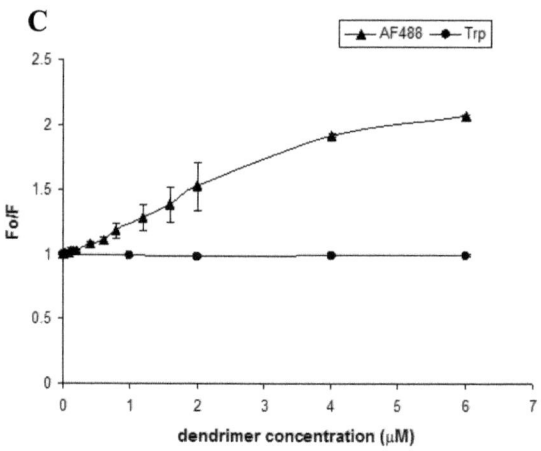

Figure 4. *(A) Changes in the polarization of labeled ODNs upon addition of dendrimer **16** c_{ODN} = 0,1 μM. (B) Changes in the polarization of labeled ODNs upon addition of their complexes with dendrimer **16** (molar ratio 10:1) to BSA of constant concentration of 10 μM. (C) Quenching of fluorescence of BSA tryptophans (C_{BSA} = 5 μM) and AF488 (C_{BSA-AF} = 0.1 μM) by dendrimer **16**. F_0 – the initial fluorescence intensity, F – the fluorescence intensity after adding dendrimer **16**.*

Moreover, dendrimers such as **16** are able to protect nucleic material against RNases. As shown in Figure 5, naked siRNA was seen to be completely degraded in the presence of RNase, while siRNA retained in the gel wells due to its union with carbosilane dendrimers manifested no signs of RNase degradation whatsoever.

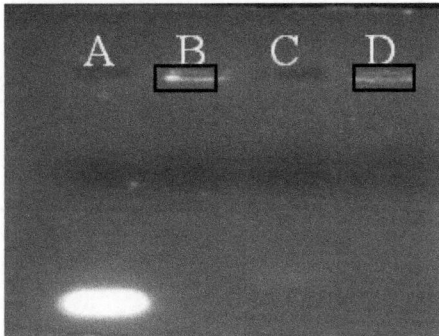

Figure 5. *Protective effect of dendrimers on siRNA in the presence of RNase: (A) siRNA only; (B) siRNA + (16); (C) siRNA + nuclease; (D) siRNA + 16 + nuclease.*

2.6 Transfection Efficiency of PBMC, CD4-T Lymphocytes, Macrophages and Dendritic Cells

Transfection efficiency experiments have been carried out with the carbosilane dendrimers mainly with the more representative **16** dendrimer in buffer (OPTIMEN I) which was analysed in different cell cultures by flow cytometry. Delivery of antisense oligonucleotides and siRNA, complexed with **16** dendrimer was made by dendrimer interaction with the different cells tested. Efficiency of fluorochrome-labelled SNA (anti HIV oligonucleotide as Rev, Gem91, anti-TAR) entry by means of **16** was measured by the percentage of viable cell population that exhibited fluorescence in the cell cytosol. This percentage represents successful uptake of fluorochrome-labelled SNA. Primary isolated cells such as PBMC, purified CD4 T lymphocytes, macrophages or dendritic cells, showed approximately 40% uptake as shown in Figure 6. For the case of immortalized cell lines like Sup T1, the transfection efficiency was around 80% (Figure 6).

Confocal studies were used to further analyze the results obtained by flow cytometry and the delivery of fluorochrome-labelled SNA by **16** was visualised for a variety of different immune system primary cells. For instance, cellular uptake of dendriplexes formed by siRNA and **16** dendrimer into T lymphocytes is shown in Figure 7. It can be seen that the siRNA alone is remarkably internalised in a 80% while complexed with **16** such percentage can be maintained or even increased to almost 100% depending on the +/- ratio (Figure 7). Macrophages showed a fluorescence pattern as aggregated, probably in relation to a very active endocytosis process (Figure 7). In addition, it consists of a cytoplasmatic pattern instead of a nuclear one, opposite to that observed previously in the CD4 T-cells.

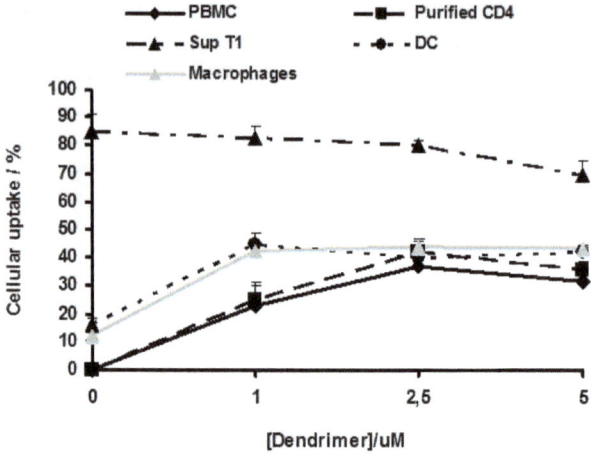

Figure 6. *Assays of transfection of the SNA–16) complex. Results are expressed as percentage of cellular uptake measured by flow cytometry relative to 2G-NN16 (range 0–5 μM), in different types of cells (PMBCs, purified CD4+ cells, DC, SupT1 lymphocyte cell line and macrophages). Data represent the mean ± SEM; n=3.*

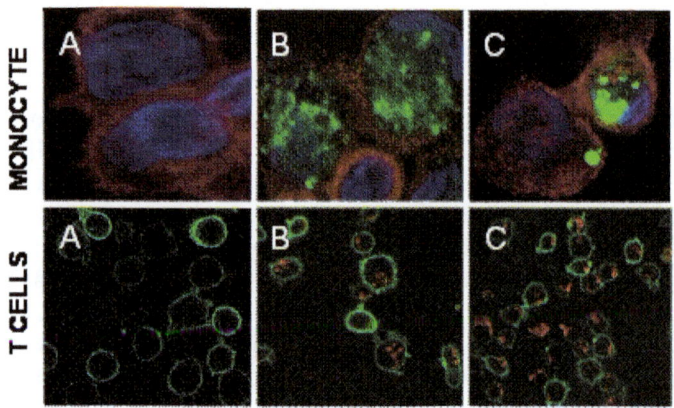

Figure 7. *Internalization of ODN into monocyte cells or siRNA into T cells. Confocal microscopy images of monocytes after 18 h incubation with mock treated (A) or with FITC-labeled ODN (B) or dendriplex (ODN-FITC/16) (C). T cells after 20 h incubation with mock treatment (A) or with Cy3-labeled siRNA (red) alone (B) or complexed with 16 (C). Cell membranes are labeled with αCD14-PE antibodies (red) for monocyte and αCD45-FITC antibodies (green) for T cells.*

2.7 Down Regulation of Gene Expression

Targeting regions that are critical for HIV replication such as TAR, which is essential for activation of HIV-1 transcription, REV, which is critical for viral replication or GEM91, which affects viral entry and reverse transcription, may disrupt the viral cycle and present new options for HIV therapy. HIV inhibition assays were performed using antisense oligonucleotides alone or complexed with **16** (also called 2G-NN16). Evaluation of the HIV p24 antigen release via ELISA was performed using culture supernatants of primary isolated PBMC and purified CD4 T lymphocytes that were incubated with different treatments. Antisense oligonucleotides TAR and GEM91 alone were able to reduce *ca.* 40% of p24 antigen release that was further improved by the dendriplex **16** /TAR&GEM91 reaching a reduction of *ca.* 60% in PBMC (Figure 8A). The same combination of dendriplex tested in purified CD4 T lymphocytes led to a p24 antigen level reduction of *ca.* 20% (Figure 8B), and a similar effect was observed when the dendriplex was composed of only the TAR or GEM91 oligonucleotide (data not shown). However, when the dendriplex was composed of **16** /TAR&sREV, p24 antigen levels were reduced by 60% compared to 20% achieved by the oligonucleotides alone (data not shown). Therefore, **16** dendrimers specifically enhanced the reduction of p24 antigen release by antisense oligonucleotides due to the improvement of transfection efficiency.

Dendriplexes containing anti HIV *nef* gene (siNEF) and a cocktail mixture of the three siRNAs siP24, siGAG1 and siNEF (siCOCKTAIL) and **16** were also tested for biological effect and compared with naked siRNA (siNEF or siCOCKTAIL) (Figure 8). An inhibition of 25% was seen for siNEF and nearly 40% for siCOCKTAIL in HIV infected PBMC when bound to **16** at a +/− charge ratio of 2 compared to control PBMC (Figure 8A). Analogously, in the case of purified CD4 T lymphocytes, more than 20% was seen for siNEF/**16** and more than 40% for siCOCKTAIL/**16** (Figure 8B). Moreover, LDH assays for these experiments show that the treatments cause minimal toxicity (data not shown).

3 CONCLUSION

We are working on new approaches to develop a novel non-viral vector for HIV inhibition based on the use of carbosilane dendrimers. Synthetic approaches have been developed for ammonium-terminated carbosilane dendrimers consisting of the alcoholysis or hydrosilylation of well-known chloro- or hydride-terminated carbosilane dendrimer respectively affording the dendrimers in high yield.[15,16,24] Dendrimers based on the presence of Si-O bonds decomposed slowly via hydrolysis of those bonds while those based on Si-C bonds are completely water-stable.

In spite of their low generation, ammonium-terminated carbosilane dendrimers mainly represented for the second generation dendrimers **16** are able to form dendriplexes with SNA.[16]

In addition, dendrimers protect ODN from binding to serum proteins or siRNA from RNases and degradation in this way.[17-20] Such protection could provide a meaningful advance for therapies based on SNA not only *in vitro* but also *in vivo*. This could translate into a reduction in the dose of the SNA needed to achieve the biological effect. When a nude ODN is administered, it is necessary to saturate all the possible binding sites within serum proteins to have a fraction of free ODN able to reach the extravascular space and perform the required activity. If these interactions could be prevented by the formation of a complex, presumably the saturation of binding sites would no longer be needed, resulting in the possibility of administering smaller amounts of SNA. In addition, this could reduce the toxic effects related to these unspecific unions of the SNA to serum proteins. Moreover, the dendrimers capability of protecting the siRNA from RNase is of fundamental importance for the siRNA to be able to exert an effect once in the interior of the cell.[25]

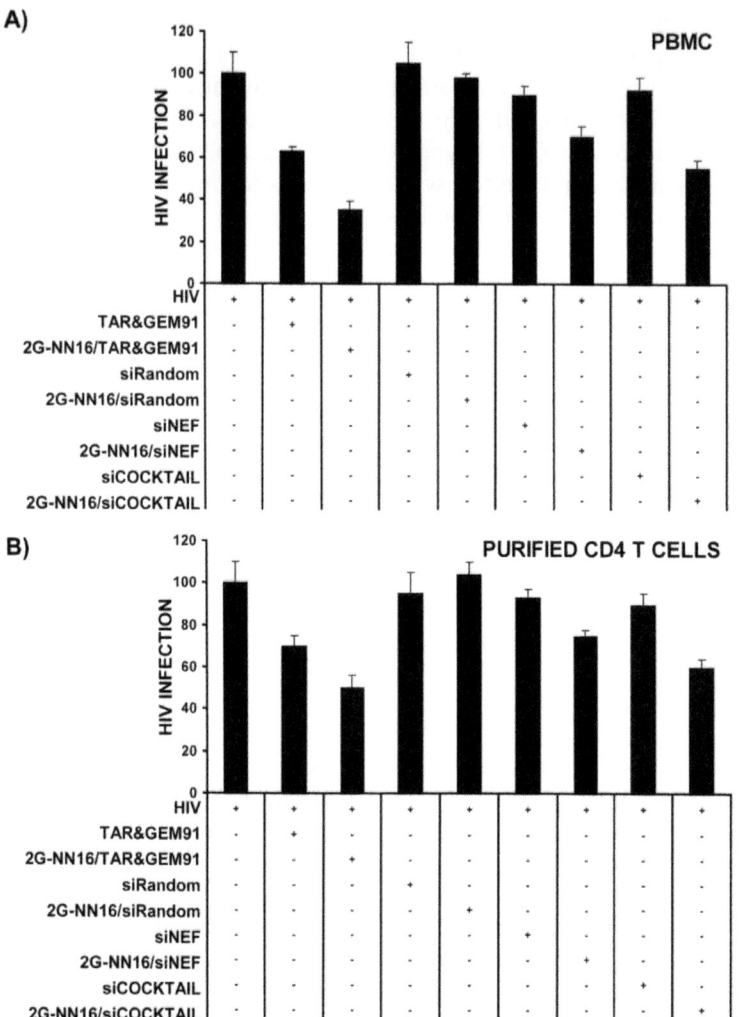

Figure 8. *Inhibition of HIV replication by **16** (also called 2G-NN16-mediated cell delivery of ODN or siRNA to HIV-infected PBMCs (A) and HIV-infected purified CD4+ T lymphocytes (B) via measurement of levels of p24 antigen release.*

Carbosilane dendrimers in general but in particular **16** showed good biocompatibility profiles in *in vitro*. The cytotoxicity assays with the dendriplex clearly show its low toxicity at concentrations needed for immune cell treatment. [16,26] Moreover, the cytotoxicity studies show that the dendriplex causes less toxicity than the dendrimer alone. Non-complexed dendrimer without the neutralizing presence of ODN or siRNA has all of its positively charged groups exposed. This indicates that the toxicity is most likely a result of the high positive charge density, a feature that can be shielded through the use of stabilizing moieties like PEG.[27] Si-O based dendrimers are able to release the ODNs progressively in a time-dependent way when they are dissolved in water. This feature could be a good evidence for their potential use in controlled release of nucleic materials and perhaps other polyanionic drugs that it is worth developing.[16]

Carbosilane dendrimers represented by **16** were found to be a successful and efficient vehicle for the transport and delivery of genetic material (ODN or siRNA) to a wide range of immune cells including PBMC, purified CD4 T-lymphocytes, macrophages and dendritic cells which all play a key role in the infection or pathology of HIV.[19,21] An important problem in researching gene therapy or ODN or RNAi in the fight against HIV lies in the fact that practically all HIV-susceptible cells are very difficult to transfect. To overcome the inherent difficulties in transfecting primary cell cultures such as PBMC or CD4 T-lymphocytes, researchers have used innovative techniques such as nucleofection or antibody fused proteins.[28] Confocal microscopy images indicate uptake of siRNA by CD4 T-cells using our transfection method with carbosilane dendrimers. The similarity of the compartmentalised fluorescent siRNA with perinuclear endosomes in terms of morphology and spatial localization suggest the possibility of entrance via endocytosis. Even though the exact internalization pathway has not yet been studied, it is most likely that the pathway is mediated by internal vesicle formation. On the other hand, the ODNs/**16** dendriplex would be kidnapped in the endosome-lysosome compartment of macrophages. It consists of a cytoplasmatic pattern instead of a nuclear one, opposite to that observed previously in the CD4 T-cells treated with siRNA/**16** dendriplex. Therefore, monocytes or macrophages behave differently in dendriplex uptake than CD4 T-cells.

The fact that we observed complete entrance of naked siRNA in CD4 T-cells within 20 hours merits special attention.[29] It can be assumed that the small size of the siRNA and ODN is the determining factor in their uptake since we have not witnessed the entrance of larger plasmids by themselves (data not shown). Regardless of their uptake by CD4 T-cells, naked siRNA and ODN would face more significant obstacles in the *in vivo* setting, precisely for which our dendrimers are designed to overcome. The design of the carbosilane dendrimers not only intends to improve transfection efficiency, stability and protection *in vivo*, but also to possess a time-dependent release capability.[16,19] This is a fundamental advantage that has enabled dendrimers to make the transition to *in vivo* scenarios.

More interestingly, **16** was found to facilitate the entry of the genetic material into immune cells, enhancing the specific reduction of HIV p24 antigen release by HIV ODN or siRNA due to improved transfection efficiency. Currently the HIV latency is a significant problem when addressing treatment for HIV infection.[2] Gene therapy with ODN or RNAi could potentially improve this weakness in HIV treatment by attacking different specific targets of the HIV cycle, reducing the opportunities for the emergence of resistant strains, and making use of a cocktail of siRNA to attack the HIV on multiple fronts. Our results suggest that a mixture of several siRNA targeted specifically to the HIV achieved an inhibitory effect of 40%. This inhibition was achieved by only targeting a mixture of HIV genes, however the possibility of combining siRNA targeted to HIV with other siRNA designed to down-regulate endogenous cellular genes essential for HIV replication could feasibly improve our results. Therefore, taking into account all these results, the carbosilane dendrimers presented here are in general good candidates for non-viral vectors in the context of biological applications of SNA, and in particular, they may present a new interesting approach for the treatment of HIV infection.

Acknowledgment

This work was supported by the COST Action (TD0802) and grant ERA-NET MNT 2007 (Spain and Poland). Also, by grants from Fondo de Investigación Sanitaria (FIS) of

Ministerio de Ciencia e Innovación (INTRASALUD PI09/02029; PS09/02669); Fundación para la Investigación y la Prevención del SIDA en España (FIPSE); MNT-ERA NET 2007 (ref. NAN2007-31198-E), Red RIS RD06-0006-0035 and INDISNET S-2010-BMD2332 (CM), and Comunidad de Madrid (S-SAL-0159-2006) by MAMF. MNT-ERA NET 2007 (ref. NAN2007-31135-E), Fondo de Investigación Sanitaria (PI080222), MINECO (CTQ2011-23245) and NANODENDMED S2011/BMD2351(CM) by RGR and UA. JLJF is supported by FIS PI081495 and Programa de Investigación de la Consejería de Sanidad de la Comunidad de Madrid. M. M. and J. M. acknowledges Czech national Cost project OC10053.

References

1 T. W. Chun, J. S. Justement, S. Moir, C. W. Hallagan, J. Maenza, J. I. Mullins, A. C. Collier, L. Corey, A.S. Fauci. *J. Infect Dis.* 2007, **195**, 1734-1736.

2 a) J. B. Dinoso, S. Y. Kim, A. M. Wiegand, S. E. Palmer, S. J. Gange, L. Cranmer, A. O´Shea, M. Callender, A. Spivak, T. Brennan, M. F. Kearney, M. A. Proschan, J. M. Mican, C. A. Rehm, J. M. Coffin, J. W. Mellors, R. F. Siciliano, F. Mandarelli. *PNAS*, 2009, **106**, 9403-9408. b) M. J. Buzon, M. Massanella, J. M. Llibre, A. Esteve, V. Dahl, M. C. Puertas, J. M. Gatall, P. Domingo, R. Paredes, M. Sharkey, S. Palmer, M. Stevenson, B. Clotet, J. Blanco, J. Martínez-Picado. *Nat. Med.* 2010, **16**, 460-465.

3 A. S. Fauci, M. I. Johnston, C. W. Dieffenbach, D. R. Burton, S. M. Hammer, J. A. Hoxie, M. Martin, J. Overbaugh, D. I. Watkins, A. Mahmoud, W. C. Greene. *Science* 2008, **321**, 530-532.

4 a) P. A. Sharp. *Genes Dev.* 2001, **15**, 485-490. b) G. A. Coburn, B. R. Cullen. *J. Antimicrob. Chemother.* 2003, **51**, 753-756.

5 P. L. Felgner, T. R. Gadek, M. Holm, R. Roman, H. W. Chan, M. Wenz, J. P. Northrop, G. M. Ringold, M. Danielsen. *Proc. Natl. Acad. Sci. U.S.A.*, 1987, **84**, 7413-7417.

6 G McLachlan, B. J. Stevenson, D. J. Davidson, D. J. Porteous. *Gene Ther.* 2000, **7**, 384-392.

7 T. V. Chirila, P. E. Rakoczy, K. L. Garrett, X. Lou, I I. Constable. *Biomaterials* 2002, **23**, 321-342.

8 a) *Dendrimers and other dendritic polymers*. Eds. J. M. J. Fréchet, D. A. Tomalia. Wiley Series in Polymer Science 2001. J. Wiley & Sons, Ltd. b) *Dendrimers and Dendrons: Concepts, Syntheses, Applications*. Ed. G. R. Newkome, C. N. Moorefield, F. Vögtle, Wiley-VCH, 2001.

9 a) S. Svenson, D. A. Tomalia. *Adv. Drug Deliv.* 2005, **57**, 2106-2109. b) R. Duncan, L. Izzo. *Adv. Drug Deliv.* 2005, **57**, 2215-2237. c) M. Guillot-Nieckowski, S. Eisler, F. Diederich. *New. J. Chem.* 2007, **31**, 1111-1127. d) O. Rolland, C. –O. Turrin, A. –M. Caminade. J. –P. Majoral. *New J. Chem.* 2009, **33**, 1809-1824.

10 J. Haensler, F. C. Szoka Jr.. *Bioconjugate Chem.* 1993, **4**, 372-379.

11 *For some examples see*: a) A. U. Bielinska, C. Chen, J. Johnson, J. R. Baker Jr.. *Bioconjugate Chem.* 1999, **10**, 843-850. b) J. Dennig, E. Duncan. *Rev. Mol. Biotech.* 2002, **90**, 339-347. c) J. Dennig. *Top. Curr. Chem.* 2003, **228**, 227-236. d) X. Liu, J. Wu, M. Yammine, J. Zhou, P. Posocco, S. Viel, C. Liu, F. Ziarelli, M. Fermeglia, S. Pricl, G. Victorero, C. Nguyen, P. Erbacher, J. P. Behr, L. Peng. *Bioconjugate Chem.* 2011, **22**, 2461-2473.

12 a) C. Loup, M. A. Zanta, A. M. Caminade, J. P. Majoral, B. Meunier. *Chem. Eur. J.* 1999, **5**, 3644-3650. b) A. M. Caminade, J. P. Majoral. *Progr. Polym. Sci.* 2005, **30**, 491-505.

13 B. H. Zinselmeyer, S. P. Mackay, A. G. Schatzlein, I. F. Uchegbu. *Pharm. Res.* 2002, **19**, 960-967.

14 a) T. Niidome, M. Wakamatsu, A. Wada, T. Hirayama, H. Aoyagi. *J. Pep. Sci.* 2000, **6**, 271-279. b) M. Ohsaki, T. Okuda, A. Wada, T. Hirayama, T. Nidome, H. Aoyagi. *Bioconjugate Chem.* 2002, **13**, 510-517.

15 P. Ortega, J. F. Bermejo, L. Chonco, E. de Jesús, F. J. de la Mata, G. Fernández, J. C. Flores, R. Gómez, Mᵃ J. Serramía, Mᵃ A. Muñoz-Fernández. *Eur. J. Inorg. Chem.* 2005 1388-1396.

16 J. F. Bermejo, P. Ortega, L. Chonco, R. Eritja, R. Samaniego, M. Müller, E. de Jesus, F. J. de la Mata, J.C. Flores, R. Gómez, Mᵃ A. Muñoz-Fernandez. *Chem. Eur J.* 2007, **13**, 483-495.

17 L. Chonco, J. F. Bermejo, P. Ortega, D. Shcharbin, E. Pedziwiatr, B. Klajnert, F. J. de la Mata, R. Eritja, R. Gómez, M. Bryszewska, Mᵃ A. Muñoz-Fernandez. *Org. & Biomol. Chem.* 2007, **5**, 1886-1893.

18 D. Shcharbin, E. Pedziwiatr, L. Chonco, J. F. Bermejo, P. Ortega, F. J. de la Mata, R. Eritja, R. Gómez, B. Klajnert, M. Bryszewska, Mᵃ A. Muñoz-Fernandez. *Biomacromolecules* 2007, **8**, 2059-2062.

19 N. Weber, P. Ortega, M. I. Clemente, D. Shcharbin, M. Bryszewska, F. J. de la Mata, R. Gómez, Mᵃ A. Muñoz-Fernandez. *J. Control. Release,* 2008, **132**, 55-64.

20 E. Pedziwiatr, D. Shcharbin, L. Chonco, P. Ortega, F. J. de la Mata, R. Gómez, B. Klajnert, M. Bryszewska, Mᵃ A. Muñoz-Fernandez. *J. Fluoresc.* 2009, **19**, 267-275.

21 T. Gonzalo, M. I. Clemente, L. Chonco, N. D. Weber, L. Díaz, M. J. Serramía, R. Gras, P. Ortega, F. J. de la Mata, R. Gómez, L. A. López-Fernández, Mᵃ A. Muñoz-Fernandez, J. L. Jiménez. *ChemMedChem.* 2010, **5**, 921-929.

22 a) A. W. van der Made, P. W. N. M. van Leeuwen. *J. Chem. Soc., Chem. Commun.* 1992, 1400-1401. b) A. W. van der Made, P. W. N. M. van Leeuwen. J. C. de Wilde, R. A. C. Brandes. *Adv. Mater.* 1993, **5**, 466-468. c) L. L. Zhou, J. Roovers. *Macromolecules* 1993, **26**, 963-968. d) D. Seyferth, D. Y. Son, A. L. Rheingold, R. L. Ostrander. *Organometallics* 1994, **13**, 2682-2690. e) I. Cuadrado, M. Morán, J. Losada, C. M. Casado, C. Pascual, B. Alonso, F. Lobete. *Advances in Dendritic Macromolecules*; Eds. G. R. Newkome, JAI press Inc: Greenwich CT, 1996, **3**, 151-195.

23 E. Pedziwiatr-Werbicka, D. Shcharbin, J. Maly, M. Marek, M. Zaborski, B. Gabara, P. Ortega, F. J. De la Mata, R. Gómez, M. A. Muñoz-Fernández, M. Bryszewska. *J. Biomed. Nanotech,* 2012, **8**, 57-73.

24 I. Posadas, B. López-Hernández, M. I. Clemente, J. L. Jiménez, P. Ortega, F. J. de la Mata, R. Gómez, Mᵃ A. Muñoz-Fernandez, V. Ceña. *Pharm. Res.* 2009, **26**, 1181-1191.

25 S. Mao, M. Neu, O. Germershaus, O. Merkel, J. Sitterberg, U. Bakowsky, T. Kissel. *Bioconjugate Chem.* 2006, **17**, 1209-1218.

26 a) R. Jevprasesphant, J. Penny, R. Jalal, D. Attwood, N. B. McKeown, A. D'Emanuele. *Int. J. Pharm.* 2003, **252**, 263-266. b) D. Fischer, Y. Li, B. Ahlemeyer, J. Krieglstein, T. Kissel. *Biomaterials* 2003, **24**, 1121-1131.

27 O. Germershaus, S. Mao, J. Sitterberg, U. Bakowsky, T. Kissel. *J. Control. Release,* 2008, **125**, 145-154.

28 a) J. Yin, Z. Ma, N. Selliah, D. K. Shivers, R. Q. Cron, T. H. Finkel. *J. Immunol. Methods,* 2006, **312**, 1-11. b) D. Peer, P. Zhu, C. V. Carman, J. Lieberman, M. Shimaoka. *Proc. Natl. Acad. Sci. U. S. A.,* 2007, **104**, 4095-4100.

29 J. F. Bermejo, L. Chonco, R. Samaniego, G. Fernandez, R. Eritja, M. A. Munoz-Fernandez. *Eur. J. Sci. Res.,* 2006, **15**, 113-121.

ANIONIC DENDRITIC POLYMERS FOR BIOMEDICAL APPLICATIONS

A. Sousa-Herves,[1§] D. Gröger,[1§] M. Calderón,[1] E. Fernandez-Megia,[*, 2] and R. Haag[*, 1]

[1] Institut für Chemie und Biochemie, Freie Universität Berlin, Takustrasse 3, 14195 Berlin, Germany. Tel: +49 30 838 52633
[2] Department of Organic Chemistry and Center for Research in Biological Chemistry and Molecular Materials (CIQUS), University of Santiago de Compostela, Jenaro de la Fuente s/n, 15782 Santiago de Compostela, Spain. Tel: +34 8818 15727

E-mail: ef.megia@usc.es, haag@chemie.fu-berlin.de
§ Both authors contributed equally to this work

1 INTRODUCTION

Since the mid of the 1980s dendritic architectures have gained increasing interest for biomedical applications because of their unique and well-defined structure, tunable size, charge, and functionality which allow for the design of well-defined, tailor-made molecules.[1-4] Special emphasis has been given to anionic dendritic polymers due to their hydrophilicity and enhanced circulation time in vivo.[5,6] While the structure of cationic dendritic polymers is,[7-9] in terms of functionality, dominated by tertiary and quaternary amines, neutral and polyanionic structures display more structural diversity and, in most of the cases, a superior biocompatibility profile.[10]

Structural features such as high functional surface, low polydispersity, superior biocompatibility, and enhanced circulation time in the blood stream make anionic dendritic polymers ideal candidates in the biomedical field.[1,3,11-13] Reported applications as drug carriers, anti-inflammatory, and antiviral agents highlight the potential of such polyanionic architectures. Moreover, their high negative surface allows for the formation of functional electrostatic complexes, such as soft nanoparticles, micelles, and layer-by-layer assemblies.

Anionic dendritic polymers have been shown to have low cytotoxicity profiles, hemolytic rates, and cell adhesion, amongst other beneficial properties compared to their cationic counterparts. Their reduced toxicity arises from the non-adhesive nature of their surface toward plasma proteins and cellular membranes.[6,14-19] Moreover, their high anionic functionality and nanosized dimensions (2-20 nm) enable their use in therapeutic applications involving multivalent interactions. Other features that make them especially suitable for a variety of applications within the biomedical field relate to their extremely high serosal transfer rates[20] and their particular extra- and intracellular fate.[21]

We herein revise the utilization of anionic dendritic polymers for biomedical applications ranging from drug delivery to anti-viral and anti-inflammatory drugs. This chapter will discuss the great potential of polyanionic dendritic architectures in nanomedicine, with a focus on some recent examples.

2 DRUG DELIVERY AND ANTICANCER THERAPY

One of the most common bio-applications of dendritic polymers is for targeted drug delivery, particularly in cancer therapy and diagnosis. Anionic dendritic polymers are especially promising because the negative charges on their surface provide a highly biocompatible profile in vivo.[10] In addition, the higher hydrophobicity of their cores compared to the polyanionic surface allows one to encapsulate or covalently bind several bioactive molecules such as cytostatic drugs, metals ions, diagnostic probes, etc.

In the non-covalent approach, the encapsulation of drugs can take place at the inner sphere through hydrophobic interactions, leading to supramolecular host-guest complexes, or on the surface of the macromolecule mediated, for instance, by ionic interactions. Chemical bonds link a drug to the macromolecule in the covalent approach, which creates dendrimer-drug conjugates. In this chapter we will highlight the potential of such systems with an example for each binding modality. For a more comprehensive overview, including neutral and positively charged dendritic scaffolds, the reader is referred to alternative chapters in this book and to other recent reviews.[2,12,22,23]

As an example for the encapsulation of hydrophobic guest molecules under formation of supramolecular aggregates, Grinstaff and coworkers have described a biodegradable polyester dendrimer made of succinic acid/glycerol and carrying terminal carboxylates, which was able to encapsulate various anticancer drugs such as camptothecin (Figure 1a). The cytotoxicity expressed in inhibition concentration (IC_{50}) was in the low nanomolar range against human cancer cell lines (MCF-7, HT-29, NCI-H460, SF-268). Up to 16-fold increased cellular uptake and enhanced retention was found for the dendrimer-drug complex in comparison to the free drug.[24]

(a) (b)

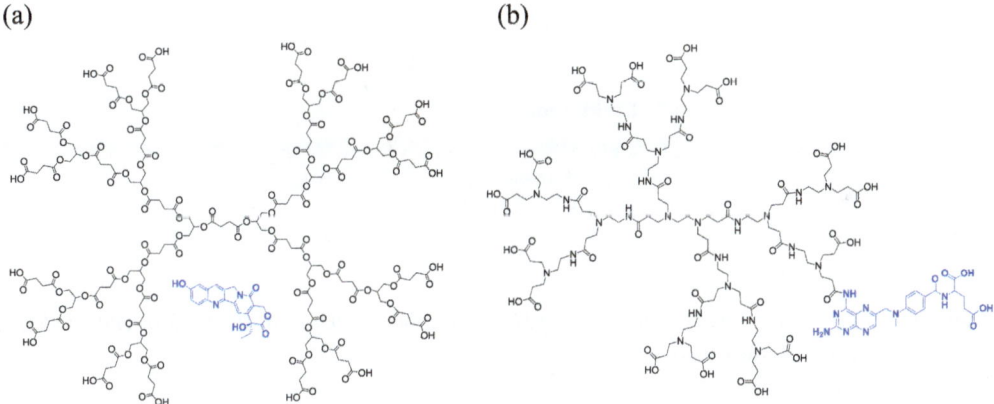

Figure 1 *(a) Representative illustration of a G3-PGLSA-COOH polyester dendrimer with encapsulated 10-hydroxycamptothecin.[24] (b) Chemical structure of a carboxyl-terminated G2.5-PAMAM dendrimer with methotrexate conjugated via amide linkages adapted with permission from ref. 21. Lower generations of the original scaffolds are illustrated.*

Collins and coworkers used electrostatic interactions between anionic carboxyl-terminated G3.5 to G6.5 PAMAM dendrimers and positively charged platinum (II) and ruthenium(II) complexes to form non-covalent dendrimer-drug complexes.[25] A therapeutic utilization of such systems, however, is hardly possible due to relatively weak binding constants of 10^4-10^5 M^{-1}, determined by NMR titration. In general, complexation within the dendritic structure or on the surface of a dendrimer often suffers from uncontrolled release while covalent attachment allows better control over payload and release profiles. In an innovative approach, the group of Kataoka has developed supramolecular micelles by electrostatic interaction between oppositely charged polyion copolymers (PIC micelles, details on the methodology are provided in the next section).[26] This kind of supramolecular aggregates utilizing electrostatic interactions are in general promising, as can be seen from the work by Kono and coworkers introducing dual responsive liposomes for temperature and pH controlled cytoplasmic delivery (Figure 2).[27] The authors applied water soluble, arylsulfonate dye (pyranine) loaded liposomes on HeLa cells and triggered the endosomal release with a temperature increase from 28 to 45 °C. This destabilization was achieved by introducing N-isopropylacryl amide (NIPAM) functions and alkyl chains on a carboxylated hyperbranched polyglycerol (HPG) scaffold. The dual signal responsive properties are based on a temperature-mediated dehydration of NIPAM groups and the pH-dependent protonation of carboxylic acid functionalities.

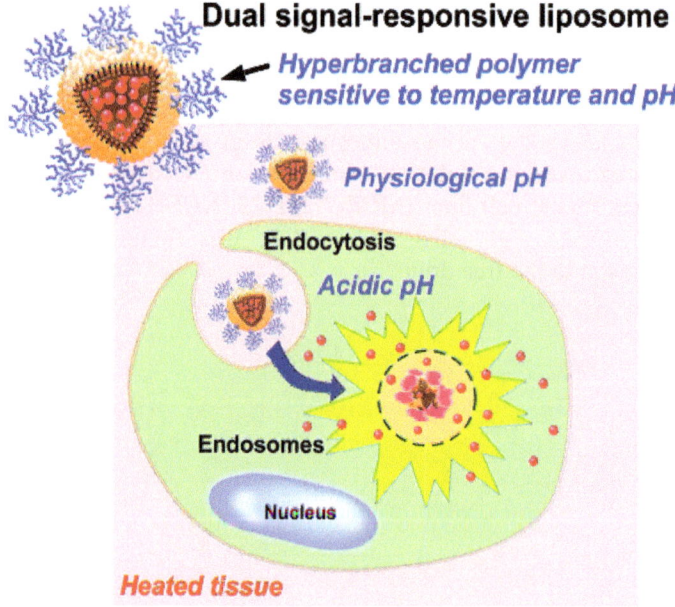

Figure 2 *Design of temperature and pH-responsive liposomal drug delivery systems, adapted with permission from ref 27.*

Among covalent dendrimer-drug conjugates, those using carboxylate terminated G2.5 and G3.5 PAMAM dendrimers are the most frequently used anionic systems. Due to their high biocompatibility and low cytotoxicity,[28] conjugates with enzymes,[29] cytostatics like methotrexate (Figure 1 b)[21] or cisplatin[30] have been extensively investigated. In general, advantages like increased water solubility, less unspecific toxicity, and higher drug efficacy due to passive accumulation through the enhanced permeability and retention (EPR) effect,[31] have been achieved. Polyesters are the most prominent biodegradable systems. As an example, carboxyl terminated G1 and G2 dendrimer/cis-platinum (II) (cis-diaminedichloroplatinum, CDDP) conjugates were proven to have an efficient cytotoxicity against HT1080, CT26, and SKOV3 cancer cells with minimum hemolysis in vitro.[32] Another dendritic anionic polyester that showed promising properties comprises a triblock copolymer of polyethylene glycol (PEG) with citrate dendrons (CPEGC) that bears carboxylate groups at the surface.[33] These anionic polymers had low cytotoxicity towards HT1080 cells over 24 h at high concentrations up to 1 mg/mL and allowed the development of pH-sensitive β-cyclodextrin conjugates. [34,35,36]

Due to a limited recognition and clearance by the reticuloendothelial system (RES), low generation anionic dendritic polymers provide adequate blood circulation times for drug delivery purposes, as representatively shown by Porter and coworkers utilizing sulfonate functionalized poly-*L*-lysine dendrimers for i.v. pharmacokinetic studies.[37] In another example, Gu and coworkers used a carboxylate terminated dendrimer, carrying a biocompatible oligomeric silsesquioxane core, for targeted delivery of doxorubicin.[38]

Further approaches range from the use of anionic dendrimers for the construction of oligodeoxynucleotide-dendrimer conjugates as antisense reagents for gene silencing[39] to anionic dendrimer-antibody conjugates for targeting,[40] and poly(glutamic acid) (PGA) dendrimer encapsulating metalloporphyrins as a photoactive light harvesting systems.[41] Further examples are a G3.5 PAMAM glucosamine conjugate preventing scar tissue formation[42] and glycosylated, carboxyl-terminated polypropyletherimine (PETIM) dendrimers preventing acute gut wall damage in infectious diarrhoeas.[43] As discussed in various reviews,[11,23,44-46] it must be noted that anionic dendrimer-drug conjugates provide an altered chemical environment that, besides the linking chemistry, can immensely influence the drug release that therefore should be optimized case by case.

3 DENDRITIC ARCHITECTURES FOR PHOTODYNAMIC THERAPY

As previously mentioned, another interesting application of anionic dendrimers is their employment on the preparation of supramolecular nanostructures, such as polyion complex (PIC) micelles.[47] Firstly described by the groups of Kataoka and Kabanov,[48,49] PIC micelles are formed by electrostatic interaction between oppositely charged polyions, normally in a stoichiometric charge ratio. Similar to classical polymeric micelles, PIC micelles have a core-shell structure with a core of ionic blocks surrounded by a neutral hydrophilic corona, typically of PEG (Figure 3 a). PIC micelles have numerous potential applications in biomedicine, including the transport of ionic drugs and biomolecules such as proteins and nucleic acids. In particular, PIC micelles containing anionic dendritic photosensitizers have been reported for photodynamic therapy (PDT) and as light-harvesting sensitizers.[26,50-55] PDT is a very promising approach for anticancer therapies that comprises the accumulation of photosensitizers in solid tumors, followed by the local photoirradiation with light of a specific wavelength. Upon irradiation, photosensitizers convert normal triplet oxygen to the highly reactive singlet oxygen ($^1O_2$), which leads to the photochemical destruction of tumoral tissues. In recent years, several approaches have been employed for the incorporation of photosensitizers into new drug delivery systems in order to increase the selectivity and efficacy of PDT, and to reduce undesirable side effects such as skin hyperphotosensitivity.

In this context, Kataoka and coworkers have developed PIC micelles from anionic dendrimers encapsulating porphyrin or phthalocyanine photosensitizers at the core (Figure 3b). In vivo studies have shown that these PIC micelles had a remarkably superior efficacy in PDT compared to the FDA-approved Photofrin®.[52] Recently, PIC micelles formed from an anionic phorphyrin dendrimer were successfully employed in vivo for the photodynamic treatment of neovascular disease, one of the major causes of legal blindness in developed countries.[56] Such in vivo results highlight the potential of these dendritic micelles as new formulations for the treatment of ophthalmic diseases.

Similarly, Kim, Jang, and coworkers, have described the preparation of a different type

(a)   (b)

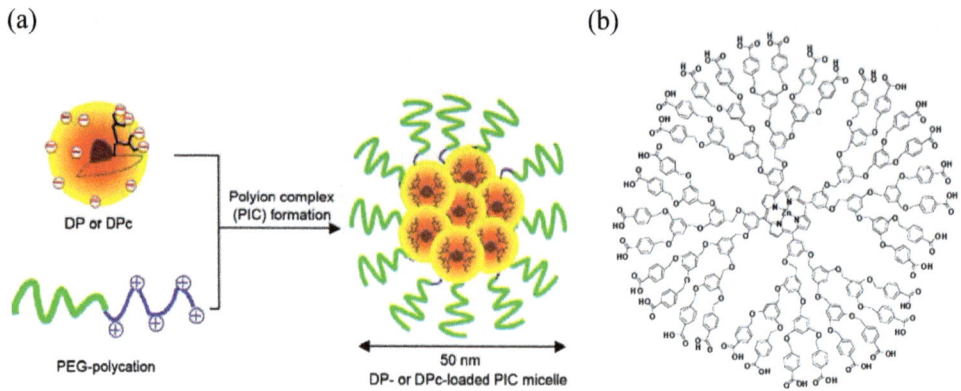

Figure 3 *(a) Schematic representation of PIC micelles for photodynamic therapy. (b) Chemical structure of the porphyrin dendrimer. Adapted with permission from ref. 53.*

of polymeric micelle, so-called polymer–metal complex micelles (PMCMs) that contain the anticancer drug cisplatin for combined sustained drug release and PDT.[57] PMCMs were formed by coordination of the cis-platinum (II) complexed CDDP with an anionic dendrimer encapsulating phthalocyanine and PEG-*b*-poly(*L*-aspartic acid). These micelles showed a sustained release of cisplatin under physiological saline conditions and could generate singlet oxygen under light irradiation, therefore constituting promising nano-devices for combination therapy. The same group has also employed an anionic dendrimer phthalocyanine for the preparation of layer-by-layer (LbL) hollow capsules for combined cancer therapy applications.[58] The anionic dendritic phthalocyanine was employed as a component in the LbL assembly, and the resulting hollow capsules were filled with the anticancer drug doxorubicin. Cell viability studies showed that combined treatment resulted in higher toxicity than either chemotherapy or PDT alone. Complementary, the group of Fernandez-Megia and Riguera has reported the preparation of remarkably stable PIC micelles from a sulfated PEG-dendritic block copolymer of the gallic acid-triethylene glycol (GATG)[59-61] family and an oppositely charged poly(amino acid).[62] An important feature of these micelles is their high stability towards dilution and ionic strength compared to conventional, non-dendritic PIC micelles, which has been attributed to the more rigid dendritic architecture. These micelles are promising vehicles for low-molecular weight drugs, proteins, nucleic acids, and imaging agents. Following a similar approach, the same group has more recently developed related pH-sensitive PIC micelles from carboxylated PEG-GATG block copolymers, with significant potential for the controlled release of pharmaceuticals in cancer therapy.[63]

4 INFLAMMATION

Targeting and treatment of inflammation with anionic dendrimers and dendritic polymers has become of great interest since many diseases go in hand with inflammatory processes. Heparin, a sulfated linear glucosaminoglycan (GAG) with a molecular weight of approximately 17 kDa, derived from bovine lung or porcine intestine, provides anti-inflammatory activity but also acts as a strong anticoagulant. Due to the risk of bleeding, the use of heparin as an anti-inflammatory agent is limited and, accordingly, synthetic, inflammation specific macromolecules with fewer anticoagulant properties are required.

Unfortunately, anticoagulant effects are a characteristic feature for the majority of intravenously administered linear and branched anionic polymers, and is one of the most important drawbacks of nanoscaled anionic macromolecules in vivo.

In an approach to develop an anionic dendritic system with potential anti-inflammatory properties and low anticoagulant effects, Haag and coworkers developed dendritic polyglycerol sulfate (dPGS, Figure 4 a) as a fully synthetic heparin analog. dPGS showed up to 25-fold increased anti-inflammatory potential (determined by the inhibition of classical and alternative complement activation) while only up to 35% anticoagulant activity (determined by the prolongation of the activated partial thromboplastin and thrombin time) in comparison to unfractionated heparin.[64]

(a)

(b)

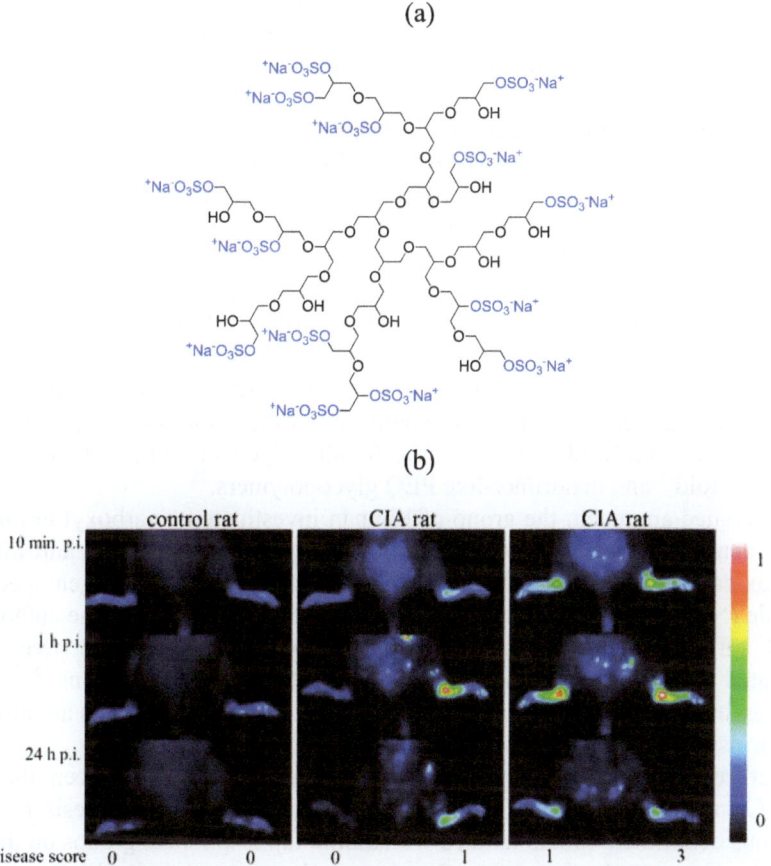

Figure 4 *(a) Idealized chemical structure of dendritic polyglycerol sulfate (dPGS). (b) Application of a dPGS-cyanine dye conjugate as an inflammation-specific diagnostic in a collagen induced arthritis rat mode. Reprinted with permission from ref.65.*

The inflammation specificity of dPGS proved to be partly based on the interaction with complement factors and on multivalent binding towards L- and P-selectin, glycoproteins that are responsible for the initial capture of leukocytes on an activated endothelium upon an inflammatory response.[66] Selectin binding was found to be the most efficient in the case of dPGS compared to alternative dendritic polyglycerol anions, namely, carboxylate, sulfonate, phosphonate, phosphate, and bisphosphonate in a competitive, concentration-dependent surface plasmon resonance (SPR) based L-selectin binding assay. By increasing the size and surface charge of dPGS, the concentrations required for L-selectin inhibition could be lowered several orders of magnitude. Due to strong multivalent binding towards inflamed topologies, fluorescently labeled dPGS were utilized as imaging agents for inflammation, as was shown in rats with collagen induced arthritis (Figure 4 b).[65] As can be seen in the image, legs in a healthy control animal showed no accumulation of the dPGS-dye conjugate, while a strong and spatially defined signal was observed in the right or both legs, respectively, in the arthritic animals. This inflammation specificity was also confirmed for sulfated polyglycerol carbohydrate architectures in vitro.[67,68] In a structure-biocompatibility relationship, dPGS and dPG phosphate were compared with cationic dPG-amine, hydroxyl terminated PAMAM dendrimers, poly(ethyleneimine) (PEI), and dextran, which showed that anionic dendritic polyglycerols are as safe as PEG in terms of cellular compatibility.[14]

Another example of inflammation-targeted anionic dendrimers was described by Diwan and coworkers using a G3.5 PAMAM-PEG-folate conjugate.[69,70] By investigating the biodistribution in arthritic rats, an elongated half-life, increased targeting efficiency, and significantly less uptake by the stomach were found. In another example, the group of Davignon investigated inflammation targeting as well as osteoclastogenesis for an azabisphosphonate-capped dendrimer in an experimental arthritis model, by examining the suppression of the disease by the reduction of cartilage destruction, bone erosion, and reduced levels of pro-inflammatory cytokines.[71] In their study, a dendrimer that was originally shown to target monocytes could be directed toward anti-inflammatory activation and exhibited anti-osteoclastic activity. Further examples for promising anionic, anti-inflammatory scaffolds are oligosaccharide glycodendrimers based on a G2.5 PAMAM scaffold[72] and dendrimer-like PEO glycopolymers.[73]

In a combined approach, the group of Kannan investigated a carboxyl terminated G3.5 PAMAM dendrimer-N-acetyl cysteine (NAC)-conjugate that showed anti-inflammatory and anti-oxidant properties based on a reduced level of reactive oxygen species (ROS), nitric oxide (NO), and TNF-α released in activated microglial cells.[74] The authors found an improved efficacy at low doses for the conjugate, compared to free NAC, and demonstrated the potential for neuroinflammation targeting applications.[75,76] It is worth mentioning that positively charged full generation PAMAM dendrimers are also known to exhibit intrinsic neuroinflammation-targeting properties.[77,78]

Another relevant example in the field is the collaboration between the groups of Majoral, Caminade, and Poupot.[71,79-82] They have reported the synthesis of a series of phosphorous dendrimers functionalized with amino diphosphonate groups on the periphery (Figure 5). The introduction of a fluorescent dye into the dendrimers allowed the visualization of their selective binding to the surface of monocytes. Video images obtained by confocal microscopy showed that dendrimers were rapidly internalized by the monocytes, which resulted in some morphological changes of the monocytes after 3-6 days of exposure, indicating that they were activated by the dendrimer. They also remained viable over longer periods than control monocytes.[80] Comparison of the gene expression of monocytes activated by the dendrimer with untreated monocytes showed that 78 genes were up-regulated, whereas 62 genes were down-regulated. Examination of these genes directed the hypothesis of an anti-inflammatory activation of human monocytes.[81] The group of Majoral has also published the synthesis of dendrimers based on a phosphorus skeleton with anionic phosphonate groups on their surface.[83] These dendrimers showed high activity in the activation and multiplication of natural killer cells (NK). Such data are promising as they pave the road to the use of antiviral or anticancer immune-therapies, where a large number of NK cells might be desirable.

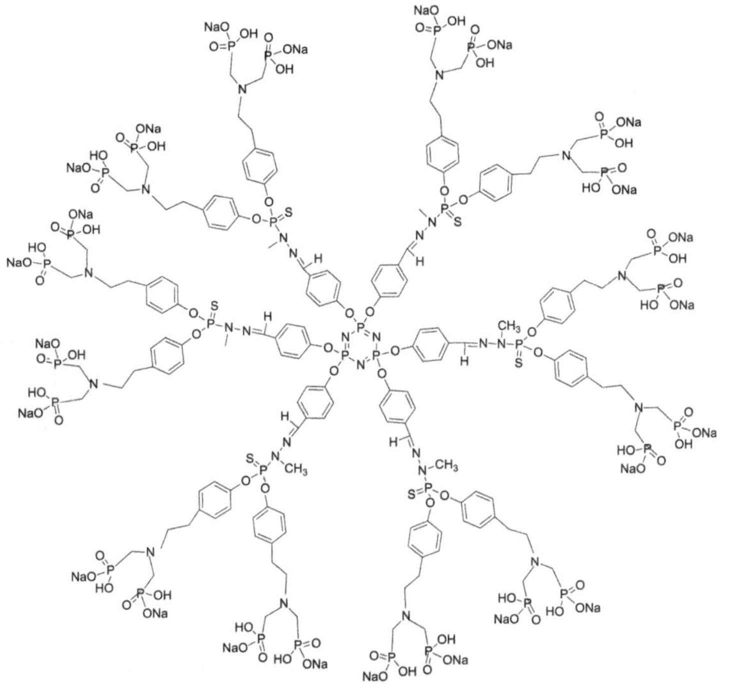

Figure 5 *Chemical structure of one of the Majoral's group phosphorous dendrimers. Adapted with permission from ref.82.*

5 ANTIVIRAL ACTIVITY

Dendrimers have also been investigated for their antiviral properties, in particular against the human immunodeficiency virus (HIV) and herpes simplex virus (HSV-1 and HSV-2).[84,85] It is possible to find in the literature examples of anionic dendrimers containing sulfate, sulfonate, or carboxylate groups with the ability to inhibit cell binding and, in some cases, even the replication of these viruses in vitro.[86-89] In the case of HSV, its cell binding mechanism has been quite precisely determined. It is known that viral entry is a complex process, involving interaction between HSV binding proteins and some cell surface receptors composed of glycosaminoglycans (heparin sulfate), followed by the fusion of the viral envelope and the plasma membrane of the host cell.

In this context, Gong and coworkers have succeeded in inhibiting the entrance and, in some cases, the replication of HSV in cells by using an anionic sulfonated dendrimer.[88] The mechanism of inhibition is based on the affinity of the virus for the sulfonate groups of the periphery of the dendrimer, which mimic the cellular receptors. HIV, on the other hand, has a glycoprotein on its surface called gp120 that is responsible for binding to CD4 receptors on human cells. The presence of positively charged amino acid residues in gp120 results in a great affinity for polyanionic dendrimers which ultimately prevent interaction of the virus with CD4 receptors of human T cells. On this basis, Witvrouw and coworkers prepared polysulfonate and polycarboxylate PAMAM derivatives, which were capable of inhibiting the replication of HIV-1 (anti-retroviral activity) and binding to different HIV strains (inhibitory activity).[87] Probably the most successful example in this field is VivaGel®, a G4 Poly-*L*-Lysine based dendrimer decorated with 32 naphthalene disulfonate groups (Figure 6).[85,90-93] VivaGel® (SPL7013, developed by Starpharma) is a topical vaginal microbicide that inhibits replication and, in some cases, the infection of HIV-1 and HSV.[89,91,92] Nowadays, microbicides are considered a very promising approach to avoid the expansion of HIV and there are several examples currently in clinical trials.[84,94,95]

(a)   (b)

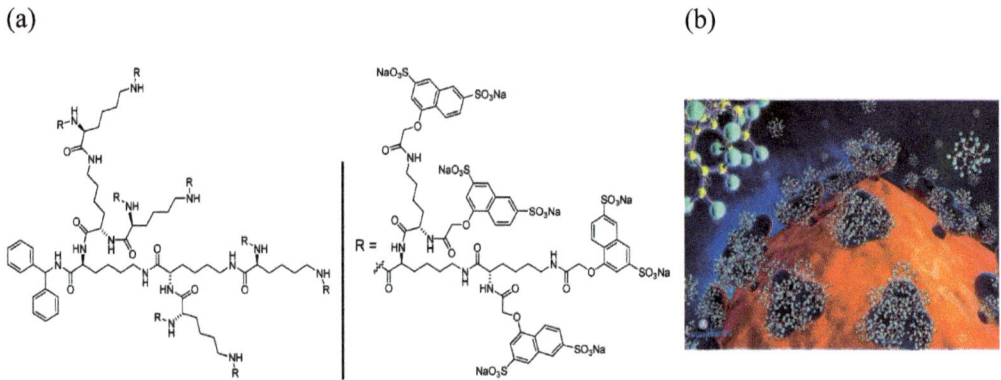

Figure 6 *(a) Chemical structure of VivaGel®, adapted with permission from ref. 85. (b) Binding of VivaGel® to the trimeric receptor on the HIV surface, with courtesy of Starpharma.*

VivaGel® has already completed phase I clinical trials, and shown very positive data in terms of safety, tolerance, and pharmacokinetics. In fact, when applied vaginally to sexually abstinent women, once a day for seven days at concentrations of 0.5–3.0 % dendrimer, no evidence of toxicity or absorption was observed. Adverse effects were slight and included abdominal pain or discomfort.[96] Moreover, when the 3% SPL7013 gel was daily applied to the penis of either circumcised or uncircumcised men for seven days, no toxicity or absorption was observed. In this case, secondary effects consisted on irritation and redness at the application site.[97] However, some limitations were still detected for VivaGel®, such as a lack of large spectrum microbicide against HIV-1 strains using CCR5 as co-receptor or against other viral types. VivaGel® is currently completing phase II trials. It is worth mentioning that VivaGel® is also being developed for treatment and prevention of bacterial vaginosis and as a coating for condoms.

Another worth mentioning work in this field is from the groups of De la Mata/Gómez and Muñoz-Fernández. In a joint effort, these authors have developed a series of anionic carbosilane dendrimers with carboxylate and sulfonate peripheral groups that showed broad-spectrum anti-HIV activity.[84,98] In particular, it was found that a second-generation dendrimer with sulfonate peripheral groups (2G-S16, Figure 7a) showed the most effective activity against a wide range of HIV-1 clades, HIV-2, and other enveloped viruses. Indeed, this dendrimer was not toxic in epithelial cell lines, CD4 lymphocytes, macrophages, and dendritic cells, and therefore can be considered as a promising microbicide for in vivo evaluation.[99]

(a)

(b)

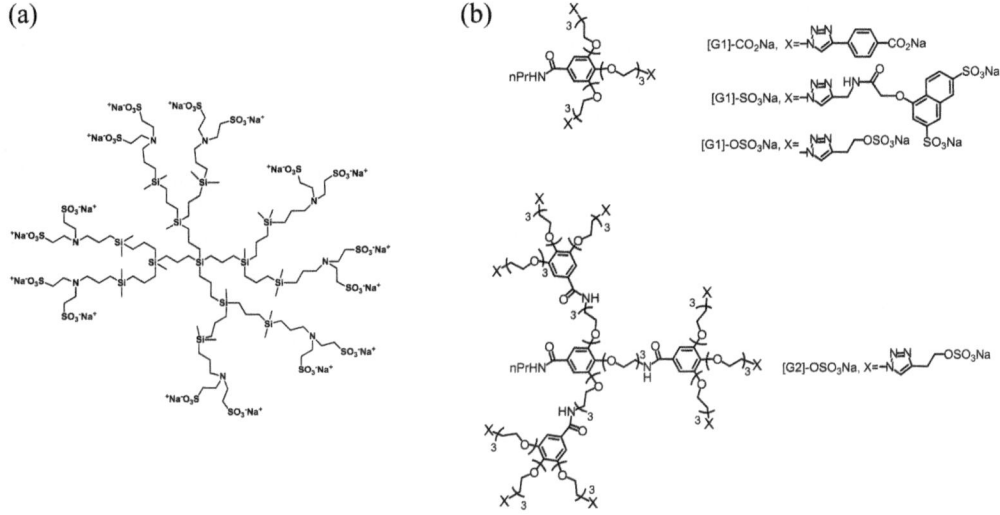

Figure 7 *(a) Structure of 2G-S16, with 16 sulfonate peripheral groups, adapted with permission from ref. 99. (b) Anionic GATG structures assessed for inhibition of the dimerization of the capsid protein CA of HIV-1, adapted with permission from ref. 100.*

Other dendritic structures that have also been successful as antiviral agents are those prepared by Blanzat, Turrin, and coworkers.[101] These authors synthesized dendrimers of poly (phosphor hydrazone) equipped with terminal phosphonic acid moieties and lateral alkyl chains at the periphery, and assessed their activity against HIV-1 in CEM-SS cells and MT-4. After 30 min of exposition to the virus, cells were treated with different concentrations of dendrimers and, after 5 days, the inhibition of HIV infection was assessed. The authors found that one of the dendrimers, containing an alkyl chain of 3 carbon atoms, showed a higher antiviral activity than dendrimers with no alkyl chain or a chain of 10 carbons. This difference in activity was attributed to the ability of short alkyl chains to interact with the lipophilic portion of gp120.

In a joint effort by the groups of Neira, Velázquez-Campoy, and Fernandez-Megia, the ability of GATG dendrimers to inhibit the dimerization of the capsid protein CA of HIV-1 was assessed (Figure 7b).[100] It was found that first-generation GATG dendrimers bound to the C-terminal domain of CA (CTD) with a dissociation constant in the micromolar range, as shown by isothermal titration calorimetry (ITC). Furthermore, the affinity of some of the dendrimers for CTD was similar to that of synthetic peptides capable of binding to the dimerization region, and of comparable magnitude to the homodimerization affinity of both CTD and CA. Moreover, a G1 dendrimer decorated with peripheral benzoate groups, was able to hamper the assembly in vitro of the HIV capsid. These results have opened the possibility of considering dendrimers as lead compounds for the development of anti-HIV drugs targeting the capsid assembly.

In this context a number of alternative HIV inhibiting dendrimers are also being investigated. Besides VivaGel®, several anionic glycodendrimers have been reported. However, many of them only interact with individual viral proteins and lack the potential for real multivalency[102,103] which requires virus-size dimensions. Therefore these early concepts of dendritic multivalent approaches need to be extended to higher multiplicity and longer length scales to compete with pathogenic viruses or bacteria in the 100 nm to 10 µm range.[5] In an effort to bring the dendritic polymers to a higher dimensional scale (20-100 nm), Haag and coworkers recently highlighted the systematic analysis of multivalent glycoarchitectures based on dendritic polyglycerol nanogels in the inhibition of the influenza virus.[104] In their study, particle sizes were varied along with the degree of functionalization to match the corresponding virus size and receptor multiplicity in order to achieve maximum binding efficiency. It was shown that the inhibitory activities of the polymeric glycoconjugates drastically increased with the particle size. Comparing the inhibition of binding and fusion to influenza virus, PG nanogels with 60 nm diameter were 7×10^3-fold more effective than dPG with diameters of 3 nm at comparable sugar concentrations. Moreover, it was demonstrated that the nanogel reduced viral infection up to 80%. This emphasizes the importance of matching sizes and multiplicity for biological surface interactions, which is achieved by the particle dimensionality of the dPG-based nanogels.[102,103]

6 OTHER APPLICATIONS

Beside the examples discussed in the previous sections, anionic dendritic polymers have been used in several other application areas. In a review from Bosch, current developments in the area of rheumatoid arthritis using phosphorus-containing dendrimers capped with anionic azabisphosphonate (ABP) end groups have been discussed in detail.[105]
Bone targeting has also become of interest, but these structures predominantly only have a low degree of anionic targeting moieties,[106] mainly bisphosphonates. Satchi-Fainaro, Pasut, and coworkers investigated the role of a bifunctional PEG–dendrimer, H_2N–PEG–dendrimer–$(COOH)_4$, as carrier for a combination of paclitaxel (PTX) and alendronate (ALN). The PTX-PEG-$(ALN)_4$ conjugate was designed to exploit active targeting by the ALN molecule and passive targeting through the EPR effect.[107]
Tissue engineering and surface modification appear to be of interest, because of a carboxyl-terminated G1.5 PAMAM dendrimer that has only shown a negligible cytotoxicity towards mouse fibroblasts (L929) and at the same time allowed cells to adhere to its surface.[108] Anionic amphiphilic dendrimers have also found application as antibacterial agents, as demonstrated by Grinstaff and coworkers.[109] So far, however, the majority of reports in this field comprise the employment of cationic dendritic species, which are limited by the toxicity inherent to their cationic nature.[110]
Another interesting application of polyanionic dendritic structures is the coating of positively charged surfaces through electrostatic interactions for charge-mediated layer by layer modification. Some first examples of imaging probes based on anionic macromolecules[65] as well as theranostic approaches[111,112] have been described but the majority of macromolecular imaging agents are still based on the conjugation of tracers to neutral dendritic polymers. Lastly, highly anionic dendritic polymer systems have great potential for the stabilization of hard matter nanoparticles and the synthesis of hard-soft matter hybrid systems in general, e.g. stabilized carbon nanotubes.[113]

7 BIODISTRIBUTION

Understanding biophysicochemical interactions of dendritic macromolecules with biological systems is of greatest importance in order to engineer nanomaterials with defined properties and desired distribution, metabolism, and excretion profiles. In a review from Nel and coworkers current proceedings are described with a focus on biophysicochemical influences on the interface between nanomaterials and proteins, cells, membranes, etc.[114] Determination of biological binding partners of certain dendritic macromolecules can indeed be accessed in vitro, e.g., via ITC, size exclusion chromatography (SEC), SPR, or quartz crystal microbalance (QCM). However, due to the complexity of biological systems, in vivo experiments, e.g., with radio labeled compounds, are usually preferred in order to get a first idea of a candidate biodistribution. The interaction of intravenously administered nanoparticles with biological systems is strongly dependent on the particles surface functionalization, size, shape, charge density, and roughness.[114] These properties dictate the speed of formation of a protein corona, immunoglobulin binding, and hence complement activation. Since recognition by the RES is hardly desired, neutral dendritic architectures are usually the preferred ones for therapeutic applications. Blood circulation times of neutral "stealth" macromolecules, e.g., PEG or hydroxyl terminated polyglycerols,[115,116] generally increase with molecular weight and size. For charged macromolecules, however, a faster clearance with increasing size is usually found.[114] While polycationic dendritic architectures bind to negatively charged cell surfaces, e.g., endothelial and epithelial, and are rapidly cleared from the circulation, polyanionic structures benefit from their negative charge and show much longer circulation times and lower cytotoxic profiles than polycations. In regard to anionic dendritic architectures, carboxyl-terminated half generation PAMAM dendrimers are the most widely explored.[19] Duncan and coworkers investigated G2.5, G3.5, and G5.5 PAMAM dendrimers after i.v. administration in rats, and recovered 20–40% of the dose after one hour from blood while accumulation occurred predominantly in liver.[6] Besides excretion via the liver, dendritic polyanions with molecular weights or hydrodynamic diameters below the renal threshold (approximately 40 kDa), are generally excreted via the kidneys within a few hours.[117,118] A different example is the approved MRI contrast agent Gadomer-17, which is based on a dendritic polylysine core and 24 Gd^{3+} chelating, carboxylic acid containing macrocyclic ligands with a total molecular weight of 17 kDa. Complete elimination from the body, mainly via glomerular filtration, was found after a single i.v. dose within several hours. It must be noted that the net charge of Gadomer-17 is neutral, if all chelating ligands are occupied with gadolinium ions.[119] Besides degradable systems such as polyesters,[120] another approach to overcome undesired deposition is topical administration, where applicable. This route has emerged as an effective way for local delivery, for instance in the case of VivaGel®, which is applied as vaginal gel against viral infections, and also other routes should be considered in the future. In summary, today only a few anionic, dendritic polymers have been intensively investigated with respect to their biodistribution, nevertheless, general trends are known. Even though dendritic polyanions exhibit advantageous properties compared to polycations, neutral, "inert" dendritic architectures are still even more suitable for most applications.

8 CONCLUSIONS

Anionic dendritic polymers have conquered the biomedical field. Although these negatively charged nanosystems are clearly outnumbered compared to neutral architectures in the field, their versatile applicability allows new design principles for the synthesis of targeted and bioactive compounds. Until now, only systems of a simple rational design, such as VivaGel®, have reached the clinical development stage. Even though many examples provide promising targeting and inhibition properties in vitro, the application of highly anionic nanostructures in vivo is often limited by interaction with hepatic tissue or proteins leading to problems in metabolism and biochemical interference. With a large number of biocompatible dendritic structures and anionic functionalities in hand, finding a balance between anticoagulant properties, selective targeting, biological activity, acceptable pharmacokinetics, and undesired interference with biochemical processes will be the main challenge in the near future. However, compared to cationic systems, anionic scaffolds are, in terms of cytotoxicity and hemolytic activity, much more biocompatible[10,30,121] which broadens the scope immensely. Nevertheless, localization in kidney for lower generation anionic dendrimers and in liver and spleen for higher generations is an important factor to be considered. It should be noted that besides many promising in vitro studies, the transfer to the corresponding in vivo situations was already successful in some cases. Nevertheless intense research is needed to demonstrate the clinical potential of these polyanionic dendritic structures.

9 APPENDIX

The European CMST COST Action TD0802 Dendrimers in Biomedical Applications has been strongly involved in the development of dendritic anionic polymers for biomedical applications. This chapter has highlighted the work realized within such network in the following references: 3, 4, 5, 10, 14, 28, 44, 71, 79-84, 93, 98-102, 104, 112, 113.

Acknowledgements

We gratefully thank the COST Action (TD0802). R. H. and D. G. would like to acknowledge the collaborative research center SFB 765 of the German Science Foundation (DFG) for financial support. E. F.-M. thanks the Spanish government (CTQ2012-34790 and CTQ2009-10963) and the Xunta de Galicia (10CSA209021PR and CN2011/037) for financial support. M. C. and D. G. acknowledge the FU Focus area ''Nanoscale''. A. S.-H. is grateful for a Marie Curie Intra-European Fellowship. Furthermore, we thank Dr. Pamela Winchester for careful proofreading.

References

1   M. A. Mintzer, M. W. Grinstaff, *Chem. Soc. Rev.* 2011, **40**, 173.
2   Y. Cheng, L. Zhao, Y. Li, T. Xu, *Chem. Soc. Rev.* 2011, **40**, 2673.
3   M. Calderón, M. A. Quadir, S. K. Sharma, R. Haag, *Adv. Mater.* 2010, **22**, 190.
4   E. Fleige, M. A. Quadir, R. Haag, *Adv. Drug Delivery Rev.* 2012, **64**, 866.
5   M. A. Quadir, R. Haag, *J. Control. Release* 2012, **161**, 484.
6   N. Malik, R. Wiwattanapatapee, R. Klopsch, K. Lorenz, H. Frey, J. W. Weener, E. W. Meijer, W. Paulus, R. Duncan, *J. Control. Release* 2000, **65**, 133.
7   S. Malhotra, H. Bauer, A. Tschiche, A. M. Staedtler, A. Mohr, M. Calderón, V. S. Parmar, L. Hoeke, S. Sharbati, R. Einspanier, R. Haag, *Biomacromolecules* 2012, **13**, 3087.
8   A. Barnard, P. Posocco, S. Pricl, M. Calderon, R. Haag, M. E. Hwang, V. W. T. Shum, D. W. Pack, D. K. Smith, *J. Am. Chem. Soc.* 2011, **133**, 20288.
9   W. Fischer, M. Calderón, A. Schulz, I. Andreou, M. Weber, R. Haag, *Bioconjugate Chem.* 2010, **21**, 1744.
10   J. Khandare, M. Calderon, N. M. Dagia, R. Haag, *Chem. Soc. Rev.* 2012, **41**, 2824.
11   S. El Kazzouli, S. Mignani, M. Bousmina, J.-P. Majoral, *New J. Chem.* 2012, **36**, 227.
12   D. Astruc, E. Boisselier, C. Ornelas, *Chem. Rev.* 2010, **110**, 1857.
13   C. C. Lee, J. A. MacKay, J. M. J. Frechet, F. C. Szoka, *Nat. Biotech.* 2005, **23**, 1517.
14   J. Khandare, A. Mohr, M. Calderón, P. Welker, K. Licha, R. Haag, *Biomaterials* 2010, **31**, 4268.

15 S. Fuchs, T. Kapp, H. Otto, T. Schöneberg, P. Franke, R. Gust, A. D. Schlüter, *Chemistry – A European Journal* 2004, **10**, 1167.

16 E. R. Gillies, E. Dy, J. M. J. Fréchet, F. C. Szoka, *Mol. Pharm.* 2005, **2**, 129.

17 M. T. Morgan, M. A. Carnahan, C. E. Immoos, A. A. Ribeiro, S. Finkelstein, S. J. Lee, M. W. Grinstaff, *J. Am. Chem. Soc.* 2003, **125**, 15485.

18 O. L. Padilla De Jesús, H. R. Ihre, L. Gagne, J. M. J. Fréchet, F. C. Szoka, *Bioconjugate Chem.* 2002, **13**, 453.

19 U. Boas, J. B. Christensen, P. M. H. Heegaard, Dendrimers in Medicine and Biotechnology: New Molecular Tools, Royal Society of Chemistry, 2006.

20 R. Wiwattanapatapee, B. Carreño-Gómez, N. Malik, R. Duncan, *Pharm. Res.* 2000, **17**, 991.

21 S. Gurdag, J. Khandare, S. Stapels, L. H. Matherly, R. M. Kannan, *Bioconjugate Chem.* 2006, **17**, 275.

22 A. R. Menjoge, R. M. Kannan, D. A. Tomalia, *Drug Discov. Today* 2010, **15**, 171.

23 R. K. Tekade, P. V. Kumar, N. K. Jain, *Chem. Rev.* 2009, **109**, 49.

24 M. T. Morgan, Y. Nakanishi, D. J. Kroll, A. P. Griset, M. A. Carnahan, M. Wathier, N. H. Oberlies, G. Manikumar, M. C. Wani, M. W. Grinstaff, *Cancer Res.* 2006, **66**, 11913.

25 M. J. Pisani, N. J. Wheate, F. R. Keene, J. R. Aldrich-Wright, J. G. Collins, *J. Inorg. Biochem.* 2009, **103**, 373.

26 W. D. Jang, N. Nishiyama, G. D. Zhang, A. Harada, D. L. Jiang, S. Kawauchi, Y. Morimoto, M. Kikuchi, H. Koyama, T. Aida, K. Kataoka, *Angew. Chem., Int. Ed.* 2005, **44**, 419.

27 T. Kaiden, E. Yuba, A. Harada, Y. Sakanishi, K. Kono, *Bioconjugate Chem.* 2011, **22**, 1909.

28 A. Janaszewska, K. Maczynska, G. Matuszko, D. Appelhans, B. Voit, B. Klajnert, M. Bryszewska, *New J. Chem.* 2012, **36**, 428.

29 X. Wang, R. Inapagolla, S. Kannan, M. Lieh-Lai, R. M. Kannan, *Bioconjugate Chem.* 2007, **18**, 791.

30 N. Malik, E. G. Evagorou, R. Duncan, *Anti-Cancer Drugs* 1999, **10**, 767.

31 H. Maeda, J. Wu, T. Sawa, Y. Matsumura, K. Hori, *J. Control. Release* 2000, **65**, 271.

32 I. Haririan, M. S. Alavidjeh, M. R. Khorramizadeh, M. S. Ardestani, Z. Z. Ghane, H. Namazi, *Int. J. Nanomed.* 2010, **5**, 63.

33 N. Hassan, M. Sanaz, N. Mina, *BioImpacts* 2011, **1**, 63.

34 H. Namazi, M. Adeli, *Biomaterials* 2005, **26**, 1175.

35 H. Namazi, M. Adeli, *Eur. Polym. J.* 2003, **39**, 1491.

36 N. Hassan, H. Yousef Toomari, *Adv. Pharm. Bull.* 2011, **1**, 40.

37 L. M. Kaminskas, B. J. Boyd, P. Karellas, S. A. Henderson, M. P. Giannis, G. Y. Krippner, C. J. H. Porter, *Mol. Pharm.* 2007, **4**, 949.

38 H. Yuan, K. Luo, Y. Lai, Y. Pu, B. He, G. Wang, Y. Wu, Z. Gu, *Mol. Pharm.* 2010, **7**, 953.

39 M. Hussain, M. Shchepinov, M. Sohail, I. F. Benter, A. J. Hollins, E. M. Southern, S. Akhtar, *J. Control. Release* 2004, **99**, 139.

40 T. Miyano, W. Wijagkanalan, S. Kawakami, F. Yamashita, M. Hashida, *Mol. Pharm.* 2010, **7**, 1318.

41 V. Rozhkov, D. Wilson, S. Vinogradov, *Macromolecules* 2002, **35**, 1991.

42 S. Shaunak, S. Thomas, E. Gianasi, A. Godwin, E. Jones, I. Teo, K. Mireskandari, P. Luthert, R. Duncan, S. Patterson, P. Khaw, S. Brocchini, *Nat. Biotech.* 2004, **22**, 977.

43 I. Teo, S. M. Toms, B. Marteyn, T. S. Barata, P. Simpson, K. A. Johnston, P. Schnupf, A. Puhar, T. Bell, C. Tang, M. Zloh, S. Matthews, P. M. Rendle, P. J. Sansonetti, S. Shaunak, *EMBO Molecular Medicine* 2012, **4**, 866.

44 M. Calderón, M. A. Quadir, M. Strumia, R. Haag, *Biochimie* 2010, **92**, 1242.

45 C. Kojima, *Expert Opin. Drug Deliv.* 2010, **7**, 307.

46 W. Gao, J. M. Chan, O. C. Farokhzad, *Mol. Pharm.* 2010, **7**, 1913.

47 Y. Lee, K. Kataoka, *Soft Matter* 2009, **5**, 3810.

48 A. V. Kabanov, T. K. Bronich, V. A. Kabanov, K. Yu, A. Eisenberg, *Macromolecules* 1996, **29**, 6797.
49 A. Harada, K. Kataoka, *Macromolecules* 1995, **28**, 5294.
50 H. R. Stapert, N. Nishiyama, D. L. Jiang, T. Aida, K. Kataoka, *Langmuir* 2000, **16**, 8182.
51 W. D. Jang, Y. Nakagishi, N. Nishiyama, S. Kawauchi, Y. Morimoto, M. Kikuchi, K. Kataoka, *J. Control. Release* 2006, **113**, 73.
52 N. Nishiyama, Y. Nakagishi, Y. Morimoto, P. S. Lai, K. Miyazaki, K. Urano, S. Horie, M. Kumagai, S. Fukushima, Y. Cheng, W. D. Jang, M. Kikuchi, K. Kataoka, *J. Control. Release* 2009, **133**, 245.
53 N. Nishiyama, Y. Morimoto, W. D. Jang, K. Kataoka, *Adv. Drug Delivery Rev.* 2009, **61**, 327.
54 N. Nishiyama, W. D. Jang, K. Kataoka, *New J. Chem.* 2007, **31**, 1074.
55 Y. Li, W. D. Jang, N. Nishiyama, A. Kishimura, S. Kawauchi, Y. Morimoto, S. Miake, T. Yamashita, M. Kikuchi, T. Aida, K. Kataoka, *Chem. Mater.* 2007, **19**, 5557.
56 R. Ideta, F. Tasaka, W.-D. Jang, N. Nishiyama, G.-D. Zhang, A. Harada, Y. Yanagi, Y. Tamaki, T. Aida, K. Kataoka, *Nano Lett.* 2005, **5**, 2426.
57 J. Kim, H.-J. Yoon, S. Kim, K. Wang, T. Ishii, Y.-R. Kim, W.-D. Jang, *J. Mater. Chem.* 2009, **19**, 4627.
58 K. J. Son, H.-J. Yoon, J.-H. Kim, W.-D. Jang, Y. Lee, W.-G. Koh, *Angew. Chem. Int. Ed.* 2011, **50**, 11968.
59 S. P. Amaral, M. Fernandez-Villamarin, J. Correa, R. Riguera, E. Fernandez-Megia, *Org. Lett.* 2011, **13**, 4522.
60 E. Fernandez-Megia, J. Correa, I. Rodríguez-Meizoso, R. Riguera, *Macromolecules* 2006, **39**, 2113.
61 E. Fernandez-Megia, J. Correa, R. Riguera, *Biomacromolecules* 2006, **7**, 3104.
62 A. Sousa-Herves, E. Fernandez-Megia, R. Riguera, *Chem. Commun.* 2008, 3136.
63 A. Sousa-Herves, R. Riguera, E. Fernandez-Megia, *PCT Int. Appl. (2010) WO 2010018286 A1 20100218.*
64 H. Türk, R. Haag, S. Alban, *Bioconjugate Chem.* 2004, **15**, 162.
65 K. Licha, P. Welker, M. Weinhart, N. Wegner, S. Kern, S. Reichert, I. Gemeinhardt, C. Weissbach, B. Ebert, R. Haag, M. Schirner, *Bioconjugate Chem.* 2011, **22**, 2453.
66 J. Dernedde, A. Rausch, M. Weinhart, S. Enders, R. Tauber, K. Licha, M. Schirner, U. Zügel, A. von Bonin, R. Haag, *Proc. Natl. Acad. Sci. U.S.A.* 2010, **107**, 19679.
67 I. Papp, J. Dernedde, S. Enders, R. Haag, *Chem. Commun.* 2008, 5851.
68 J. Dernedde, I. Papp, S. Enders, S. Wedepohl, F. Paulus, R. Haag, *J. Carbohydr. Chem.* 2011, **30**, 347.
69 D. Chandrasekar, R. Sistla, F. J. Ahmad, R. K. Khar, P. V. Diwan, *J. Biomed. Mat. Res.* 2007, **82A**, 92.
70 A. S. Chauhan, S. Sridevi, K. B. Chalasani, A. K. Jain, S. K. Jain, N. K. Jain, P. V. Diwan, *J. Control. Release* 2003, **90**, 335.
71 M. Hayder, M. Poupot, M. Baron, D. Nigon, C.-O. Turrin, A.-M. Caminade, J.-P. Majoral, R. A. Eisenberg, J.-J. Fournié, A. Cantagrel, R. Poupot, J.-L. Davignon, *Sci. Transl. Med.* 2011, **3**, 81ra35.
72 J. L. de Paz, C. Noti, F. Böhm, S. Werner, P. H. Seeberger, *Chem. Biol.* 2007, **14**, 879.
73 S. M. Rele, W. Cui, L. Wang, S. Hou, G. Barr-Zarse, D. Tatton, Y. Gnanou, J. D. Esko, E. L. Chaikof, *J. Am. Chem. Soc.* 2005, **127**, 10132.
74 B. Wang, R. S. Navath, R. Romero, S. Kannan, R. Kannan, *Int. J. Pharm.* 2009, **377**, 159.
75 R. Iezzi, B. R. Guru, I. V. Glybina, M. K. Mishra, A. Kennedy, R. M. Kannan, *Biomaterials* 2012, **33**, 979.
76 S. Kannan, H. Dai, R. S. Navath, B. Balakrishnan, A. Jyoti, J. Janisse, R. Romero, R. M. Kannan, *Sci. Transl. Med.* 2012, **4**, 130ra46.
77 H. Dai, R. S. Navath, B. Balakrishnan, B. R. Guru, M. K. Mishra, R. Romero, R. M. Kannan, S. Kannan, *Nanomedicine* 2010, **5**, 1317.

78 A. S. Chauhan, P. V. Diwan, N. K. Jain, D. A. Tomalia, *Biomacromolecules* 2009, **10**, 1195.
79 A.-M. Caminade, C.-O. Turrin, J.-P. Majoral, *New J. Chem.* 2010, **34**, 1512.
80 M. Poupot, L. Griffe, P. Marchand, A. Maraval, O. Rolland, L. Martinet, F.-E. L' Faqihi-Olive, C.-O. Turrin, A.-M. Caminade, J.-J. Fournié, J.-P. Majoral, R. Poupot, *FASEB J.* 2006, **20**, 2339.
81 S. Fruchon, M. Poupot, L. Martinet, C.-O. Turrin, J.-P. Majoral, J.-J. Fournié, A.-M. Caminade, R. Poupot, *J. Leukoc. Biol.* 2009, **85**, 553.
82 D. Portevin, M. Poupot, O. Rolland, C.-O. Turrin, J.-J. Fournié, J.-P. Majoral, A.-M. Caminade, R. Poupot, *J. Transl. Med.* 2009, **7**, 1.
83 L. Griffe, M. Poupot, P. Marchand, A. Maraval, C.-O. Turrin, O. Rolland, P. Métivier, G. Bacquet, J.-J. Fournié, A.-M. Caminade, R. Poupot, J.-P. Majoral, *Angew. Chem. Int. Ed.* 2007, **46**, 2523.
84 J. L. Jimenez, M. Pion, F. J. d. l. Mata, R. Gomez, E. Munoz, M. Leal, M. A. Munoz-Fernandez, *New J. Chem.* 2012, **36**, 299.
85 T. D. McCarthy, P. Karellas, S. A. Henderson, M. Giannis, D. F. O'Keefe, G. Heery, J. R. A. Paull, B. R. Matthews, G. Holan, *Mol. Pharm.* 2005, **2**, 312.
86 R. D. Kensinger, B. C. Yowler, A. J. Benesi, C.-L. Schengrund, *Bioconjugate Chem.* 2004, **15**, 349.
87 M. Witvrouw, V. Fikkert, W. Pluymers, B. Matthews, K. Mardel, D. Schols, J. Raff, Z. Debyser, E. De Clercq, G. Holan, C. Pannecouque, *Mol. Pharmacol.* 2000, **58**, 1100.
88 Y. Gong, B. Matthews, D. Cheung, T. Tam, I. Gadawski, D. Leung, G. Holan, J. Raff, S. Sacks, *Antiviral Res.* 2002, **55**, 319.
89 N. Bourne, L. R. Stanberry, E. R. Kern, G. Holan, B. Matthews, D. I. Bernstein, *Antimicrob. Agents Chemother.* 2000, **44**, 2471.
90 *Further Information under: http://www.starpharma.com.*
91 R. Rupp, S. L. Rosentha, L. R. Stanberry, *Int. J. Nanomed.* 2007, **4**, 561
92 Y.-H. Jiang, P. Emau, J. S. Cairns, L. Flanary, W. R. Morton, T. D. McCarthy, C.-C. Tsai, *AIDS Res. Hum. Retroviruses* 2005, **21**, 207.
93 R. Haag, F. Kratz, *Angew. Chem. Int. Ed.* 2006, **45**, 1198.
94 V. Pirrone, B. Wigdahl, F. C. Krebs, *Antiviral Res.* 2011, **90**, 168.
95 Q. Abdool Karim, S. S. Abdool Karim, J. A. Frohlich, A. C. Grobler, C. Baxter, L. E. Mansoor, A. B. M. Kharsany, S. Sibeko, K. P. Mlisana, Z. Omar, T. N. Gengiah, S. Maarschalk, N. Arulappan, M. Mlotshwa, L. Morris, D. Taylor, o. b. o. t. C. T. Group, *Science* 2010, **329**, 1168.
96 J. O'Loughlin, I. Y. Millwood, H. M. McDonald, C. F. Price, J. M. Kaldor, J. R. A. Paull, *Sexually Transmitted Diseases* 2010, **37**, 100.
97 M. Y. Chen, I. Y. Millwood, H. Wand, M. Poynten, M. Law, J. M. Kaldor, S. Wesselingh, C. F. Price, L. J. Clark, J. R. A. Paull, C. K. Fairley, *J. Acquir. Immune Defic. Syndr.* 2009, **50**, 375.
98 B. Rasines, J. Sanchez-Nieves, M. Maiolo, M. Maly, L. Chonco, J. L. Jimenez, M. A. Munoz-Fernandez, F. J. de la Mata, R. Gomez, *Dalton Trans.* 2012, **41**, 12733.
99 L. Chonco, M. Pion, E. Vacas, B. Rasines, M. Maly, M. J. Serramía, L. López-Fernández, J. De la Mata, S. Alvarez, R. Gómez, M. A. Muñoz-Fernández, *J. Control. Release* 2012, **161**, 949.
100 R. Doménech, O. Abian, R. Bocanegra, J. Correa, A. Sousa-Herves, R. Riguera, M. G. Mateu, E. Fernandez-Megia, A. Velázquez-Campoy, J. L. Neira, *Biomacromolecules* 2010, **11**, 2069.
101 A. Perez-Anes, G. Spataro, Y. Coppel, C. Moog, M. Blanzat, C.-O. Turrin, A.-M. Caminade, I. Rico-Lattes, J.-P. Majoral, *Org. Biomol. Chem.* 2009, **7**, 3491.
102 C. Fasting, C. A. Schalley, M. Weber, O. Seitz, S. Hecht, B. Koksch, J. Dernedde, C. Graf, E.-W. Knapp, R. Haag, *Angew. Chem. Int. Ed.* 2012, **51**, 10472.
103 B. D. Gates, Q. Xu, J. C. Love, D. B. Wolfe, G. M. Whitesides, *Annu. Rev. Mater. Res.* 2004, **34**, 339.

104 I. Papp, C. Sieben, A. L. Sisson, J. Kostka, C. Böttcher, K. Ludwig, A. Herrmann, R. Haag, *ChemBioChem* 2011, **12**, 887.

105 X. Bosch, *ACS Nano* 2011, **5**, 6779.

106 S. Zhang, J. E. I. Wright, N. Özber, H. Uludağ, *Macromol. Biosci.* 2007, **7**, 656.

107 C. Clementi, K. Miller, A. Mero, R. Satchi-Fainaro, G. Pasut, *Mol. Pharm.* 2011, **8**, 1063.

108 S. T. Khew, Q. J. Yang, Y. W. Tong, *Biomaterials* 2008, **29**, 3034.

109 S. R. Meyers, F. S. Juhn, A. P. Griset, N. R. Luman, M. W. Grinstaff, *J. Am. Chem. Soc.* 2008, **130**, 14444.

110 J. Rojo, R. Delgado, *Anti-Infect. Agents Med. Chem.* 2007, **6**, 151.

111 C. Ornelas, R. Pennell, L. F. Liebes, M. Weck, *Org. Lett.* 2011, **13**, 976.

112 S. Reichert, M. Calderón, K. Licha, R. Haag, in *Multifunctional Nanoparticles for Drug Delivery Applications*, eds. S. Svenson, R. K. Prud'homme, Springer US, 2012, pp. 315.

113 A.-M. Caminade, J.-P. Majoral, *Chem. Soc. Rev.* 2010, **39**, 2034.

114 A. E. Nel, L. Madler, D. Velegol, T. Xia, E. M. V. Hoek, P. Somasundaran, F. Klaessig, V. Castranova, M. Thompson, *Nat. Mater.* 2009, **8**, 543.

115 R. Chapanian, I. Constantinescu, D. E. Brooks, M. D. Scott, J. N. Kizhakkedathu, *Biomaterials* 2012, **33**, 3047.

116 K. Saatchi, P. Soema, N. Gelder, R. Misri, K. McPhee, J. H. E. Baker, S. A. Reinsberg, D. E. Brooks, U. O. Häfeli, *Bioconjugate Chem.* 2012, **23**, 372.

117 S. H. Medina, M. E. H. El-Sayed, *Chem. Rev.* 2009, **109**, 3141.

118 S. S. Nigavekar, L. Y. Sung, M. Llanes, A. El-Jawahri, T. S. Lawrence, C. W. Becker, L. Balogh, M. K. Khan, *Pharm. Res.* 2004, **21**, 476.

119 B. Misselwitz, H. Schmitt-Willich, W. Ebert, T. Frenzel, H.-J. Weinmann, *Magn. Reson. Mater. Phys., Biol. Med.* 2001, **12**, 128.

120 J.-F. Stumbé, B. Bruchmann, *Macromol. Rapid Commun.* 2004, **25**, 921.

121 R. Duncan, L. Izzo, *Adv. Drug Delivery Rev.* 2005, **57**, 2215.

POLY(AMIDOAMINE) (PAMAM) DENDRIMERS AS NON-VIRAL VECTORS FOR THE DELIVERY OF RNA THERAPEUTICS

X. Liu,[1,3,4,5,6] P. Posocco,[2] C. Liu,[1,7] T. Yu,[1,7] Q. Wang,[1] V. Dal Col,[1,2] C. Chen,[1,7,8] Y. Wang,[1] P. Rocchi,[3,4,5,6] S. Pricl,[2] and L. Peng[1,*]

[1] Centre Interdisciplinaire de Nanoscience de Marseille, CNRS UMR 7325, 163, avenue de Luminy, 13288 Marseille, France

[2] Molecular Simulation Engineering (MOSE) Laboratory, Department of Industrial Engineering and Information Technology (DI3), University of Trieste, Via Valerio 10, 34127 Trieste, Italy

[3] Centre de Recherche en Canérologie de Marseille, Inserm, U1068, 13009 Marseille, France

[4] Institut Paoli-Calmettes, 13009 Marseille, France

[5] Aix-Marseille Université, 13284 Marseille, France

[6] CNRS, UMR7258, 13009 Marseille, France

[7] State Key Laboratory of Virology, Wuhan University, 430072 Wuhan, P. R. China

[8] Aix-Marseille Université, Institut de Chimie Radicalaire, UMR 7273, 13390 Marseille, France

1 INTRODUCTION

RNA interference (RNAi), first reported by Fire and Mello in 1998,[1] denotes a sequence-specific gene silencing process triggered by small interfering RNAs (siRNAs).[2] On the basis of RNAi, synthetic siRNA can be designed and applied to target any gene with known sequence, hence it can be harnessed to silence disease genes with a therapeutic aim.[3] This has created a completely new era of RNA therapeutics. However, RNAi technology for therapeutic application requires safe and easy-to-handle siRNA delivery systems able to protect the siRNA during extra- and intra-cellular delivery and take it safely to the site of interest.[4] Both viral and non-viral vectors have been explored as siRNA carriers.[4] While viral vectors show high efficacy, they are hampered by serious concerns over safety, high production costs and short shelf life etc. While the non-viral alternatives do overcome the limitations concerning safety risk and manufacturing costs, they are less effective than the viral vectors. These non-viral vectors are usually divided into two main classes – cationic lipids and polymers.[4-6] In both cases, the positively charged vectors are able to assemble the siRNA into nanoparticles via electrostatic interactions, which can protect the siRNA from degradation and promote cellular uptake by endocytosis. After internalization, the siRNA/vector complexes first escaped from the endosomes and then the siRNA is released into the cytoplasm to undergo the RNAi process and consequently silence the targeted gene (Figure 1).

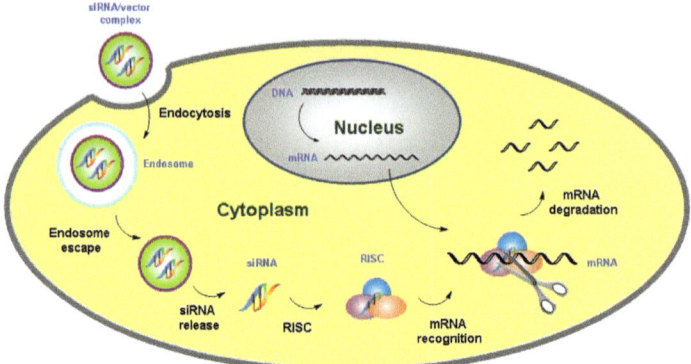

Figure 1 *Non-viral vectors mediated siRNA delivery and gene silencing in mammalian cells.*

One special family of polymers, the cationic dendrimers, are emerging as promising non-viral vectors for siRNA delivery.[7, 8] Unlike traditional polymers, dendrimers are composed of three distinct domains: 1) a central core, 2) repetitive branch units organized in geometrically radiated progression, and 3) a large number of terminals on the outer surface. Most importantly, the structures of dendrimers can be precisely controlled during their stepwise synthesis achieved either *via* divergent or *via* convergent strategies. Consequently, the obtained dendrimers have well-defined structures and narrow polydispersity in addition to their unique structural geometry and multivalency, and are thus expected to make an ideal drug delivery platform. Up to now, a multitude of dendrimers have been explored for siRNA delivery, in particular, poly(amidoamine) (PAMAM) dendrimers.[9] These dendrimer vectors bear positively charged amine functionalities at the dendrimer surface and are responsible for ionic condensation with negaively charged siRNA molecules under physiological conditions. They also harbor tertiary amines in the interior and can thus preferentially promote siRNA release *via* the "proton sponge" effect.[10] The released siRNA molecules eventually join the RNAi machinary to regulate gene silencing process. In this chapter, we will focus on the structurally flexible and amphiphilic poly(amidoamine) (PAMAM) dendrimers developed in our group as non-viral vectors for siRNA delivery.

2 STRUCTURALLY FLEXIBLE PAMAM DENDRIMERS

Poly(amidoamine) (PAMAM) dendrimers were first synthesized by Tomalia[11] and have been extensively investigated as non-viral vectors for DNA delivery.[12] The active ingredient for DNA delivery is fractured and degraded PAMAM dendrimers, which are obtained from the intact dendrimers either by thermal degradation or by alkaline hydrolysis.[13] Not only is the precise control over structure lost during this degradation process but it is neither chemically rational nor economical, as the preparation of intact dendrimers is time-consuming, and requires strictly controlled stepwise synthesis and laborious purification. With this in mind, we have developed the structurally flexible triethanolamine (TEA) core PAMAM dendrimers (Figure 2A) as non-viral vectors for nucleic acid delivery, in particular siRNA delivery.[14] The TEA core is considerably more extended compared to the conventional NH_3 core (Figure 2B), and we therefore expected that the corresponding PAMAM dendrimers would have more space to accommodate the branching units and thus be structurally more flexible. In other words, TEA-core based dendrimers would be more readily available to interact with siRNA because of having branching units less densely packed with their terminal groups when compared to their NH_3-core molecular counterparts. Our prediction was confirmed by multiscale molecular modeling investigation.[15, 16]

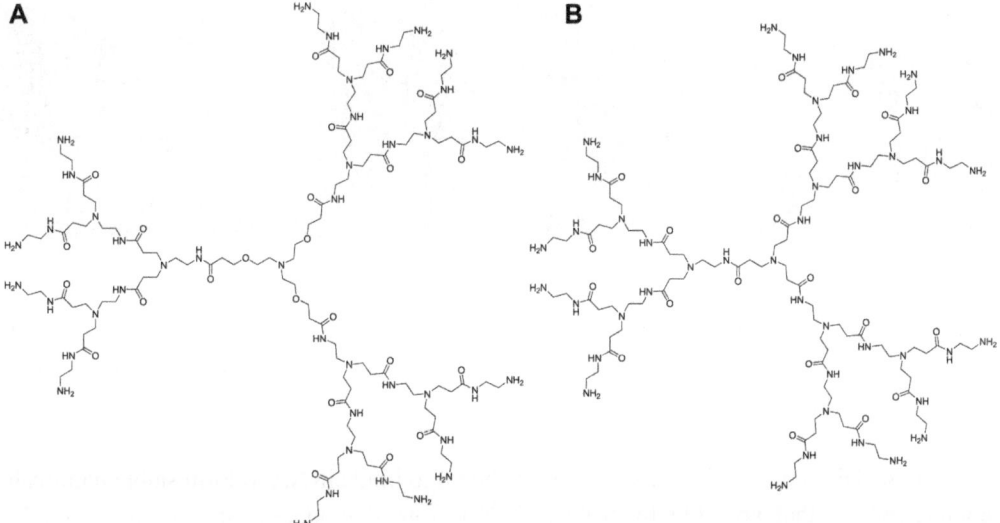

Figure 2 *Structurally flexible triethanolamine (TEA) core PAMAM dendrimer (A) and traditional amine (NH_3) core PAMAM dendrimer (B) of generation 2.*

Indeed, the conformation of the TEA-core dendrimers is such that the outer branches can readily move towards the phosphate backbone of RNA during complex formation, and the surface amino groups can arrange themselves *via induced-fit* for optimal binding with the nucleic acid. In contrast, the more rigid and compact structure of the alternative NH_3-core PAMAM molecule prevents it from undergoing a significant conformational rearrangement as required by *induced-fit*; as a consequence, less amine groups are available with which to self-orient towards the best siRNA binding. In detail, the more compact the conformation and higher the level of backfolding, the higher the intrinsic rigidity of the NH_3-core PAMAM dendrimers resulting in a lower density of terminal amines on the molecular surface, ultimately preventing this molecule from undergoing the substantial conformational readjustment required for optimal RNA binding. A compact confirmation was further confirmed by evidence of a partial penetration of the nucleic acid within the molecular structure of the NH_3-core dendrimer. In contrast, by virtue of its larger core, greater flexibility, and hence higher mobility of its outer arms, the prevailing location of terminal groups in the case of the TEA-core dendrimers is shifted towards the molecular periphery with respect to that in same generation of NH_3-core dendrimer. Consequently, the charged end-groups of the TEA-core PAMAM dendrimer are able to reposition themselves for optimal binding with the nucleic acid more efficiently than those of the NH_3-core PAMAM molecule (Figure 3).

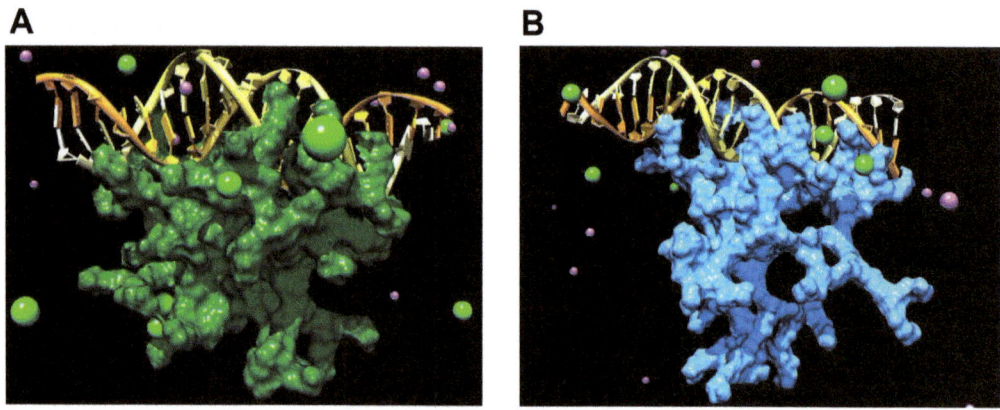

Figure 3 *Equilibrium molecular dynamics snapshots of TEA-core (A) and NH_3 -core (B) PAMAM dendrimers of generation 5, taken as a proof of concept. The dendrimer molecule is encased using its van der Waals surface. The nucleic acid is depicted as a yellow ribbon. Cl^- and Na^+ ions are shown as green and purple spheres, respectively. Water is not shown for clarity.*

These TEA-core dendrimers have been shown to bind siRNA to form stable nanoscale complexes[14, 17] that are able to protect siRNA from degradation and promote cellular uptake. A higher generation of these flexible PAMAM dendrimers (generation 7) was effective in the delivery of siRNA to induced gene silencing of the luciferase gene in A549Luc cells which stably express the GL3 luciferase gene.[7] The excellent siRNA delivery capacity of these dendrimers was further confirmed by their effective delivery of an siRNA targeting heat shock protein 27 (Hsp27) in human castration-resistant prostate cancer PC-3 cells which led to potent down-regulation of Hsp27 (Figure 4). Hsp27 is a molecular chaperone playing an important role in drug resistance and has been recently considered as a novel target for treating drug-resistant prostate and other cancers.[18-20] Following the gene silencing with Hsp27 siRNA/dendrimer complexes, an effective anti-proliferation effect was achieved, alongside the observation of apoptosis induced by caspase activation in the prostate cancer models.[21]

However, the large-scale chemical synthesis of this higher generation dendrimer with good quality is technically demanding and it would be potentially difficult to meet the purity and quality control standards required by clinical applications. Accordingly, the possibility of developing low generation dendrimers for the effective delivery of siRNA therapeutics constitutes *per se* a challenging but worthwhile goal.

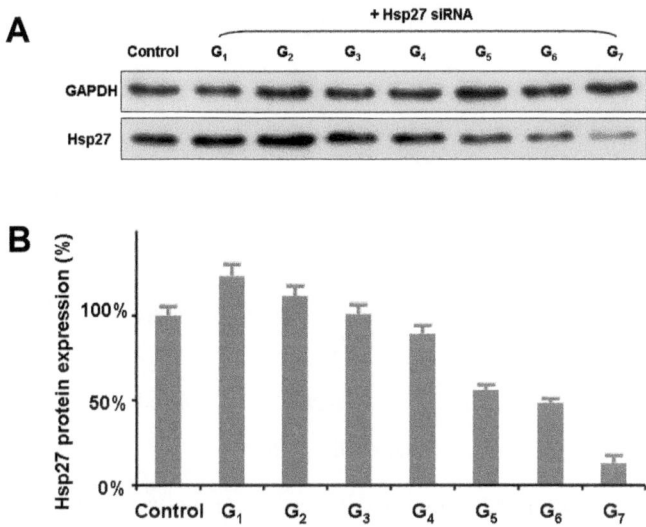

Figure 4 *TEA core PAMAM dendrimer-mediated siRNA delivery and gene silencing of heat shock protein 27 (Hsp27) revealed by Western Blot (A) and related quantification profile (B) is strongly dependent on the dendrimer generation.*

Our earlier study indicated that the size of the RNA molecules and the generation of the dendrimers both play a critical role on the construction of stable and uniform nanoscale RNA/dendrimer complexes:[17] higher generation dendrimers are required for a better interaction and efficient delivery of smaller siRNA molecules, whereas lower generation dendrimers may be sufficient to allow a strong interaction with larger RNA molecules. We demonstrated this using sticky siRNA molecules[22] with complementary A_n/T_n overhangs (n = 5 or 7), which are able to self-assemble into "gene-like" longer double-stranded RNAs (Figure 5). Indeed, the lower generation G_5 TEA-core PAMAM dendrimer was shown to effectively deliver siRNA to achieve potent gene silencing of Hsp27 and significant anticancer activity in the castration-resistant prostate cancer models *in vitro* and *in vivo* (Figure 6).[23]

We wondered whether in addition to the hypothesized formation of "gene-like" longer double strand RNA molecules, the two complementary A_n/T_n overhangs of the sticky siRNAs might also act as a pair of protruding molecular arms, allowing the siRNA molecule to enwrap the spherical, low generation dendrimers with higher binding affinity compared with a conventional siRNA with two short T_2/T_2 overhangs. To this end, we studied the complex formation of TEA-core PAMAM dendrimer G_5 with different siRNA molecules (conventional siRNA with T_2/T_2 overhangs, and sticky siRNAs with either A_5/T_5 or A_7/T_7 overhangs) by atomistic molecular dynamics techniques (Figure 7). The structural differences between the complexes were obvious: both longer overhangs (A_5/T_5 and A_7/T_7) significantly enhanced the binding of the sticky siRNAs to the G_5 dendrimer by forming more compact complexes.

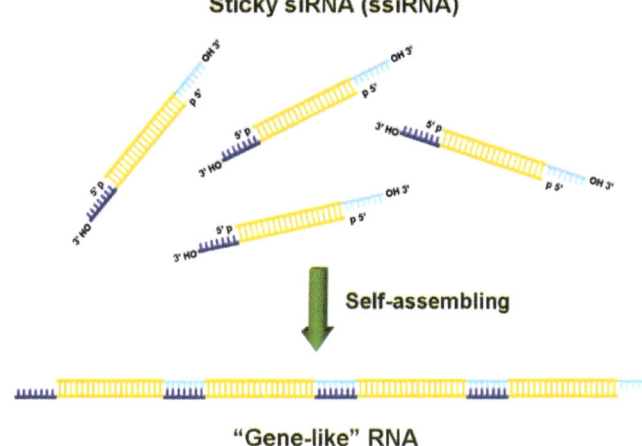

Figure 5 *Cartoon presentation of self-assembly of sticky siRNA into "gene-like" longer double stranded RNA.*

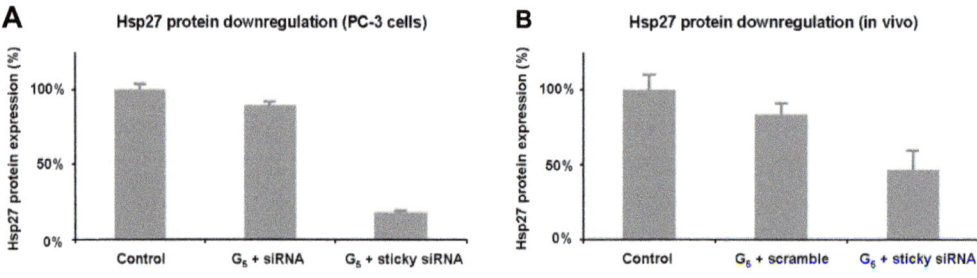

Figure 6 *Triethylamine (TEA) core dendrimer G_5-mediated delivery of sticky siRNA targeting Hsp27 induced potent gene silencing of Hsp27 (A) in vitro in comparison with conventional siRNA and (B) in vivo in a tumor-xenograft mice model.*

In both cases (Figures 7B and 7C), not only did the unmatched nucleotide sequences act as anchoring points for the siRNA onto the dendrimer surface, but also the double-stranded portion of the siRNA was able to better adapt its overall conformation for a more efficient nucleic acid/nanovector interaction. In contrast, the presence of the short T_2/T_2 overhangs has no substantial beneficial impact on dendrimer binding by the relevant siRNA (Figure 7A). Based on these results, we hypothesized that, in addition to the possible formation of "gene-like" longer double strand RNA molecules, such stronger binding to dendrimer of sticky siRNAs over conventional siRNAs might also contribute towards the enhanced delivery activity of G_5.[23]

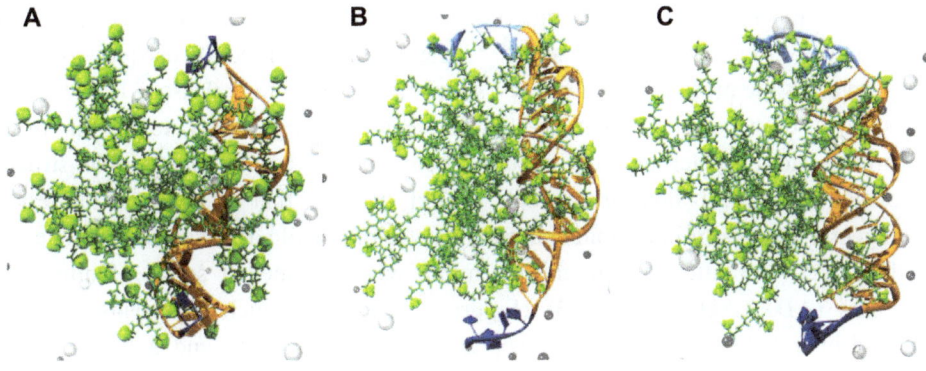

Figure 7 *Selected equilibrated molecular dynamics snapshots of the complexes between the TEA-core G$_5$ dendrimer with siRNA bearing an overhang of T$_2$/T$_2$ (A) A$_5$/T$_5$ (B) and A$_7$/T$_7$ (C) In all panels, the dendrimer is in forest green sticks, the terminal charged amine groups highlighted as light green sticks-and-balls. The siRNA is portrayed as an orange ribbon, the two overhangs depicted in light blue for A$_n$ and navy blue for T$_n$ (n=2, 5, and 7). Some Cl$^-$ and Na$^+$ ions and counter ions are shown as big light gray and small dark gray spheres, respectively. Water is omitted for clarity.*

Recently, the **G$_5$** dendrimer has been demonstrated to efficiently deliver dicer substrate siRNA (dsiRNA)[24] into human T cells and primary PBMC cells, resulting in effective gene silencing.[25] Moreover this dendrimer was able to deliver a cocktail of dsiRNA molecules targeting both HIV replication and host HIV infection in an HIV-infected humanized RAG-hu mice model. The resulting gene silencing led to extraordinary anti-HIV activity, with significant suppression of viral loads by several orders of magnitude, as well as the effective prevention of host CD4 T-cell depletion and of viral escape.[25]

Furthermore, the **G$_5$** dendrimer has been shown to successfully deliver the mature miR-124 RNA duplexes into glioblastoma stem cells (GSC1)[26]. The delivered miR-124 RNA efficiently down-regulated the expression of NRAS, a small guanine-nucleotide binding protein belonging to one of the three RAS (KRAS, NRAS, HRAS) isoforms,[27] with the RAS signaling pathway playing a crucial role in many cancers by regulating cell proliferation, differentiation, and survival.[26] Collectively, all these results demonstrate the extremely promising potential of this family of dendrimers for further clinical applications to deliver a variety of RNA therapeutics. We are currently developing targeting strategies to decorate our dendrimer with various targeting components such as antibodies, peptides and small molecular ligands in order to deliver RNA therapeutic molecules specifically into tumor tissue and cancer cells for safe and efficacious cancer treatment.

3 AMPHPHILIC PAMAM DENDRIMERS

As mentioned in the introduction section, cationic lipids and polymers are the most common non-viral vectors.[4-6] Compared to viral vectors, the inadequate release of siRNA into the cytosol often constitutes one of the main obstacles hindering efficient non-viral delivery. The mechanism used by lipid vectors to achieve endosome release of siRNA is presumed to involve membrane fusion,[5, 6] whereas that commonly used by polymeric vectors involves the proton sponge effect[10] shown to facilitate the release.[28] However, both vectors have drawbacks to their use, lipid vectors being highly toxic for *in vivo* applications and polymer delivery systems being plagued with undefinable structural composition. An ideal non-viral vector would be one that is able to harness the advantageous features of both lipid and polymer vectors, while at the same time overcome or reduce their limitations. With this in mind, we developed a series of amphiphilic dendrimers (**AD1, AD2**, and **AD3**) (Figure 8) each of which represents a kind of lipid/dendrimer hybrids bearing a hydrophobic long alkyl chain and a low generation hydrophilic PAMAM dendron. The amphiphilic dendrimer (**AD1**) composed of a C18 alkyl chain and a hydrophilic PAMAM dendron with 8 amine terminals, is capable of combining the advantageous features of lipid and dendrimer vectors, and can efficiently deliver siRNA to target heat shock protein 27 in human castration-resistant prostate cancer PC-3 cells, leading to potent down-regulation at both the mRNA and protein levels and effective anticancer activity *in vitro* and *in vivo* (Figure 9).[29]

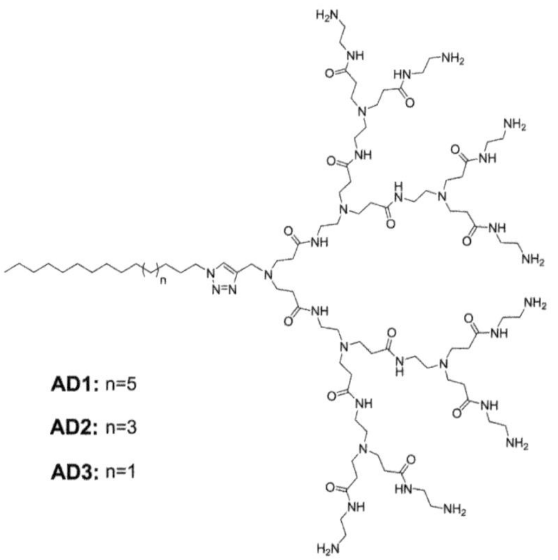

AD1: n=5

AD2: n=3

AD3: n=1

Figure 8 *Amphiphilic dendrimers (AD1, AD2 and AD3) featuring a low generation hydrophilic PAMAM dendron and a hydrophobic alkyl chain with length of C14, C16 and C18, respectively.*

Using a combination of theoretical and experimental approaches, a preliminary analysis revealed that this amphiphilic dendrimer possesses optimal siRNA binding strength allowing it to safely carry the nucleic acid cargo along its journey into the cell and efficiently discharge the siRNA payload upon reaching its final destination (Figure 10). The presumed molecular rationale for this finding is that an optimal balance is reached between the hydrophobic chain length and the hydrophilic dendron structure thus conferring the vectors with the ability to firstly efficiently assemble the siRNA and later effectively disassemble from it during endosome release, ultimately resulting in an optimal siRNA delivery and potent gene silencing. Our preliminary results suggest that such optimal balance between the length of the hydrocarbon tails and the dimensions of the dendron head play a crucial role in the transfection activity and that the length of the hydrocarbon tail is a key factor allowing efficient and stable self-assembly of structures for effective siRNA binding and delivery.

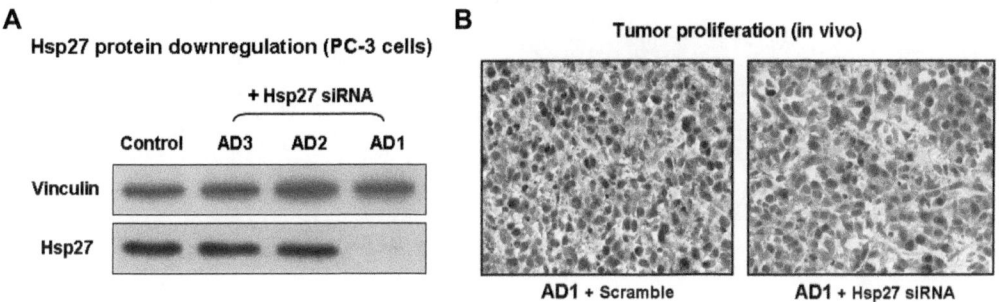

Figure 9 *(A) Amphiphilic dendrimers mediated Hsp27 siRNA delivery and gene silencing of Hsp27 is strongly dependent on the alkyl chain length. (B) In vivo antiproliferative effect resulted from amphiphilic dendrimer AD1-mediated Hsp27 siRNA delivery in a prostate cancer xenograft mice model.*

To our knowledge, this is the first report of an amphiphilic dendrimer able to successfully deliver siRNA and produce potent gene silencing *in vitro* and *in vivo*. It may therefore constitute a promising non-viral system for siRNA delivery in therapeutic applications. We are currently focusing our efforts on performing a detailed structure/activity relationship analysis to gain a better insight into and understanding of this amphiphilic dendrimer vector. This knowledge will be applied in testing the vector in various disease models based on siRNA therapeutics.

4 CONCLUSION AND PERSPECTIVES

Over the past decade, dendrimers have attracted increasing amount of attention for their potential use as non-viral vectors for siRNA delivery. Their nanometric size (1-10 nm) and well-defined structure with spherical architecture bearing unique radiating branching units in the interior and numerous end groups on the surface make them ideal drug delivery platforms. We have developed structurally flexible and amphiphilic PAMAM dendrimers for siRNA delivery. They have proven to be excellent vectors for siRNA delivery in various disease models *in vitro* and *in vivo*. Collaboration with computer scientists has enhanced our understanding of the siRNA/dendrimer interaction and formation of the related complex as well as the release of siRNA from these complexes. While considerable basic knowledge has been acquired and significant advances made in this regard, further translation to the clinical setting represents a challenging road ahead. Our structurally flexible dendrimer has been scheduled for a Phase I clinical trial this year. Our goal is to develop multifunctional biodegradable dendrimeric delivery platforms for siRNA delivery while respecting the need to maximize the efficacy and specificity of delivery and minimize the complicated side effects.

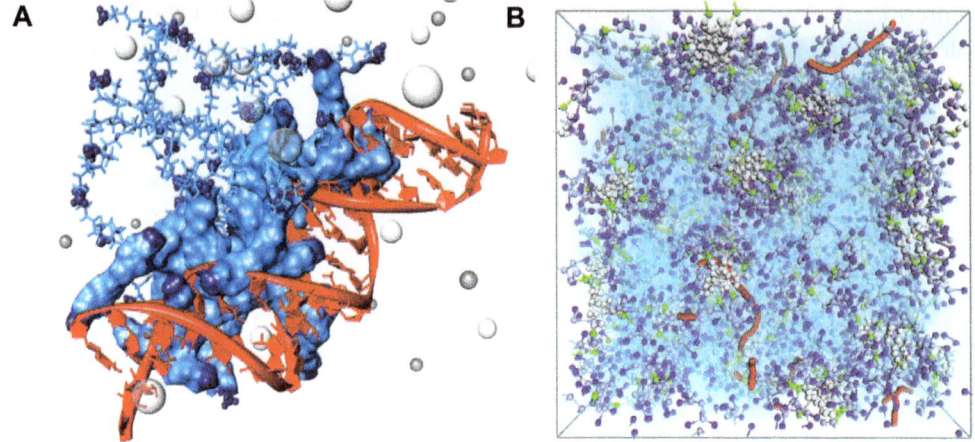

Figure 10 *Atomistic (A) and mesoscale (B) equilibrium snapshots of the amphiphilc PAMAM dendrimer bearing a C18 alkyl chain and 8 terminal amine groups in complex with siRNA. The dendrimer is considered in its self-assembled form. Legend: (A) The dendrimer is in light blue sticks, the terminal charged amine groups highlighted as navy blue sticks-and-balls. The siRNA is portrayed as a red ribbon. Some Cl⁻ and Na⁺ ions and counter ions are shown as big light gray and small dark gray spheres, respectively. Water is omitted for clarity. The binding interface region between siRNA and each micelle formed with the dendrimers is also emphasized. (B) Purple and lilac, hydrophilic dendron moieties; light grey, hydrophobic tail; green, linker connecting hydrophilic/hydropofibic parts. Water and counterions are portrayed as a light blue field, siRNA molecules as red thick sticks.*

5. ACKNOWLEDGEMENTS

We acknowledge financial support from the international ERA-Net EURONANOMED European Research project DENANORNA, Association pour la Recherche sur les Tumeurs de la Prostate, Association Française contre les Myopathies, Canceropôl PACA, CNRS and INSERM. This work was carried out under the auspice of European COST Action TD0802 "Dendrimers in Biomedical Applications".

References

1. A. Fire, S. Xu, M. K. Montgomery, S. A. Kostas, S. E. Driver and C. C. Mello, *Nature*, 1998, **391**, 806.
2. G. J. Hannon, *Nature*, 2002, **418**, 244.
3. D. Castanotto and J. J. Rossi, *Nature*, 2009, **457**, 426.
4. K. A. Whitehead, R. Langer and D. G. Anderson, *Nat. Rev. Drug Discovery*, 2009, **8**, 129.
5. Y. C. Tseng, S. Mozumdar and L. Huang, *Adv. Drug Deliv. Rev.*, 2009, **61**, 721.
6. A. Schroeder, C. G. Levins, C. Cortez, R. Langer and D. G. Anderson, *J. Intern. Med.*, 2010, **267**, 9.

7. J. Zhou, J. Wu, N. Hafdi, J. P. Behr, P. Erbacher and L. Peng, *Chem. Commun.*, 2006, 2362.

8. M. Ravina, P. Paolicelli, B. Seijo and A. Sanchez, *Mini-Rev. Med. Chem.*, 2010, **10**, 73.

9. X. Liu, P. Rocchi and L. Peng, *New J. Chem.*, 2012, **36**, 256.

10. O. Boussif, F. Lezoualc'h, M. Zanta, M. Mergny, D. Scherman, B. Demeneix and J. Behr, *Proc. Natl. Acad. Sci. U. S. A.*, 1995, **92**, 7297.

11. D. A. Tomalia, A. M. Naylor and W. A. Goddard III, *Angew. Chem.Int. Ed. Engl.*, 1990, **29**, 138.

12. M. Guillot-Nieckowski, S. Eisler and F. Diederich, *New J. Chem.*, 2007, **31**, 1111.

13. M. X. Tang, C. T. Redemann and F. C. Szoka, Jr., *Bioconjugate Chem.*, 1996, **7**, 703.

14. J. Wu, J. Zhou, F. Qu, P. Bao, Y. Zhang and L. Peng, *Chem. Commun.*, 2005, 313.

15. X. Liu, J. Wu, M. Yammine, J. Zhou, P. Posocco, S. Viel, C. Liu, F. Ziarelli, M. Fermeglia, S. Pricl, G. Victorero, C. Nguyen, P. Erbacher, J. P. Behr and L. Peng, *Bioconjugate Chem.*, 2011, **22**, 2461.

16. K. Karatasos, P. Posocco, E. Laurini and S. Pricl, *Macromol. Biosci.*, 2012, **12**, 225.

17. X. C. Shen, J. Zhou, X. Liu, J. Wu, F. Qu, Z. L. Zhang, D. W. Pang, G. Quéléver, C. C. Zhang and L. Peng, *Org. Biomol. Chem.*, 2007, **5**, 3674.

18. P. A. Cornford, A. R. Dodson, K. F. Parsons, A. D. Desmond, A. Woolfenden, M. Fordham, J. P. Neoptolemos, Y. Ke and C. S. Foster, *Cancer Res.*, 2000, **60**, 7099.

19. P. Rocchi, A. So, S. Kojima, M. Signaevsky, E. Beraldi, L. Fazli, A. Hurtado-Coll, K. Yamanaka and M. Gleave, *Cancer Res.*, 2004, **64**, 6595.

20. Y. Xia, P. Rocchi, J. L. Iovanna and L. Peng, *Drug Discov. Today*, 2012, **17**, 35.

21. X. X. Liu, P. Rocchi, F. Q. Qu, S. Q. Zheng, Z. C. Liang, M. Gleave, J. Iovanna and L. Peng, *ChemMedChem*, 2009, **4**, 1302.

22. A. L. Bolcato-Bellemin, M. E. Bonnet, G. Creusat, P. Erbacher and J. P. Behr, *Proc. Natl. Acad. Sci. U. S. A.*, 2007, **104**, 16050.

23. X. Liu, C. Liu, E. Laurini, P. Posocco, S. Pricl, F. Qu, P. Rocchi and L. Peng, *Mol. Pharmaceutics*, 2012, **9**, 470.

24. D. H. Kim, M. A. Behlke, S. D. Rose, M. S. Chang, S. Choi and J. J. Rossi, *Nat. Biotechnol.*, 2005, **23**, 222.

25. J. Zhou, C. P. Neff, X. Liu, J. Zhang, H. Li, D. D. Smith, P. Swiderski, T. Aboellail, Y. Huang, Q. Du, Z. Liang, L. Peng, R. Akkina and J. J. Rossi, *Mol. Ther.*, 2011, **19**, 2228.

26. M. F. Lang, S. Yang, C. Zhao, G. Sun, K. Murai, X. Wu, J. Wang, H. Gao, C. E. Brown, X. Liu, J. Zhou, L. Peng, J. J. Rossi and Y. Shi, *PLoS One*, 2012, **7**, e36248.

27. L. Ma, J. Teruya-Feldstein and R. A. Weinberg, *Nature*, 2007, **449**, 682.

28. E. Wagner, *Acc. Chem. Res.*, 2012, **45**, 1005.

29. T. Yu, X. Liu, A. L. Bolcato-Bellemin, Y. Wang, C. Liu, P. Erbacher, F. Qu, P. Rocchi, J. P. Behr and L. Peng, *Angew. Chem. Int. Ed.*, 2012, **51**, 8478.

DENDRIMERIC ANTIGENS. NEW APPROACHES TOWARDS DETECTION OF IgE-MEDIATED DRUG ALLERGY REACTIONS

M.I. Montañez[1,2], C. Mayorga[1,2], M.J. Torres[1,2], A.J. Ruiz-Sanchez[2,3], M. Malkoch[4], A. Hult[4], M. Blanca[1,2] and E. Perez-Inestrosa[2,3]

[1] Research Laboratory, FIMABIS-Carlos Haya Hospital, 29009 Malaga, Spain.
[2] BIONAND-Andalusian Centre for Nanomedicine and Biotechnology, Parque Tecnologico de Andalucía, 29590 Malaga, Spain
[3] Department of Organic Chemistry, Faculty of Science, University of Malaga, 29071 Malaga, Spain.
[4] KTH Royal Institute of Technology, School of Chemical Science and Engineering, Department of Fibre and Polymer Technology, SE-100 44, Stockholm, Sweden.

1 INTRODUCTION

1.1 The Hapten Model in Drug Allergy Reactions

The immune system protects the host from a variety of foreign substances by producing components (antibodies and cells) capable of specifically interacting with these substances. An "antigen" or "immunogen" is the name given for a substance which is able to both elicit an immune response and interact with the products of that response (sensitized cells and antibodies).[1] Antigens are usually macromolecules that contain different epitopes that can interact with the diverse components of the immune system. Antigens are parts of microbial structures among other possibilities.[2] As antigens are macromolecular structures, this all suggests that drugs would be too small to elicit allergic reactions by themselves. Accordingly, immunological activation induced by drugs has been explained by several mechanisms, though the most commonly accepted mechanism is based on the "hapten hypothesis" formulated by Landsteiner.[3] Haptens are low molecular weight substances which normally are able to interact with the products of an immune response (e.g. antibodies) but cannot cause a response on their own. Haptens can only cause a response after covalent binding to carrier proteins.[4] Chemically reactive drugs or their metabolites can act as haptens and form covalent adducts with extracellular or intracellular proteins (Figure 1). The resulting hapten-carrier (drug-protein) conjugate can be immunogenic and can thus induce an allergic reaction.[5]

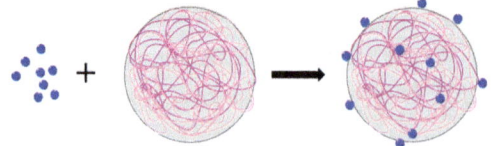

Hapten Molecules   Carrier Molecule   Hapten-Carrier Conjugate
Complete Antigen

Figure 1 *Schematic representation of how hapten molecules can become immunogenic*

Benzylpenicillin is the classical hapten that has been studied in detail and has traditionally been considered as the model hapten to understand drug allergy reactions. The conjugation of penicillins to carrier proteins occurs through reaction of the electrophilic β-lactam ring with the nucleophilic free amino groups on proteins (Figure 2).[5] As a result, and in the case of benzylpenicillin, the ring in its chemical structure becomes opened once coupled to the protein. This entire moiety, called benzylpenicilloyl (BPO), corresponds to the major antigenic determinant or epitope responsible for the allergic response to benzylpenicillin.[6] In general, the open form of other penicillin antibiotics, the penicilloyl group, is also assumed to be the major determinant responsible for the allergic response to these drugs.

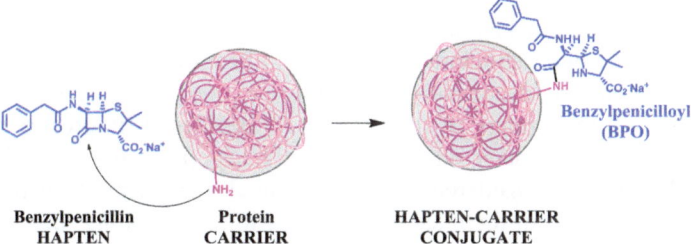

Benzylpenicillin   Protein   HAPTEN-CARRIER
HAPTEN   CARRIER   CONJUGATE

Figure 2 *Formation of BPO, the antigenic determinant of benzylpenicillin*

1.2 In Vitro Diagnosis of β-lactam Allergy

Allergic reactions to β-lactams represent the primary cause of drug reactions mediated by specific immunological mechanisms. To identify penicillin Immunoglobulin E (IgE)-mediated allergy, *in vitro* immunoassays have been employed as a complementary diagnostic method to *in vivo* tests (skin testing and drug provocation tests). *In vitro* testing has the advantage of being exempt from risk for the patient, although the sensitivity is not as optimal as with the *in vivo* tests.[7] In this chapter we will focus on and mention repeatedly the same kind of immunoassay: the radioallergosorbent test (RAST). RAST is a test tube that measures IgE antibodies directed against a hapten (drug), which may indicate whether the patient is allergic to a specific drug. This technique employs solid supports covalently bonded to hapten-carrier conjugates as materials to incubate with patient sera. After such incubation, followed by appropriate washing, only IgE specific to the targeted drug, recognizing specifically the hapten-carrier conjugate, is quantified by using radiolabelled mouse anti-human IgE. A typical support for RAST to benzylpenicillin consists of activated cellulose or agarose surfaces coupled to conventional carrier molecules, which are conjugated to benzylpenicilloyl (BPO) groups.[8]

Conventional peptide carrier conjugates are human serum albumin (HSA) or poly-L-lysine (PLL). These have the disadvantage of an imprecise density of amine groups and thereby haptens in their structure and the haptens are randomly distributed in the large protein or peptide carriers. On one hand, HSA, traditionally considered the natural globular carrier, has the limitation of its intrinsic low hapten-carrier density, in addition to which not all the haptens are exposed in the periphery of the protein.[8] On the other hand, though PLL conjugates increase hapten-carrier ratios, the polydisperse nature of PLL means that their conjugates have low reproducibility and reliability in antibody recognition tests.[9] Furthermore, the random coil of the flexible polymer chains makes the three-dimensional structures rather variable and difficult to predict. Thus, like linear polymers but depending on their conformations, they may envelop a substantial fraction of appended ligands.

1.3. Role of Dendrimers

Unlike conventional carriers, dendrimers are characterized by their structural precision.[10] This feature can be considered the starting point of our contribution with nanotechnology in the field of drug allergy diagnosis.[11]

Dendrimers may well represent the nanosized structures that have opened up most expectations for biomedical applications.[11] They are highly branched and monodisperse macromolecules that display an exact and large number of functional groups distributed with unprecedented control on the dendritic framework. Dendrimers may be visualized as consisting of three critical architectural domains: (a) the multivalent surface, containing a large number of potentially reactive and/or passive sites, (b) the interior shells surrounding the core, and (c) the core to which the regular branches are attached.[12]

Based on their globular structure, compared to linear polymers of the same molecular weight, it is foreseen that dendrimers will deliver extraordinary features for diagnostic purposes, among a broad range of applications.[13] Besides their precise and controlled structure, dendrimers offer other advantages over linear polymers; e.g., the surface and interior of dendrimers are considered segregated[14] so all the peripheral haptenic ligands of the conjugates obtained from them should be accessible for binding; dendrimers can also have a larger capture area than linear analogues with the resulting high capture likelihood.[15]

Although the interesting properties of dendrimers have prompted a great number of studies aimed at developing new synthesis approaches[16-19] and novel biomedical applications,[2, 20-22] their potential for emulating the carrier protein in hapten-carrier conjugates for IgE recognition has hardly been exploited. As well-defined, multivalent, derivatizable, stable molecules, dendrimers are ideal hapten carriers, making it possible to prepare multivalent conjugates with well-defined molecular properties.

2 DENDRIMERS AS CARRIER PROTEINS: DENDRIMERIC ANTIGENS

1.2 Preparation of Dendrimeric Antigens (DeAn)

Polyamidoamine (PAMAM) dendrimers were chosen as carriers because of their commercial availability and their potential as multivalent protein-like materials for biotechnological applications,[10] such as their generally globular shape, aqueous solubility for all molecular sizes, polyamide structure, and free primary amino groups on the surface. The general aim of this study was to design and synthesize a sequence of precisely defined molecular structures to achieve hapten–carrier conjugates of increasing BPO density at the periphery of preformed PAMAM dendrimers and to exploit their exo-receptor properties in IgE detection.[23] Chemically, our main challenge was to construct synthetic (hapten-dendrimer) conjugates capable of reproducing *in vitro* the IgE molecular recognition that happens *in vivo* with natural (hapten-protein) conjugates.

The formation of the BPO antigenic determinant structures is based on the electrophilic properties of the β-lactam ring against nucleophilic reagents, such as primary amines of lysine residues from proteins. First, a simple approach to establish the reaction rate of the formation of the BPO residue and its NMR spectral determination consisted of studying the reaction of benzylpenicillin with a simple nucleophile like butylamine (Scheme 1a).[23-24] The reaction in aqueous media was very fast and completed within 15 minutes. Furthermore, only the product corresponding to the aminolysis of the β-lactam ring (**Bu-BPO**) was detected.

The strategy to functionalize the terminal amine groups of the PAMAM dendrimers with BPO residues consisted of using the same reactivity described above with butylamine (Scheme 1b). The dendritic antigens of different generations (from G0 to G6) were obtained from the reaction between the corresponding PAMAM dendrimers and an excess of benzylpenicillin in an aqueous carbonate buffer (pH 10.8). The completion of the reaction was monitored by ^{1}H and ^{13}C NMR. The control of the temperature and time stated in each case proved to be a strongly influential factor to obtain a complete peripheral substitution (Table 1). Thus, dendrimeric antigen (DeAn) of the lowest generations (G0 and G1) were obtained at room temperature; whereas, the reaction at low temperatures (4 °C) favours the functionalization of the periphery in dendrimers of higher generations (from G2 to G6). This could be due to a reduced mobility of the substituted branches at low temperatures, which may decrease the steric hindrance in the nucleophilic primary amines. As a result, the synthesis of these BPO-containing dendrimers involved quantitative functionalization of the terminal amino groups of the seven PAMAM generations used (G0-G6). The complete functionalization of the three lower generations (G0-G2) could be proved by mass spectrometry analysis using the MALDI-TOF technique. Moreover, NMR characterization was appropriately acquired for all the generations of DeAn. These nanoconjugates show very similar homogeneous ^{1}H and ^{13}C NMR spectra for all generations, which is indicative of highly symmetric structures and a monodisperse nature.[23-24]

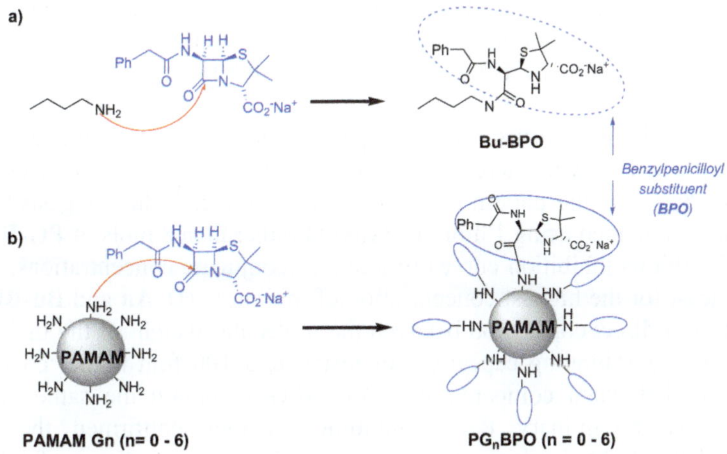

Scheme 1 *Reaction of benzylpenicillin with a) butylamine and b) PAMAM dendrimers*

Table 1 *Reaction yields and conditions for DeAn **PG$_n$BPO** (n=0-6)*

Dendrimeric Antigens	Peripheral groups	Yield	Temperature Reaction	Reaction time
PG$_0$BPO	4	73 %	20-23 °C	1 day
PG$_1$BPO	8	70 %	20-23 °C	2 days
PG$_2$BPO	16	80 %	4 °C	4 days
PG$_3$BPO	32	70 %	4 °C	5 days
PG$_4$BPO	64	82 %	4 °C	6 days
PG$_5$BPO	128	67 %	4 °C	7 days
PG$_6$BPO	256	85 %	4 °C	8 days

The conformation that an epitope adopts on the surface of a carrier macromolecule is a key aspect in the process of molecular recognition by specific ligands. In the study of how these BPO residues become exposed to interact with IgEs at the surface of artificial DeAn, the evidence from NMR (NOESY) is well supported by fully atomistic Molecular Dynamic Simulations.[24] The thiazolidine moiety of the BPO residue is projected to the outer space of the dendrimeric domain, whereas the benzyl acyl side chain mainly interacts with the branches of the dendrimer, in an inner location. The space-filling structure and the related fractal dimensionality takes account of the compactness of the dendrimer series indicating that these DeAn have a more polymeric-like structure than the PAMAM dendrimers, showing an homogeneous and densely packed structure.[24] This compact structure requires a space filling geometry that implies back-folding of these dendrimers and the aspect ratio of the dendrimers is best defined as oblate ellipsoid, except for the higher generations. These macromolecules are flexible entities, where water and the counterions can significantly penetrate the dendrimer.

2.2 IgE Recognition of DeAn: Immunoassays

The capacity of different DeAn to bind specific IgE antibodies was analyzed by RAST inhibition studies using sera from patients allergic to benzylpenicillin (with different IgE levels). These experiments were carried out using a solid phase functionalized with PLL-BPO conjugates,[25] whereas in the fluid phase the sera were incubated with the different **DeAn** and **Bu-BPO**, as inhibitors, at different concentrations. Inhibition results were positive for all conjugates of BPO suggesting that inhibition occurs, i.e. specific IgE recognition exists.

When the inhibition curves were compared using the same number of penicillin equivalents (data not shown) there were no differences between the different **DeAn** and **Bu-BPO**, showing a similar pattern in the three sera studied.[23] This suggests that the same inhibition can be obtained using 1 mol of **PG₃BPO** rather than 8 mols of **PG₀BPO**.

Figure 3 exhibits inhibition curves in terms of conjugate concentrations, which show inhibition at least for the highest concentration of inhibitors (**DeAn** and **Bu-BPO**). As can be seen, there is a direct correlation between the molecular weight of the inhibitor and the specific IgE antibody binding capacity. For instance, a 100 fold higher concentration of **Bu-BPO** is needed when compared with **PG₂BPO** to obtain the same percentage of inhibition. These preliminary RAST inhibition studies confirmed the efficacy of penicilloylated PAMAM dendrimers as conjugates for the recognition of IgE antibodies from patients allergic to penicillin. It can therefore be concluded that the hapten–carrier (dendrimer) conjugates (or DeAn) studied mimic recognition with natural hapten–carrier (protein) conjugates.

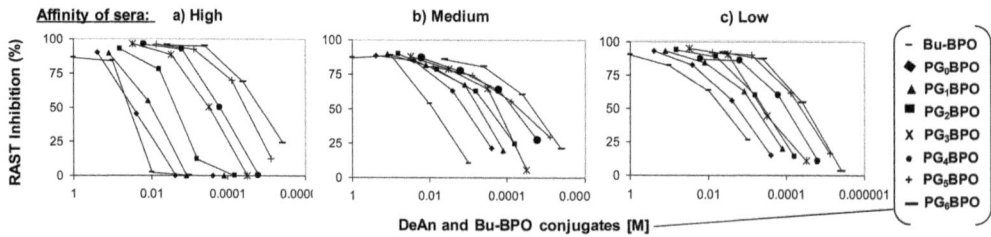

Figure 3   *RAST inhibition assays of 3 sera (a,b,c) allergic to benzylpenicillin using synthetic conjugates (**DeAn** and **Bu-BPO**) as inhibitors at different concentrations.*

3 IMMUNOASSAYS WITH DENDRIMERIC ANTIGENS

3.1 Mode of Anchoring the Dendrimeric Antigens to Solid Supports

As described in the introduction section, solid phases are employed to attach the hapten-carrier conjugates to produce a solid-phase *in vitro* immunoassay, such as RAST. Based on their shape, physical properties[10] and proven IgE specific molecular recognition,[23] dendrimers can be viewed as carrier protein mimetics. As a consequence, penicilloylated dendrimers have recently been anchored on different solid supports[26] as platforms for detecting IgE antibodies from penicillin-allergic patients. We here describe how cellulose discs are used as the solid phase given the importance of the easy handling of these materials for routine hospital assays. The linkage between the conjugate and the solid-phase is of a covalent nature and relies on direct covalent immobilization to chemically activated surfaces, or the use of a linker that mediates immobilization on an appropriately derivatised surface. Classical and novel methods have been employed to functionalize the surfaces and to immobilize the DeAn.

A proper immobilization of the conjugate as well as the reduction of non-specific protein-surface interactions is critical for the successful detection of the antibodies.[27-28] It is even more important to identify new concepts in materials that allow extensive freedom to manipulate and control the function of solid surfaces. Parameters, such as the number and nature of functional groups, hydrophobicity and hydrophilicity, spatial distribution and surface topology need to be taken into account to find the optimal conditions to control protein adsorption behaviour.[29]

3.1.1 Direct Connection by Using Traditional Activating Reagents. The use of cyanogen bromide is one of the most common activation methods for solid supports in biochemistry[30] and classically used for RAST material applications.[31] This methodology involves the conversion of hydroxyl groups of cellulose into cyanate groups (**C-OCN**). The subsequent reaction with PAMAM dendrimer primary amino groups yields the isourea derivative via which the dendrimers are anchored to the solid phase (Scheme 2a).[32] A newly developed procedure, described in Scheme 2b-c, uses haloalkanoyl halides (chloroacetyl chloride and α-bromoisobutyryl bromide), as they are bifunctional compounds and can therefore be used as a chemical linker. Both reagents are immobilized by reaction of the haloalkanoyl halide with the hydroxyl groups in the solid-support[33] to yield **C-Br** and **C-Cl** discs. Thus, the reagents are attached to the cellulose through an ester bond, whereas the other end of the reagent molecule is able to form an amine linkage with the PAMAM dendrimers.[34] To make the dendrimers antigenic and achieve the appropriate polarity and functionality in the solid-phase, focusing on immunoassays, the unreacted activated groups of all dendrimerized surfaces are neutralized by reaction with 2-aminoethanol to obtain **C(X)PG$_n$** supports (Scheme 2a-c). Finally, these dendrimerized surfaces enable the covalent immobilization of the desired hapten, benzylpenicillin, providing BPO-PAMAM conjugates on cellulose supports.

3.1.2 Use of Spacers. When using direct immobilization of conjugates, the proximity of the support may prevent the interaction of antibodies with some hapten units on the conjugate (those placed in close contact with the support surface). Hydrophilic spacers have been used as linkers to increase the hydrophilicity and flexibility of compounds at surfaces,[35] and to distance the immobilized substrate from the surface of a solid support,[27, 36-37] which can reduce steric interferences between the substrates, resulting in higher recognition efficiency with the specific biomolecule to be detected. Thus, to immobilize covalently DeAn onto cellulose surfaces, Spacer I (described in Scheme 2d) was designed considering the following: (i) a linker with a extended flexible structure allows enough distance between the nanoconjugate and the surface to avoid steric hindrance interactions, both in the covalent conjugation process (during material fabrication) and in antibody recognition (during biosensor application), (ii) a hydrophilic polyethylenglycol (PEG) spacer reduces nonspecific binding with the surface and holds the nanoconjugate suspended in aqueous solution away from the support, preventing it from flattening onto the surface, (iii) a bifunctionality bearing chloride and acylchloride groups at opposite chain termini facilitates surface conjugation.

The cellulose surfaces are activated using two different methodologies involving the spacer (Scheme 2d-e).[26] The activation in Scheme 2d involves the immobilization of **Spacer I** through the haloalkanoyl functionality with the hydroxyl groups in the solid-phase. Thus, the spacer is attached to the cellulose through an ester bond whereas the other end of the spacer molecule, the chloride functionality, is able to form an amine linkage with the PAMAM dendrimers. The Scheme 2e procedure involves the silanization of the solid support with an aminopropylsilane through ether linkage, which allows the homogeneous functionalization of the support and maximizes the density of the functional groups introduced to yield **C-APS** surfaces. The amino functionalized surface is then reacted with **Spacer I** to result in surface **C-Spacer II**, which displays the chloride functionality, and forms amine linkage with the PAMAM dendrimers. These procedures lead to the formation of a chemically activated dendritic solid support. After neutralizing the unreacted groups with 2-aminoethanol, the resulting surfaces can be used for the covalent immobilization of the desired biomolecules, such as hapten drugs. Hence, these dendronized surfaces allow the covalent immobilization of benzylpenicillin, providing BPO-PAMAM conjugates on solid-phases.

3.1.3 Direct Connection by Using Click Chemistry. The most representative example of click reactions is the copper-catalyzed azide alkyne cycloaddition (CuAAC) reaction with attractive properties such as high yields, tolerance to various reaction conditions, and the formation of a single product.[38] Other advantages can be considered in surface chemistry applications, such as chemoselectivity and stability of the 1,2,3-triazole moiety linker. The robust and chemoselective CuAAC reaction has been employed not only to explore the hybridization concept of biocompatible bis-MPA (Bis-methylol propionic acid) dendritic moieties[39] to cellulose substrates but also to exploit the resulting orthogonal functional surfaces.[40] The hydroxyl groups on the cellulose surfaces are activated by the introduction of azide groups through reaction with 4-azidomethyl benzoic anhydride, as illustrated in Scheme 2f. A series of dendron generations (G1-G5) with an acetylene core have been successfully attached to the cellulose surfaces through the robust CuAAC click reaction. The peripheral hydroxyl groups of dendrons are further reacted to AB$_2$C trifunctional monomer (A= anhydride, B= hydroxyl, C= azide), which introduces dual functionality at the surface with both azide and external acetonide group units. The deprotection of the latter group leads to a surface (**C-BG$_n$(OH)N$_3$**) expressing bifunctionality with a more hydrophilic environment.

Orthogonal postfunctionalization of these well-controlled bifunctional dendritic cellulose surfaces can be exploited to tailor selectively physical and chemical properties of surfaces to obtain sophisticated functional materials. The acetylene functional amoxicilloyl is reacted using click chemistry under aqueous conditions. To display the tunable nature of these surfaces, triethyleneglycol (TEG) moieties are successfully added to the free alcohols to change physical properties (Scheme 2f). Consequently, both TEG and amoxicillin are combined to tune the hydrophilic nature of the surface and in parallel incorporate the hapten. The dual-functionality introduced is a powerful tool for the design of sophisticated surfaces with promising applications in drug allergy testing.

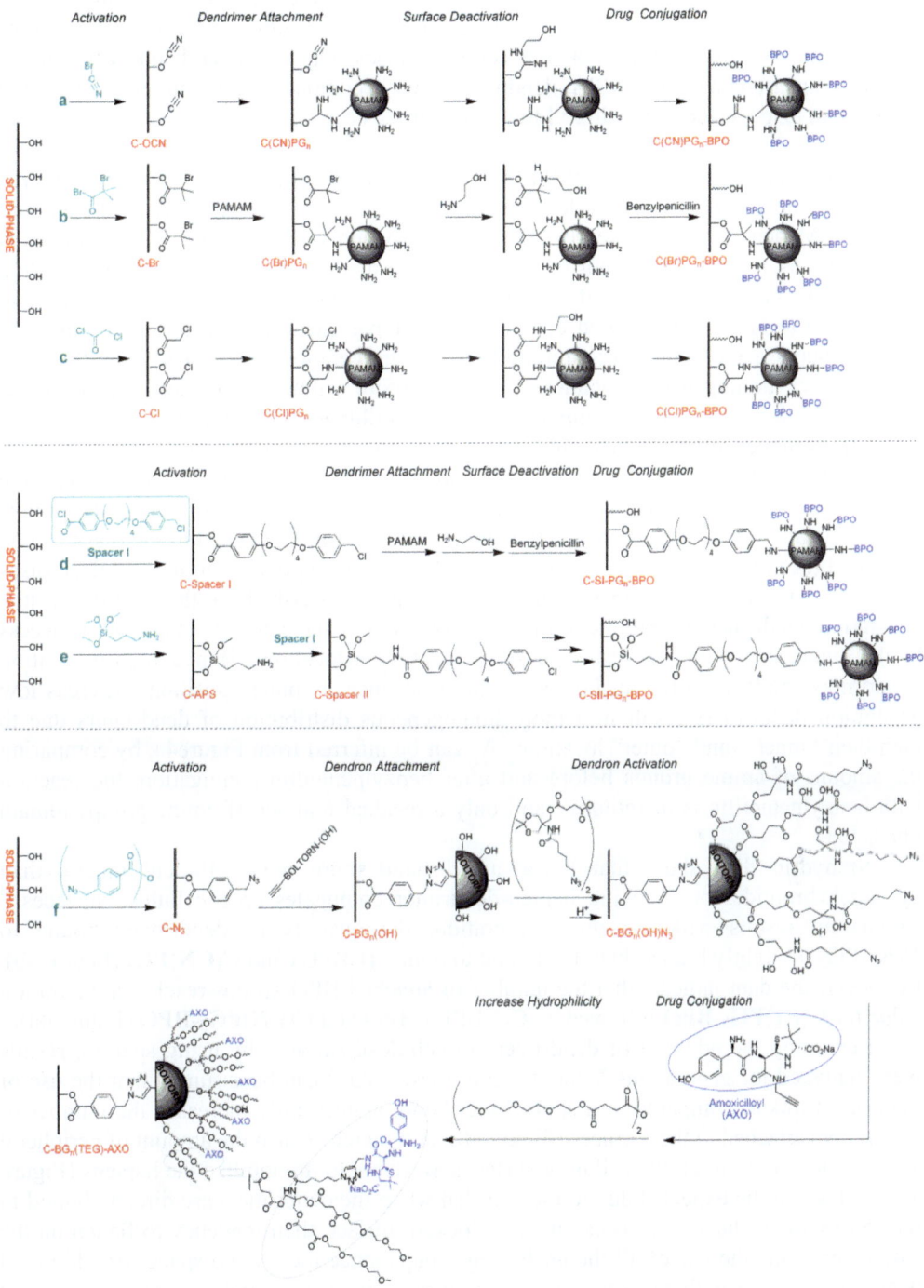

Scheme 2 *Cellulose surface modification methodologies to attach DeAn*

3.2 Dendritic Cellulose Disc Characterization.

To ensure reliability of the potential immunoassays, the quality of the developed materials was evaluated. In general the quality of the new cellulose surfaces involving amino-functionalized PAMAM dendrimers can be systematically controlled by quantification of surface primary amino groups on the cellulose discs. On the other hand, when using hydroxyl-functionalized Bis-MPA dendrons, other techniques based on monitoring the presence of azide, ester and hydroxyl functional groups can be useful.

*3.2.1 Characterization of PAMAM dendrimerized surfaces.*The number of free primary amine groups present in dendrimerized surfaces is a good measure of the amount of PAMAM dendrimers covalently bonded to activated cellulose discs. This number is determined by reacting the dendrimerized cellulose discs with ninhydrin and monitoring the resulting brightly coloured deep blue or purple compound (Ruhemann's purple) in quantitative terms.[41] This method enables the selective quantification of surface primary amine groups in the dendrimers immobilized on the cellulose discs. The overall results show very homogeneous values, and therefore almost identical degrees of functionalization, for all discs within each type and within each generation.[32]

For cyanogen bromide activated cellulose surfaces the number of amino groups is dependent on the particular dendrimer generation (n= 0-6) used: exhibiting a Gaussian-like distribution centred on generation 2 (Figure 4a). Based on the number of free amino groups present in each PAMAM dendrimer, the amount of dendrimer attached to the discs can be estimated (see Figure 4b): thus the number of dendrimers supported on the cellulose discs decreases with increasing generations.[32] This can be ascribed to the ability of low generation dendrimers to migrate to the inner locations in the cellulose tangle while access by the higher generations is restricted to the most outer locations. Hence, high generation dendrimers result in partial anchorage of the dendrimer at "outer" positions whereas low generation dendrimers result in a more homogeneous distribution of dendrimers due to both their "inner " and "outer" locations. As can be inferred from Figure4a, by comparing the amount of amine groups before and after benzylpenicillin conjugation, the reaction with benzylpenicillin is quantitative and only a residual number of amine groups remain unreacted.

Ninhydrin data show that haloalkanoyl halides are more efficient linkers than cyanogen bromide for attaching hapten-dendrimer conjugates onto cellulose surfaces.[34] Comparing results with the third generation, the quantity of dendrimers bound to **C(Br)PG₃** is slightly higher than that bound to both **C(Cl)PG₃** and **C(CN)PG₃** (Figure 4b). Moreover, the data indicate that the number of attached BPO groups reaches a maximum value for **C(Br)PG₃-BPO**,followed by **C(Cl)PG₃-BPO** and **C(CN)PG₃-BPO** (Figure 4a).

Regarding the addition of dendrimers to cellulose surfaces by using spacers, results were analyzed for generations 2 and 4. From these data it can be assumed that the use of the spaced linker, compared to a short direct bond, significantly increases the number of dendrimers attached to the surfaces (Figure 4b), and therefore also the amount of peripheral amine groups present on the cellulose surfaces available to immobilize the haptens (Figure 4a).[26] This is to be expected due to the fact that when the dendrimers are directly bound to the solid support the surface is essentially blocked. In fact, their tendency to flatten on the surface prevents the use of all the anchoring groups since there is no space for additional dendrimers to reach them. The use of a spacer to induce separation from the support surface and the flexibility that the dendrimer can adopt significantly increase the amount of dendrimers anchored. In addition, the amino silylation coupled with the use of the spacer translates into increased dendritic density on the cellulose surfaces. Concerning the generation used, when dendrimers are directly attached onto the cellulose surfaces the number of immobilized BPO with G2 is around two-fold higher than with G4. However, on surfaces activated with the spacers (**C-SI-PG$_n$** and **CSII-PG$_n$**), the amount of BPO does not depend on the dendrimer generation. This can also be attributed to the fact that dendrimers flatten on the surface when directly attached onto the solid support.

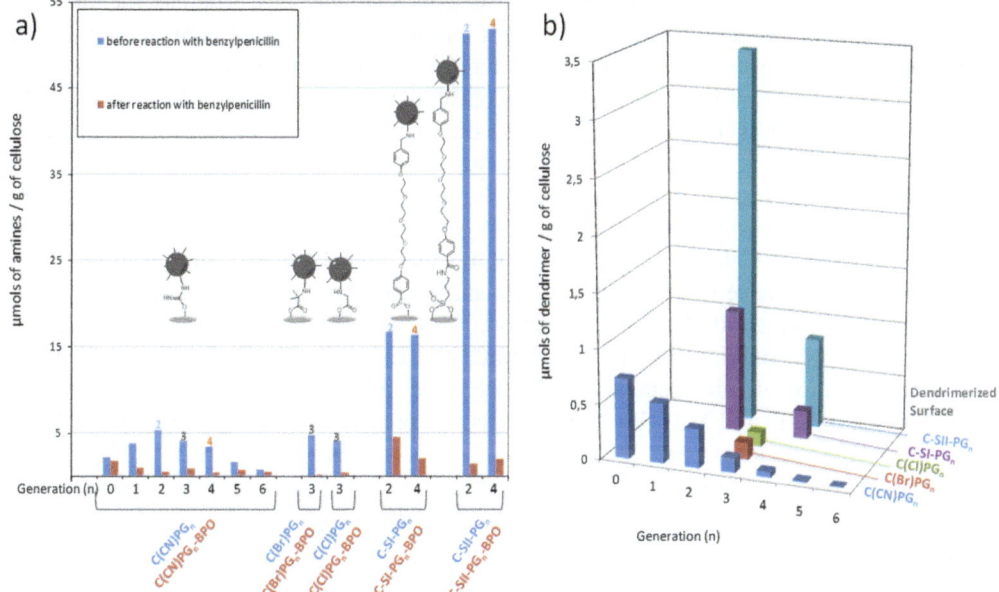

Figure 4 *Results of the determination of primary amino groups at the dendrimerized cellulose discs expressed in a) μmol amine groups before and after reaction with benzylpenicillin and b) μmol of dendrimer*

3.2.2 Characterization of Bis-MPA based Dendronized Surfaces. The development of **C-BG$_n$(TEG)-AXO** surfaces is monitored by using a click dye reagent and the resulting surfaces are well-characterized using X-ray photoelectron spectroscopy (XPS), FT-IR, and contact angle (CA) measurements.[40]

To ensure that cellulose surfaces contain covalently attached azides, these are reacted with acetylene functionalized Disperse Red (Figure 5a) via the CuAAC as a visual evaluation method of a covalent attachment of molecules. The azide-functionalized surfaces yield red surfaces whereas the non-containing azide surfaces yield white surfaces.[40] Therefore, the visual control using the colorimetric reagent (shown in Figure 5a) enables its use as a sensor not only to detect the azides present on the surface but also to determine the success of the CuAAC reaction.

To investigate the features of the dendronized surfaces, water static CA measurements were conducted to monitor the changes in hydrophobicity and hydrophilicity. Due to the inherent roughness and the absorbing nature of the cellulose surfaces,[33] these data can only be taken as qualitative changes of the surface properties. The results described in Table 2 revealed a hydrophobic surface after the activation of cellulose surfaces (**C-N$_3$**), followed by a decrease in CA for the dendronized **C-BG$_n$(OH)**, resulting in the more hydrophilic surfaces when the higher generations are involved. After the reaction with the AB$_2$C monomer, the CA increased because of the presence of acetonide groups, and after deprotection, **C-BG$_n$(OH)N$_3$**, CA decreased again. Additionally, FT-IR analysis showed the presence and amplification of the carbonyl stretch (1730 cm^{-1}) with the addition of dendrons to the surfaces, which is not seen for unmodified cellulose (Figure 5b).[40]

XPS was employed to establish the functionalization of the cellulose surfaces. Figure 5c-e shows the C 1s and N 1s spectra of the successive surfaces and atomic concentration of N 1s and C 1s. The C 1s spectrum of unmodified cellulose consists of a main peak with a binding energy of 285.5 eV attributed to C-O bonds (Figure 5c), whereas for the **C-N$_3$** surfaces the intensity of this peak decreases because of a higher contribution of the overlapping peaks corresponding to O−C=O and C−C/C−H, demonstrating the presence of esters on the surface. Both latter peaks increase for the further modified surfaces **C-BG$_n$(OH)** and **C-BG$_n$(OH)N$_3$**. The highest content of carbonyl carbon is obtained for surfaces decorated with dendrons, which is in agreement with the polyester content of the attached dendrons. Figure 5d shows the N1s spectra of the successive surfaces. The appearance of the N1s signal at 399 eV for **C-N$_3$** shows the introduction of azide groups on the surfaces. XPS of **C-BG$_n$(OH)** surfaces shows the N peak slightly shifted to 398.5 eV with a marked difference in its shape, with the single broad peak being characteristic of the triazol structure formed after the click reaction. For **C-BG$_n$-(OH)N$_3$** surfaces, the presence of azides could be established by the appearance of a shoulder at 401 eV. Figure 5e shows the relative ratio of nitrogen/carbon, which was analyzed by the relative atomic concentration of C 1s and N 1s. From the results, the presence of azide groups on **C-N$_3$** and **C-BG$_n$-(OH)N$_3$** surfaces can be concluded. For **C-BG$_n$(OH)-AXO** surfaces, the attachment of amoxicillin moieties through a triazol was shown by the change of the XPS N 1s peak shape (Figure 5d) and a higher content of nitrogen (Figure 5e).

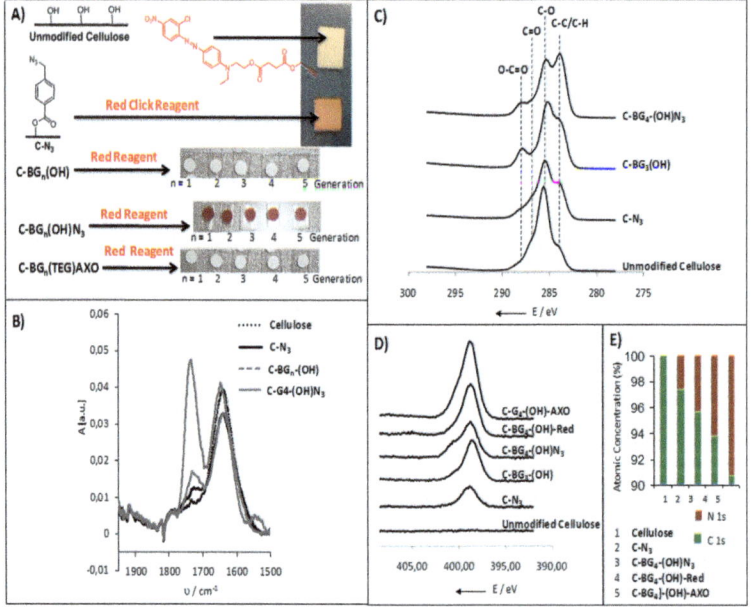

Figure 5 *A) Cellulose solid phases treated with Red-Disperse-derived and (CuPPh$_3$)$_3$Br/DIPEA in THF. B) FT-IR spectra of the unmodified and modified cellulose surfaces. XPS spectra of the C 1s (C) and N 1s (D) regions and atomic concentration of N 1s and C 1s (E).*

Table 2 *Contact Angle (CA in degree)-results obtained for modified filter paper*

n	C-N$_3$	C-BG$_n$-(OH)	C-BG$_n$-(Acet)N$_3$	C-BG$_n$-(OH)N$_3$	C-BG$_n$-(TEG)N$_3$
-	113				
1		110	111	77	68
2		108	111	73	65
3		106	113	69	65
4		89	108	67	68
5		51	101	66	54

3.3. Immunoassay evaluation

The ability of most of the surfaces described here to operate in biological samples was tested by RAST assay using sera from patients. The new materials have been successfully used to detect IgE in patients diagnosed with an immediate allergic reaction (with high and low IgE levels) to benzylpenicillin, in addition to which, the different fine-tuning techniques mentioned were used to further improve the sensitivity of the assay.

First the simpler C(CN)PGn-BPO solid-phases showed their ability to detect IgE antibodies via RAST tests; overall, the dendrimerized discs exhibited RAST levels with allergic patients, and negative RAST with controls who tolerated this drug. Therefore, these dendrimerized cellulose discs interact effectively to bind specifically IgE antibodies, indicating that the penicilloylated dendrimers mimic the antigens toward which IgE were directed.[32] Comparison of the IgE binding capacity of PAMAM dendrimers of different generations (0-6) used as carrier molecules (Figure 6a) showed no relationship with the density of haptens or conjugates on the surface, though there was some dependence on the particular generation and the corresponding RAST level for each type of serum. The lower generations of dendrimer conjugates tended to exhibit lower RAST binding levels. In fact, the RAST level increased with the increasing generation number, peaking around generation 3 or 4. However, the highest generations studied (G5 and G6) exhibited decreased or constant RAST levels. Because G2, G3 and G4 exhibited optimum RAST levels in these studies, they were chosen as the carriers to compare different discs.

RAST results acquired with discs activated by the traditional cyanogen bromide methodology were compared with those obtained from the use of haloalkanoyl halides as reagents and third generation PAMAM dendrimers (Figure 6b).[34] Selective and specific IgE recognition was observed in the different activated discs, presenting a higher percentage of positivity when α-bromoisobutyryl bromide was employed, followed by chloroacetyl chloride and cyanogen bromide. These improvements in *in vitro* sensitivity are in agreement with the higher density of nanoconjugates on the surfaces.

Figure 6c compares RAST data of discs activated by the traditional methodology with those including spacers, using PAMAM dendrimers of generation 2 and 4. The different discs produced a high percentage of RAST in high specific IgE sera from patients allergic to benzylpenicillin, with no differences in the three types of discs or the two generations. The use of spacers compared to short linkers makes no difference for the diagnosis of patients with a high IgE level. However, in sera with a low IgE level, higher detection of IgE was observed with the use of the spacers than with direct connection. In fact, **C-SI-PG$_2$-BPO** discs enabled different cases to be correctly diagnosed as allergic to benzylpenicillin. Moreover, the specificity reached with these discs is very high, as deduced from the results obtained from the controls. The accessibility on these support assays seems to be increased to a higher degree with **Spacer I** compared to **Spacer II**, when the concentration of specific IgE antibodies in the sera is low. This may be due to a higher functionalization density on surfaces with **Spacer II**, resulting in steric interferences between benzylpenicillin haptens, and preventing access to the specific IgE interaction. The less dense cellulose surfaces, although still highly functionalized with **Spacer I**, provide greater flexibility, allowing the immobilized nanoconjugates to move into position to establish the IgE-specific interaction.

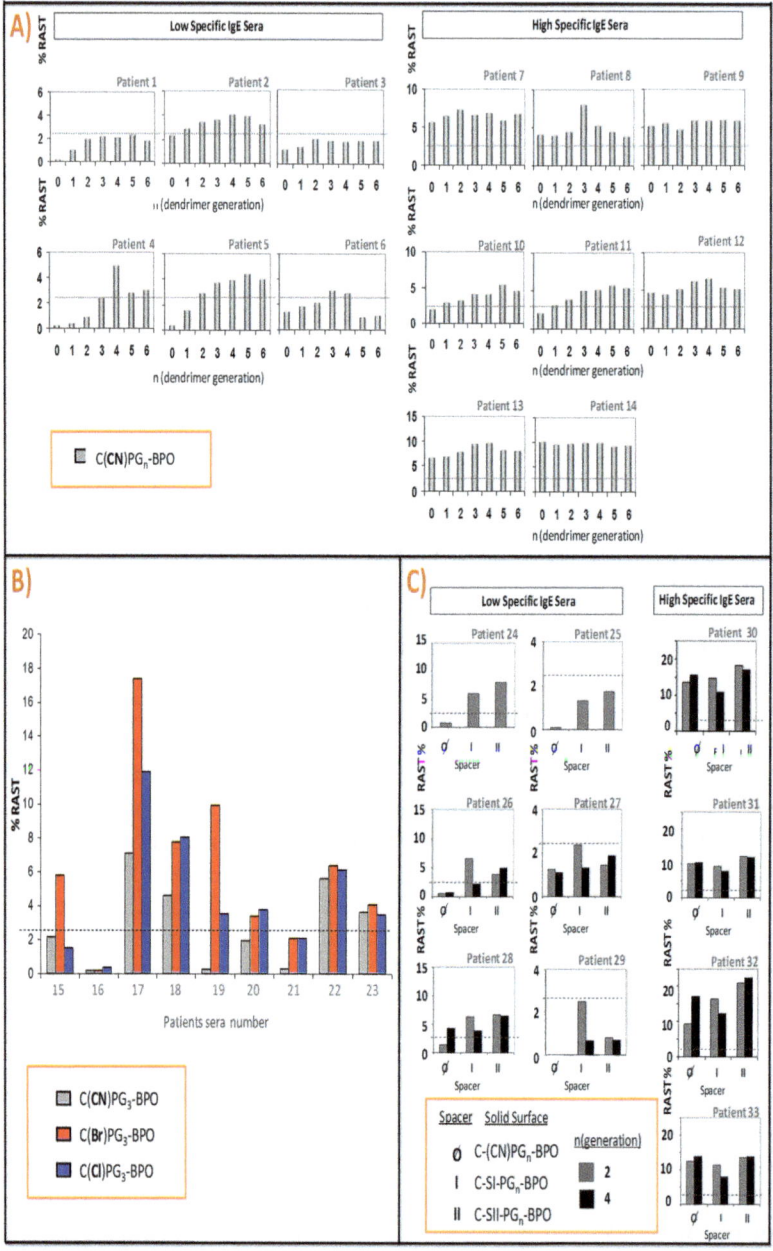

Figure 6 *RAST values (as % of RAST, y-axis) for patients' sera using different solid-phases: (A) **C(CN)PGₙ-BPO** for all generations, (B) also including **C(X)PG₃-BPO** for G3, (C) and surfaces including spacers for G2 and G4.*

4 CONCLUSIONS

The possibility of manipulating matter at the nanoscale range permits the understanding of the relationship between structures and new properties. This enables the preparation of new structures and assemblies whose intrinsic properties depend directly on their size and geometry.[42] The emergence of the recently recognized field of nanomedicine has led to useful applications in the area of immunology, and involves the search for new and tunable properties.

As a result of dendrimers unique features (a globular shape, controlled size, hollow structure and the intrinsic property of multivalency), they are often referred to as synthetic compounds able to mimic proteins in their interaction with the immune system. This success suggests dendrimers can be used for *in vitro* diagnosis of allergy, thus avoiding the use of invasive *in vivo* tests, which are usually considered as the standard in the diagnosis of hypersensitivity reactions.[11]

Different methodologies have been developed to prepare chemically controlled and reproducible dendronized and dendrimerized cellulose surfaces for their use in RAST applications. Clinical evaluation of these methodologies shows that the use of a flexible spacer provides a more available nanoconjugate for IgE molecular recognition and can therefore avoid false negative results in those patients with low but nevertheless positive IgE levels.

Acknowledgments
This research was supported by different sources: Ministerio de Ciencia e Innovacion-Spain (CTQ2010-20303), Junta de Andalucía (PI-0551-2009, PI-0545-2010, PI-0699-2011, CTS-06603, CTS-395), Fondo de Investigaciones Sanitarias- Spain (FIS/PS09/01768), COST action TD0802 and FIS-Thematic Networks and Co-operative Research Centers: RIRAAF (RD07/0064). This research was co-financed by FEDER funds. MIM acknowledges the financial support from Marie Curie IEF-300230. MM is grateful to the Swedish Research Council (VR) for its financial support (2010-453).

References

1   G.T. Hermanson, in *Bioconjugate Techniques (Second Edition)*, Academic Press, New York, 2008, ch.19. p. 743.
2   P.M.H. Heegaard, U. Boas and N.S. Sorensen, *Bioconjugate Chem.*, 2009, **21**, 405.
3   K. Landsteiner and J. Jacobs, *J. Exp. Med.*, 1935, **61**, 643.
4   J. Uetrecht, *Chem. Res. Toxicol.*, 2008, **21**, 84.
5   A. Ariza, M.I. Montañez and D. Perez-Sala, *Curr. Opin. Allergy Clin. Immunol.*, 2011, **11**, 305.
6   M.E. Weiss and N.F. Adkinson, *Clin. Allergy*, 1988, **18**, 515.
7   C. Antúnez, E. Martín, J.A. Cornejo-García, N. Blanca-Lopez, R. R-Pena, C. Mayorga, M.J. Torres and M. Blanca, *Curr. Pharm. Des.*, 2006, **12**, 3327.
8   M. Blanca, C. Mayorga, E. Perez, R. Suau, C. Juarez, J.M. Vega, M.J. Carmona, M. Perez-Estrada and J. Garcia, *J. Immunol. Methods*, 1992, **153**, 99.
9   M. Blanca, F. Moreno, C. Mayorga, J. Garcia, M. Fernandez, E. Perez, C. Juarez and R. Suau, *J. Clin. Immunoassay*, 1994, **17**, 166.
10   J.M.J. Fréchet and D.A. Tomalia, *Dendrimers and Other Dendritic Polymers*, Wiley & Sons Ltd, West Sussex, 2001.
11   M.I. Montañez, A.J. Ruiz-Sanchez and E. Perez-Inestrosa, *Curr. Opin. Allergy Clin. Immunol.*, 2010, **10**, 297.

12 V.P. Torchiling, *Nanoparticulates as drug carriers*, Imperial College Press, London, 2006.
13 D. Astruc, E. Boisselier and C.t. Ornelas, *Chem. Rev.*, 2010, **110**, 1857.
14 F. Zeng and S.C. Zimmerman, *Chem. Rev.*, 1997, **97**, 1681.
15 H.J. Han, R.M. Kannan, S. Wang, G. Mao, J.P. Kusanovic and R. Romero, *Adv. Funct. Mater.*, 2010, **20**, 409.
16 G. Franc and A.K. Kakkar, *Chem. Soc. Rev.*, 2010, **39**, 1536.
17 R. Hourani and A. Kakkar, *Macromol. Rapid Commun.*, 2010, **31**, 947.
18 A. Carlmark, C.J. Hawker, A. Hult and M. Malkoch, *Chem. Soc. Rev.*, 2009, **38**, 352.
19 M.V. Walter and M. Malkoch, *Chem. Soc. Rev.*, 2012, **41**, 4593.
20 S.-E. Stiriba, H. Frey and R. Haag, *Angew. Chem. Int. Ed.*, 2002, **41**, 1329.
21 T.D. Svenson S, *Adv. Drug Deli.v Rev.*, 2005, **57**, 2106.
22 A.-M. Caminade, C. Padié, R. Laurent, A. Maraval and J.-P. Majoral, *Sensors*, 2006, **6**, 901.
23 F. Sánchez-Sancho, E. Pérez-Inestrosa, R. Suau, C. Mayorga, M.J. Torres and M. Blanca, *Bioconjugate Chem.*, 2002, **13**, 647.
24 M.I. Montañez, F. Najera and E. Perez-Inestrosa, *Polymers*, 2011, **3**, 1533.
25 F. Moreno, M. Blanca, C. Mayorga, S. Terrados, M. Moya, E. Pérez, R. Suau, J.M. Vega, J. García, A. Miranda and M.J. Carmona, *Int. Arch. Allergy Immunol.*, 1995, **108**, 74.
26 A.J. Ruiz-Sanchez, M.I. Montañez, C. Mayorga, M.J. Torres, N. Seda Kehr, Y. Vida, D. Collado, F. Najera, L. De Cola and E. Perez-Inestrosa, *Curr. Med. Chem.*, 2012, **19**, 4942.
27 M. Fuentes, C. Mateo, R. Fernández-Lafuente and J.M. Guisán, *Biomacromolecules*, 2006, **7**, 540.
28 Y.L. Jeyachandran, J.A. Mielczarski, E. Mielczarski and B. Rai, *J. Colloid Interface Sci.*, 2009, **341**, 136.
29 R.A. Latour, *Biointerphases*, 2008, **3**, FC2.
30 H.P. Jennissen, *J. Mol. Recognit.*, 1995, **8**, 116.
31 R.G. Edwards, D.A. Spackman and J.M. Dewdney, *Int. Arch. Allergy Appl. Immunol.*, 1982, **68**, 352.
32 M.I. Montañez, E. Perez-Inestrosa, R. Suau, C. Mayorga, M.J. Torres and M. Blanca, *Biomacromolecules*, 2008, **9**, 1461.
33 A. Carlmark and E. Malmström, *J. Am. Chem. Soc.*, 2002, **124**, 900.
34 M.I. Montañez, C. Mayorga, M.J. Torres, M. Blanca and E. Perez-Inestrosa, *Nanomed. Nanotechnol. Biol. Med.*, 2011, **7**, 682.
35 M. Furuya, M. Haramura and A. Tanaka, *Bioorg. Med. Chem.*, 2006, **14**, 537.
36 B.C. Weimer, M.K. Walsh and X. Wang, *J. Biochem. Biophys. Methods*, 2000, **45**, 211
37 J.L. Zimmermann, T. Nicolaus, G. Neuert and K. Blank, *Nature Protocols* 2010, **5**, 975
38 H.C. Kolb, M.G. Finn and K.B. Sharpless, *Angew. Chem. Int. Ed.*, 2001, **40**, 2004.
39 N. Feliu, M.V. Walter, M.I. Montañez, A. Kunzmann, A. Hult, A. Nyström, M. Malkoch and B. Fadeel, *Biomaterials*, 2012, **33**, 1970.
40 M.I. Montañez, Y. Hed, S. Utsel, J. Ropponen, E. Malmström, L. Wagberg, A. Hult and M. Malkoch, *Biomacromolecules*, 2011, **12**, 2114.
41 M. Friedman, *J. Agric. Food Chem.*, 2004, **52**, 385.
42 O. Rolland, C.-O. Turrin, A.-M. Caminade and J.-P. Majoral, *New J. Chem.*, 2009, **33**, 1809.

MOLECULAR DYNAMICS OF LYSINE DENDRIMERS. COMPUTER SIMULATION AND NMR

I. Neelov[1,2], S. Falkovich[2], D. Markelov[2,3], E. Paci[4], A. Darinskii[2] and H. Tenhu[1]

[1] University of Helsinki, FIN00014, A.I.Virtasen Aukio 1, Helsinki, Finland
[2] Institute of Macromolecular Compounds of Russian Academy of Sciences, 199004, St. Petersburg, V.O., Bolshoy prospect, 31, Russia
[3] St. Petersburg State University, Department of Physics, 198504, St. Petersburg, Petrodvorets, Ulyanovskaya str., 1, Russia
[4] University of Leeds, LS2 9JT, Leeds, UK

1 INTRODUCTION

Dendrimers are tree-like macromolecules, regularly branching from a single center. The first dendrimers were synthesized in the late 70s - early 80s.[1-4] Peptide dendrimers usually consist of linear sequences of aminoacid residues combined into branched dendrimer structure by lysine residues. Thus different peptide dendrimers differ from each other by primary structure of amino acids residues in the linear fragments between neighboring branch points of the dendrimer. Peptide dendrimers are less well known than poly(amido amine) (PAMAM), poly(ethyleneimine) (PEI), carbosilane and other synthetic dendrimers; however, the first peptide (poly-L-lysine) dendrimers were synthesized in early 80s.[5,6] Due to better biocompatibility of these dendrimers they successfully compete with other synthetic dendrimers for use in different biomedical applications. Peptide (lysine) dendrimers were used for a long time as multiple antigen peptides (MAPs)[7] and could be used as carriers in drug and gene delivery.[8] They also could act themselves as antimicrobial or antiamyloid agents.[9,10]

Modeling of peptide dendrimers was conducted earlier for some dendrimers with modified functional terminal groups[11-15], designed for use in specific biomedical applications. However, no extensive systematic study of the structure and especially the mobility of non-modified lysine dendrimers have been performed. Here we describe application of method of molecular dynamics for study of basic characteristics of simplest lysine dendrimers of different generations and at different temperatures. Along with modeling, we performed an experimental study of local mobility in these dendrimers by NMR. The dendrimers used in NMR were synthesized by G.P.Vlasov and coworkers.[16]

In the beginning of the chapter we describe the model of lysine dendrimers, the modeling method and the method of preparation of initial equilibrated configurations of these dendrimers. We also briefly describe application of NMR for investigation of the mobility of lysine dendrimers and the information that can be derived from it. The next two parts contain results of the simulation of lysine dendrimers of different generations G=1-5 at room temperature and the temperature dependences of structural and dynamical characteristics of dendrimers generations G=2 and 4 obtained iusing molecular dynamics simulation and NMR methods.

2 MODEL AND METHODS

The structure of lysine dendrimer of the first generation ($G = 1$) synthesized by Vlasov *et al.* [16] is shown in Figure 1. Dendrimers usually consist of a core (center), spacers, connecting the neighboring branch points and terminal groups. The core of our lysine dendrimers is composed of two amino acid residues: core alanine, (with positively charged (protonated) NH_3^+ group) and the core lysine. In the following generation two lysine residues are attached to the core lysine residue. At the ends of these two first generation lysine residues there are four terminal lysine residues, which ends with positively charged (protonated) NH_3^+ groups. It should be noted that unlike most other symmetric dendrimers the lysine dendrimers have two different asymmetric spacers (fragments between nearest branch points) consisting of three and seven valence bonds, respectively. Short spacer is a fragment of peptide backbone and long spacer is a slightly modified side group of lysine residue (see Fig.1).

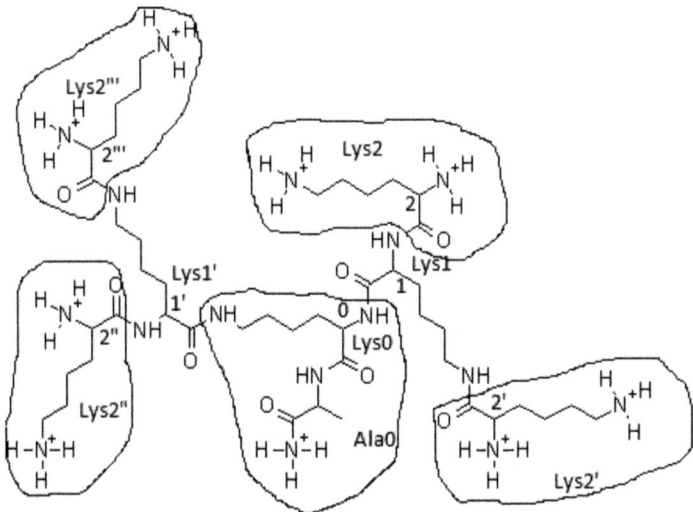

Figure 1 *Structure of lysine dendrimer of the first generation (G=1). Aminoacid residues Ala0 and Lys0 and branching point 0 belong to the core, Lys1, Lys1' and branching points 1, 1' – to the first generation of dendrimer and residues Lys2-Lys2''' form its terminal groups. Spacers between points 0-1, 1-2, 1'-2'' consist of 3 covalent bonds, and spacers 0-1', 1-2', 1'-2''' – consist of 7 covalent bonds*

2.1. Molecular dynamics method

Modeling was performed using the molecular dynamics method for systems consisting of a single dendrimer molecule, water molecules and chlorine counterions in a cubic box with periodic boundary conditions. The characteristics of the simulated systems are summarized in Table 1.

Each dendrimer was initially built by "convergent"[17] method using the software package HyperChem 5.[18] It means that the dendrimer of generation G was constructed by covalent linking of centers of the two $G/2$ generation dendrimers. Thus, for example, the second generation dendrimer was prepared by merging of two first generation dendrimers, **Table 1**

Table 1 *Parameters of simulated lysine dendrimers: G – number of generations, M – molecular mass , Q – charge, N_b – number of branching points, N_t – number of terminal groups and <a> – periodic cubic box size*

G	M, g/mol	Q, e	N_b	N_t	<a>, nm
1	958	9	7	8	6
2	2028	17	15	16	6
3	4095	33	31	32	7
4	8229	65	63	64	8.5
5	16496	129	127	128	9.4

(shown in Fig. 1) and the fourth-generation dendrimer was created by merging of two second generation dendrimers. These structures (before and after the merger) were optimized by molecular mechanics method with an all atom model *in vacuo*.

Molecular dynamics modeling was performed using the GROMACS 4.5.5 package[19] using one of the most modern Amber force fields: AMBER-99SB[20] and explicit water solvent. Some calculations were performed also in CHARMM package with forcefield CHARMM19 and FACTS[21] implicit solvent. The equilibration process consisted of three stages, because in the initial structure of the simulated systems there are many overlapping groups of atoms and, therefore, strong steric interactions between them. In systems containing peptides this leads to the possibility of transition of peptide groups from the favorable trans-conformation to energetically less favorable cis-conformation. Since the energy barrier between these conformations is very high, the reverse transition requires a great time and the time of the numerical simulation could be not sufficient for relaxation of peptide groups. To avoid freezing of the peptide bonds in these metastable cis-state the peptide groups were fixed in the trans-conformation in the first two stages of the equilibration by introducing an additional elastic potential (with a constant elasticity equal 10^6 kcal/mol) between atoms in peptide group. In the first stage of the equilibration process the dendrimer macromolecule was simulated *in vacuo*. In the second stage the water molecules and chlorine counterions (to neutralize positive charge of NH_3^+ groups in dendrimer) were added. The rigid three-center TIP3P model of water[22] was used and simulation was carried out in a cubic cell with periodic boundary conditions. The third stage of optimization, as the second, was carried out in water with counterions, but without restraining of the conformations of the peptide groups. Each of these three stages of the optimization included four stages: energy minimization for 500 steps with the steepest descent method and three short (100 steps) MD runs in the *NVT* ensemble with integration step 0.02, 0.2 and 2fs, correspondingly. During the optimization all non-bonded interactions were "truncated" at distances of 0.9 nm. The temperature was maintained by Berendsen thermostat with a time constant $\tau_T = 0.4$ ps.

After this multistage optimization the additional relaxation of system was performed during 50ns MD run. During this run exactly the same approach and parameters (*NPT* ensemble with Nosé-Hoover thermostat (with $\tau_T = 0.4$ ps) and Parrinello-Rahman barostat at normal pressure with time constant $\tau_P = 0.5$ ps, and the particle mesh Ewald (PME) method[19] to account for long range electrostatic interactions) were used as in the subsequent 150ns productive run.

2.2 NMR method

NMR relaxation method is widely used for study of the local orientational mobility of different H-H vectors in dendrimers (see, for example, papers[23-30]). One of the most common approaches is to study the spin-lattice NMR relaxation. In the case of dipole-dipole relaxation mechanism of the relaxation rate $1/T1_H$ for the hydrogen atoms can be represented by a spectral density $J(\omega, \mathbf{T})$

$$\frac{1}{T_{1H}}(\omega, \mathbf{T}) = A_0\left(J(\omega, \mathbf{T}) + 4J(2\omega, \mathbf{T})\right), \tag{1}$$

where

$$A_0 = N(S(S+1))/5\left(\gamma_H^4 \hbar^2 / r_{HH}^6\right), \tag{2}$$

γ is gyromagnetic ratio for ^1H, r_{HH} is the effective distance between the observed hydrogen atoms, S is the spin, ω is the frequency of the instrument, $\hbar = h/2\pi$ is the - reduced Planck constant.

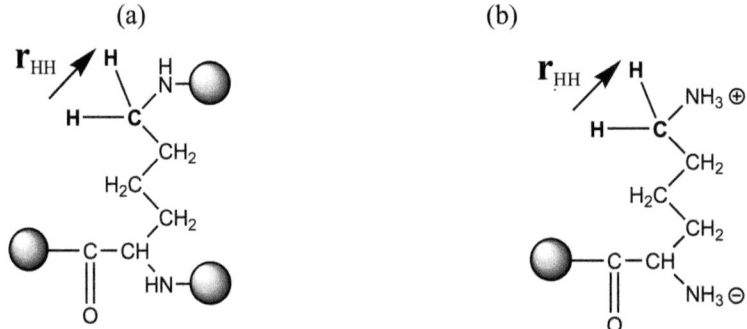

(a)   (b)

Figure 2 *The structural formula of lysine dendrimer segments. Gray circles denote the branch points. The **CH₂** group containing* r_{HH} *vector studied in the NMR experiment is marked with the bold font for the internal (a) and terminal (b) groups*

The spectral density $J_i(\omega, \mathbf{T})$ corresponds to the Fourier transform of the orientation relaxation time of autocorrelation function $P_2(t)$.

$$P_2(t) = \frac{3}{2}\left(<(r_i(t)r_i(0))^2> - \frac{1}{3}\right) \tag{3}$$

If this function is described by single exponential decline

$$P_2(t) = \exp\left(-\frac{t}{\tau_{cor}}\right) \tag{4}$$

with correlation time τ_{cor}, then $J(\omega, \mathbf{T})$ is represented as

$$J(\omega, \mathbf{T}) = \frac{\tau_{cor}(\mathbf{T})}{1 + (\omega\tau_{cor}(\mathbf{T}))^2}, \tag{5}$$

Usually the temperature dependences of the NMR correlation times are experimentally measured at a fixed frequency ω. If the temperature dependence of the correlation times exhibit a maximum then equation

$$\omega\tau_{cor}(\mathbf{T}) \approx 0.62 \tag{6}$$

allows determination of the value of τ_{cor}. For poly-L-lysine dendrimers ^1H NMR spectra of the internal (Fig. 2a) and the terminal (Fig. 2b) CH₂ groups are separated and correlation times of both types of groups could be obtained from experimental data.

Local dynamics was studied for two samples of lysine dendrimer of G = 2 and 4 generations. The chemical structures of the samples studied in NMR coincided with the structures used in the molecular dynamics simulation (see Fig.1). The synthesis of the samples was described in detail earlier.[16] The test system in NMR consisted of a strongly diluted solution of lysine dendrimer in deuterated water (D_2O). The concentration of the dendrimer in all cases does not exceed 1 wt. %. The temperature range used is limited by boiling and freezing points of D_2O. The spin-lattice relaxation time $(T_{1H)}$ for hydrogen atoms were measured on Bruker apparatus AVANCE-400 at a frequency of 400 MHz for different temperatures in the range 278K - 363K using the standard pulse sequence "inversion-recovery" (π-π / 2).

3 ROOM TEMPERATURE PROPERTIES

3.1 Structural characteristics of lysine dendrimers

The size of dendrimers can be characterized by the mean-squared gyration radius Rg

$$R_g^2 = \frac{1}{M}\sum_i m_i(r_i - r_{COM})^2$$

(7)

where M is a molecular mass of a dendrimer, m_i is the molecular mass of the i-th atom, r_i is the radius vector to the i-th atom, r_{COM} is the radius vector to the center of mass (COM) of the dendrimer and the summation is done over all atoms of the dendrimer.

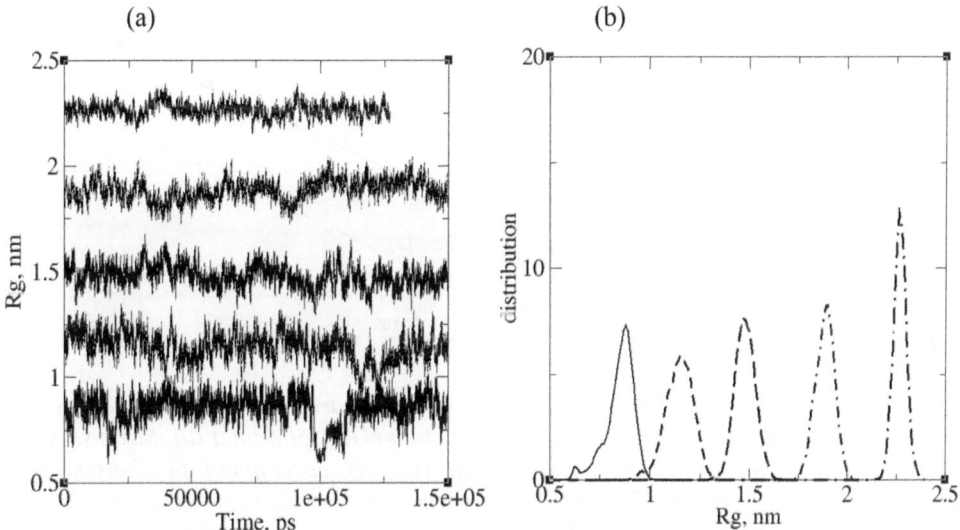

Figure 3 *The variation of the gyration radius R_g with time for dendrimers G=1-5 (from bottom to top) (a) and the distribution of gyration radius R_g for dendrimer generation G=1 (solid line), G=2 (short dashed), G=3 (long dashed), G=4 (short dash-dotted) and G=5 (long dash-dotted) (b)*

This function was calculated using the g_gyrate function of GROMACS.[19] The time dependence of R_g for dendrimers of different generation (G=1-5) is shown in Fig.3a. The distribution function of gyration radius R_g for dendrimers of different generation (G=1-5) is shown in Fig.3b. Both plots show that the average value of R_g increases with G and the fluctuation (half-width of the distribution function of R_g) decreases with size of dendrimer monotonically. It means that the size of dendrimer increases with the generation number but at the same time the larger dendrimers become more rigid (i.e. fluctuations of their size decrease).

Relaxation times for fluctuations of dendrimer size could be obtained from auto-correlation functions (ACF) for R_g^2:

$$C(t) = (<R_g^2(i)R_g^2(i+t)> - <R_g^2>^2)/((<R_g^4> - <R_g^2>^2) \qquad (8)$$

where $R_g^2(i)$ is the R_g^2 value in i-th time step, t is the time-shift (in time-step units) and $<>$ means averaging through all i.

The time dependence of this function for dendrimers of different generations is presented on Fig.4a. Relaxation times (i.e. the times corresponding to the decay of these correlation function from 1 to 1/e) increase from 0.5ns (G=1 dendrimer) to 2ns (for G=5 dendrimer). These times are essentially smaller than the length of the molecular dynamics trajectories (200 ns consisting of 50 ns equilibration run and 150ns production run) for each dendrimer in present calculations. This confirms that trajectories are sufficiently long and that the systems under investigation are properly equilibrated.

(a)   (b)

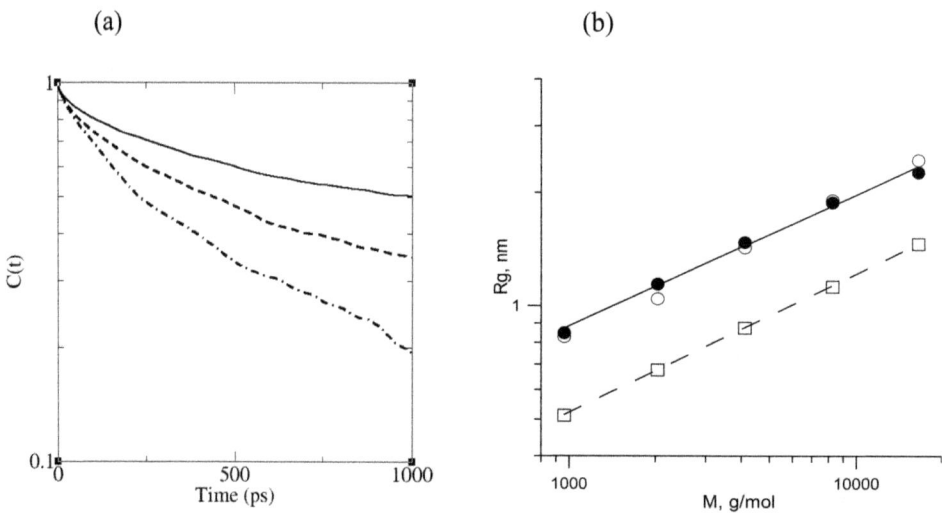

Figure 4 *Normalized autocorrelation function of the square of the gyration radius Rg of dendrimers G1 (dot-dashed line), G3 (dashed line) and G5 (solid line) (a). Mean square R_g as a function of the molecular mass. Filled symbols correspond to charged lysine dendrimers in explicit water. Hollow symbols corresponds to the same dendrimer in vacuo (circles) and uncharged lysine dendrimer in implicit solvent (squares)(b)*

The dependence of R_g on molecular weight M (Fig.4b) obtained from simulation in explicit water is well described by the power law $R_g \sim M^{0.34}$ where the exponent 0.34 is close to value 1/3 for spheres with the constant average density of monomers.[31-32] Besides the simulation of charged lysine dendrimers in the explicit water we have performed also a simulation of the same dendrimers *in vacuo* and uncharged lysine dendrimers (with deprotonated NH_2 terminal groups) in implicit solvent using the FACTS model available in CHARMM ([22]). Interestingly the sizes of charged lysine dendrimers of different generations G and the value of the exponent in power law (for R_g dependence on M) *in vacuo* is very close (see Fig.4b) to that estimated in explicit solvent. The size of uncharged lysine dendrimers is smaller than that of charged ones but the exponent in the dependence of the dendrimer size on molecular mass is equal 0.36 which is rather close to that of charged dendrimeres.

Table 2 *The values of the ratio of main components $R_{g1}:R_{g2}:R_{g3}$ of gyration radius Rg of lysine dendrimers of generations G=1-5*

G	1	2	3	4	5
$R_{g1}:R_{g2}:R_{g3}$	1:0.94:0.56	1:0.92:0.65	1:0.93:0.66	1:0.92:0.76	1:0.95:0.82

The shape of lysine dendrimers could be characterized by ratios $R_{g1}:R_{g2}:R_{g3}$ of the principal moments of the gyration tensor which could be calculated by its diagonalization (see Table 2). The ratio of the two longest components (R_{g1} and R_{g2}) is rather similar for all dendrimers while smallest component (R_{g3}) differs from them especially for dendrimers of smaller generations. Thus the dendrimer shape is similar to disk for low generations (*G*=1-3) and becomes closer to the isotropic sphere for higher generations (*G*=4-5).

Information about the internal structure of lysine dendrimer could be obtained from radial distribution function of all atoms and terminal groups relative to its center of mass (Fig.5a and Fig.5b correspondingly) These functions were calculated using the g_rdf function of GROMACS[19] and show the average number of particles inside the spherical shell of the given radius *r*. The shape of the radial distribution function of all atoms relatively to the center of mass of lysine dendrimers is similar to that for the radial distribution function of terminal groups but the maximum of the latter one is slightly shifted to larger distances. For dendrimers with symmetric branching such as PAMAM, for example (where the paths from the dendrimer center to each terminal group have the same length) the distribution of terminal groups for completely extended branches is described by the delta function. Thus the similarity in the distribution of terminal groups and all atoms of dendrimer as in Fig.5 for dendrimer with symmetric branching should be due to backfolding, i.e. due to the bending of dendrimer branches into the dendrimer interior.

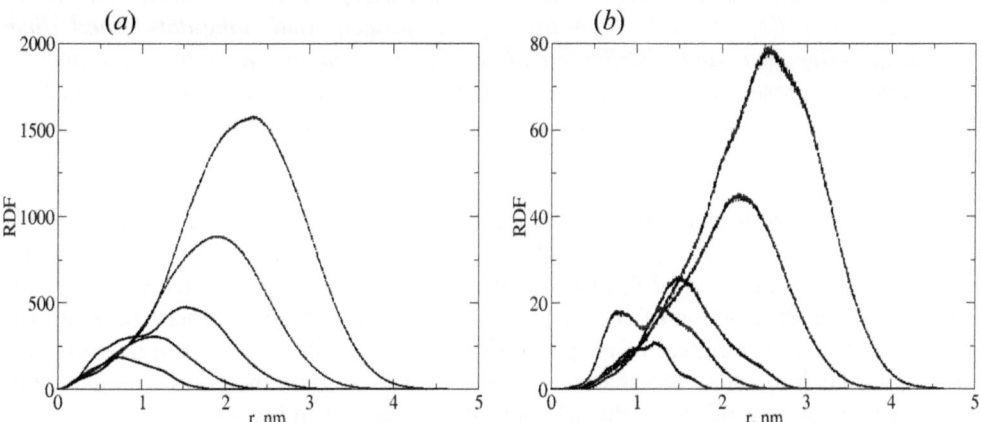

Figure 5 *Radial distribution function (not normalized) of all atoms (a) and terminal groups (b) relatively to the center of mass of dendrimer of generations G from 1 to 5*

However in lysine dendrimers with the asymmetric branching (short and long spacers) the paths (as well as length of vectors between COM and different terminal groups) are different and the distribution of these lengths is described by the Pascal triangle even in dendrimers with completely extended branches. The real distribution of length of vectors between COM and terminal groups in such asymmetric dendrimers is a result of the combination of the triangle distribution and the backfolding.

The backfolding of dendrimer branches could be realized through the bending of spacers or (and) the variation of angles between spacers of neighboring generations. Short spacers (fragment of peptide backbone consisting of three valence bonds, see Fig. 2) are rather rigid. Long spacers (modified side group of lysine, see Fig. 2) could, in principle, change their conformation and length (i.e. length of vector connecting neighboring branching points). The distribution function of the length l of long spacers is shown in Fig. 6a. Long spacers in lysine dendrimers of different generations (G=1-5) are highly stretched (the mean value of length l are between 0.79 and 0.81 nm, about 90% of the maximum possible extension (without distortion of covalent bonds and valent angles). The distribution functions of spacer lengths is rather broad for G=1 dendrimer but

(a)   (b)

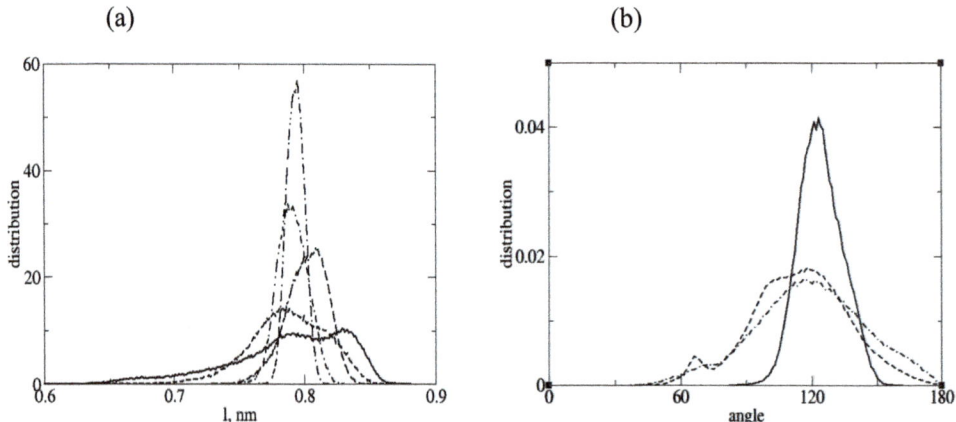

Figure 6 *Distribution of length (end-to-end distance) of long spacers for G=1-5 dendrimers (solid, dashed, long-dashed, dot-dashed and long-dot-dashed lines, correspondingly) (a), and distribution of angles between two neighboring spacers in neighboring sub-generations of lysine dendrimers. Angles between two short spacers (solid line), between short and long spacers (dashed line) and between two long spacers (dot-dashed line) (b)*

become narrower with increasing of generation number G of dendrimer. This means that long spacers become more rigid for higher generation dendrimers which is in agreement with narrowing distribution of R_g of lysine dendrimers with increasing generation number (see Fig.3). The distribution of short spacers lengths has a sharp peak near 0.38 nm (not shown) for lysine dendrimers of all generations. Thus the short spacers are significantly more rigid than long ones. The sharpness of these peaks slightly increases with generation number (not shown) similarly to the behavior of long spacers in Fig.6a.

Fig.6b shows the distribution of angles between vectors of neighboring spacers in two consecutive subgenerations of the G=4 lysine dendrimer. We calculated these functions separately for angles between two short (ss) spacers (solid line), between short and long (sl) spacers (dashed line) and between two long (ll) spacers (dot-dashed line). It is seen, that the angles between two short (ss) spacers fluctuate only in very narrow interval ($\pm 20°$) and the value of these angles >90° with maximum near 120°. On the other hand the angles between short and long as well as angles between two long spacers show the essentially wider distribution. Thus we can conclude that the main mechanism of the reorientation of neighboring spacers relatively each other in lysine dendrimers is a change of angles in *sl* and *ll* pairs of spacers.

3.2 Spacers' mobility

Global fluctuations of dendrimer size (and in particular fluctuation of R_g, see Fig.3a and Fig.3b) occur due to the fluctuations of the length and the re-orientation of its spacers. The dynamics of the fluctuations of the spacer lengths and their orientational mobility can be characterized by the autocorrelation function (ACF) for the square length (l^2) of the spacer (i.e. square of length of vector connecting two neighboring branch points)

$$C_l(t) = (<l^2(i)l^2(i+t)> - <l^2>^2)/(<l^4> - <l^2>^2) \qquad (9a)$$

and for the orientation of unit vector (l_1) directed along this vector

$$P_l(t) = <l_1(i)l_1(i+t)> \qquad (9b)$$

where $l^2(i)$ and $l_1(i)$ are the l^2 value and vector l_1 in i-th time step, correspondingly, t is the time-shift (in time-step units) and $<>$ means averaging through all i.

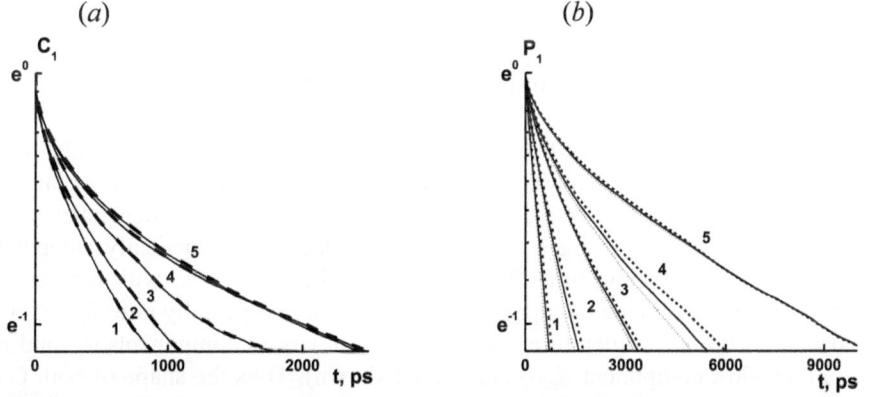

Figure 7 *Length (a) and orientation (b) ACFs of lysine dendrimers with G = 1 (1), = 2 (2), = 3 (3), = 4 (4), = 5 (5) for short (dotted line), long (dashed line), and all (solid line) internal spacers. (Length correlation function for short spacers decay quicker than 1 ps for all dendrimers and not shown on Fig.7a)*

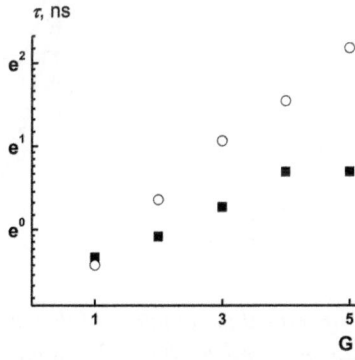

Figure 8 *Characteristic times of length (squares) and orientation (circles) fluctuations obtained from ACFs of internal spacers*

Correlation functions $C_1(t)$ and $P_1(t)$ for lysine dendrimers of generation $G1$-$G5$ are presented in Fig.7a and Fig.7b respectively. It is interesting that orientational ACF (Fig.7b) for short (dotted lines) and long (dashed lines) internal spacers calculated separately are close to each other and to curves averaged through all (short and long) internal spacers (solid lines) in Fig.7a and Fig.7b. All these functions decay with time slower as the generation number increases. Relaxation times estimated from decay of $C_1(t)$ and $P_1(t)$ correlation functions to $1/e$ for all spacers (solid lines) are shown on Fig.8. Characteristic times for relaxation of spacer length increase from near 0.7 ns for $G1$ dendrimer to 6 ns for $G5$ dendrimer while the orientational times increase from 0.9ns to about 9ns. Thus the orientational relaxation times of spacers increase with generation number more than relaxation times for fluctuation of spacer lengths. This difference reflects the fact that the behavior of the orientational correlation function $P_1(t)$ is determined not only by the local mobility of the spacer but also by the rotation of the dendrimer as a whole. It is well known that the characteristic time of this rotation strongly depends on the particle size. For example for an impenetrable sphere it increases with the radius R as R^3. [31-32]

4 EFFECT OF THE TEMPERATURE

4.1 Structural characteristics of lysine dendrimers. MD results.

Because the NMR experiments at different temperatures were performed only for lysine dendrimers of the second and fourth generations we show in this part the results of MD simulation for these dendrimers. The corresponding temperature dependences of the gyration radius are shown on Fig. 9a: the size of dendrimers is practically independent of the temperature. At the same time the shape of dendrimer change with temperature. In particular the ratio of principal components R_{g1}:R_{g2}:R_{g3} and especially ratio R_{g1}:R_{g3} become more close to 1 with the temperature due to decrease of largest components R_{g1} and R_{g2} and increase of smallest component R_{g3} (data are not shown). Thus the shape of both G=2 and G=4 dendrimers become more spherical with increase of temperature.

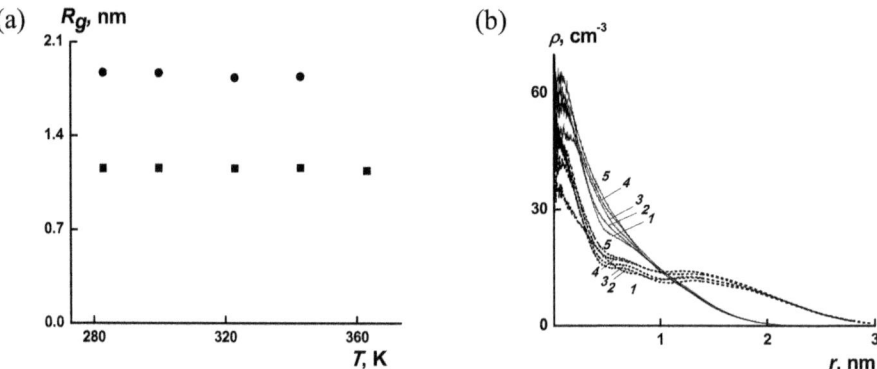

Figure 9 *The dependences of structural parameters of dendrimers obtained in the MD: the radius of gyration of the dendrimer and R_g (G = 2 - squares, G = 4 - a circles) on the temperature (a) and the density distribution function $\rho(r)$ of atoms of the dendrimer with respect to its center of mass for G = 2 (solid lines) and G = 4 (dashed lines) at temperatures T = 283K (1), 300K (2), 323K (3), 343K (4), 363K (5) (b).*

The weak effect of the temperature on the internal structure of the dendrimer is seen also from the temperature behavior of the radial density distribution function $\rho(r)$ of all atoms of the dendrimer with respect to its center of mass (see Fig.9b). The calculation of this function was done using the standard function g_rdf from the GROMACS package.[19]

4.2 Spacers' mobility

Time autocorrelation functions (ACFs) for fluctuation of spacers lengths (Eq. 9a) and orientations of spacers (Eq. 9b) calculated for $G=4$ dendrimers at different temperatures

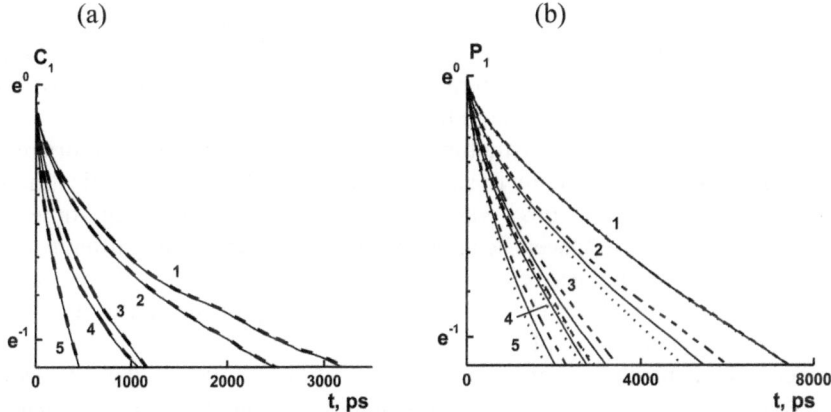

Figure 10. *Length (a) and orientational (b) ACF for G = 4-generation lysine dendrimers at T = 283 K (1), = 300 K (2), = 323 K (3), = 343 K (4), = 363 K (5) for short (dotted line), long (dashed line), and all (solid line) internal spacers. (The length autocorrelation function for short spacers decays faster than 1 ps for all dendrimers and it is not shown on Fig10a)*

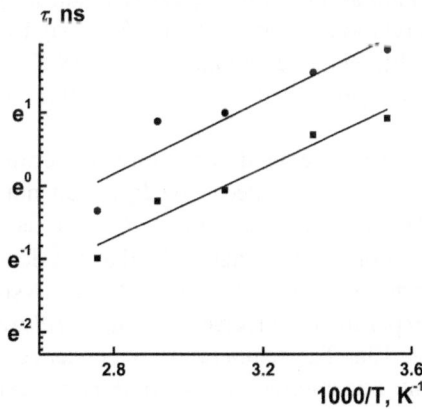

Figure 11 *Relaxation times for the length ACF (square) and orientational ACF (circle) of all internal spacers vs 1000/T. Solid lines are fitting curves by the Arrhenius equation $\ln(\tau) = A + E_a/k_BT$, where A is a constant, E_a is the activation energy and k_B is Boltzmann's constant*

Table 3 *Activation energies for relaxation times of long spacers for G=4 dendrimer, corresponding to the decay of the correlation functions from 1 to 1/e*

ACF type	E_a, kJ/mol
distance ACF	20 ± 2
orientational ACF	21 ± 4

from T=283K to 363K are presented in Fig.10. Length correlation function for short spacers decay faster than for 1 ps for all dendrimers and are not shown on Fig10a. The orientational ACF (Fig.10b) for short (dotted lines) and long (dashed lines) internal spacers calculated separately are very close to each other and to curves averaged through all internal spacers (solid lines) at all temperatures (similar behaviour was obtained for lysine dendrimer of different generation at room temperature, see Fig.7b).

The dependence of the characteristic times for fluctuation of lengths and orientations of spacers on the inverse temperature is shown in Fig.11. The characteristic times of the rotation autocorrelation functions were greater than corresponding times of the autocorrelation functions of spacers lengths at all temperatures. This difference between length and rotation correlations reflects the fact that the behavior of the orientational function $P_1(t)$ is determined not only by the local mobility of the spacer but also by the rotation of the dendrimer as a whole [27].

The temperature dependence of the relaxation times follows the Arrhenius law $\tau_{cor}(\mathbf{T}) = \tau_0 \exp(E_a / k_B \mathbf{T})$ where $\mathbf{T}$ is the temperature, k_B the Boltzmann constant, E_a the activation energy and τ_0 is a constant independent of the temperature. The activations energies obtained (see Tab.3) E_a =20 and 21kJ/mol for length and orientation correlation functions, respectively.

4.3 Local mobility. MD and NMR

For the comparison of the simulation results with NMR data we have calculated the second order orientational autocorrelation function $P_2(t)$ (Eq. (3)) for the H-H vectors in CH_2 groups of $G= 2$ and 4 dendrimers at temperatures $\mathbf{T} = 238$ K , 300 K , 323 K , 343 K and 363 K. The calculation was performed using the g_angle function from GROMACS package. [19]

Time dependences $P_2(t)$ were averaged separately for terminal (Fig.12a) and internal (Fig.12b) CH_2 groups. In all cases the decay of $P_2(t)$ can not be described by a single exponent as in equation (4). However, we use this equation as first approximation for the data analysis with the correlation time τ_{cor} determined as the decay time *of $P_2(t)$ correlation function to 1/e*. (A similar approach is used here in the analysis of experimental data for the spectral density). The experimental inverse *spin-lattice relaxation time* ($1/T_{1H}$) obtained by NMR are shown in Fig. 13a. The temperature dependences of $1/T_{1H}$ for terminal and internal groups are different. For internal groups there is a maximum on this dependence. At the same time the temperature dependence of $1/T_{1H}$ for terminal groups does not exhibit a maximum. This means that the correlation times for the terminal groups are much smaller than those for internal groups at the same temperatures. The maximum for internal groups of $G = 4$ dendrimer is shifted towards higher temperatures compared to the maximum for $G = 2$ dendrimer. Hence (from eq. (6)), the correlation times for internal groups of the $G = 4$ dendrimer are larger than for the $G = 2$ dendrimer. The presence of a maximum in the temperature dependence of $1/T_{1H}$ allows us to estimate correlation times for internal groups directly from experimental data (Fig. 13a) by using equations (1), (5) - (6). The value of the parameter A_0 was calculated from the experimental value of $1/T_{1H}$ in the maximum by use of the equation (6). The resulting value of $A_0 = 0.4 \times 10^{10}$ s^{-2} is slightly different from the value ($A_0 = 0.56 \times 10^{10}$ s^{-2}) obtained from equation (2) and tabulated constants of the bond length and bond angle for CH_2 groups. The correlation times for each temperature were calculated by using this value of A_0 and the experimental values of $1/T_{1H}$.

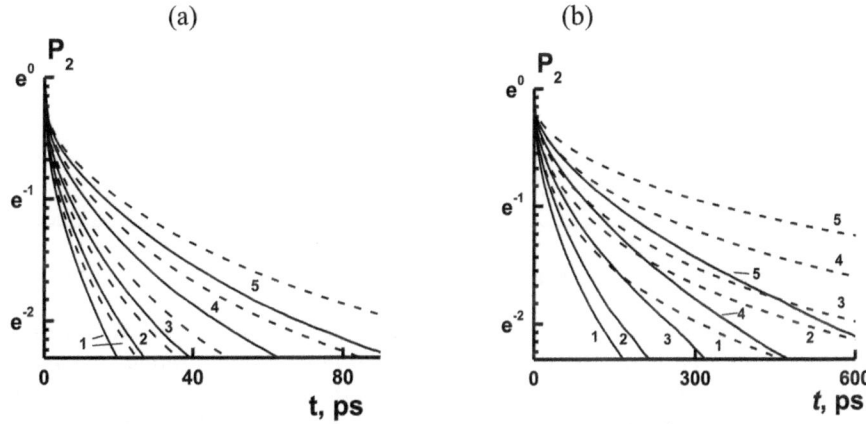

Figure 12 *Time dependence of the orientational autocorrelation function $P_2(t)$ for the terminal (a) and internal (b) CH_2 groups, shown in Fig. 2, at different temperatures, $T = 363K$ (1), $343K$ (2), $323K$ (3), $300K$ (4), $283K$ (5). The results of computer simulation for lysine dendrimers $G = 2$ (solid lines) and $G = 4$ (dashed lines)*

The values of τ_{cor} for both internal and terminal groups, obtained from simulation and from the NMR data at various temperatures are shown in Fig. 13b. For internal groups there is a semi-quantitative agreement between the results of computer simulation and experimental data. The existing difference can be attributed, at least partially, to the use of a simplified procedure to calculate the correlation time τ_{cor} based on the approximation that the correlation functions $P_2(t)$) decay single exponentially. On the other hand the slopes the correlation functions $P_2(t)$) decay single exponentially. On the other hand the slopes of temperature dependences of τ_{cor} obtained from simulation and NMR (see Fig. 13b) are close to each other. By using the Arrhenius equation the corresponding activation energies E_a were estimated (Table 4). The activation energy (19.9kJ/mol) for internal relaxation times τ_{cor} of H-H groups for G=4 dendrimer obtained by MD are close to activation energies (20 and 21 kJ/mol, (see Tab.3)) for relaxation times of autocorrelation functions of internal spacers length and orientation correspondingly (see eq. (9a) and eq. (9b)) obtained by the same method. The values of Ea for terminal groups were obtained from results of computer simulation by the same way (decay of $P_2(t)$ from 1 to $1/e$) as for internal groups. As to NMR data the absence of maximum in the temperature dependence of $1/T_{1H}$ does not allow direct calculation of the correlation times.
However, in this case, Ea can be determined by using the interval of temperatures, where

$\omega\tau_{cor}(\mathbf{T}) \ll 1$. The equation (1) can be re-written as

$$\ln(1/T_{1H}(\mathbf{T})) = \ln(B) + \ln(\tau_{cor}(\mathbf{T})) = \ln(B) + \ln(\tau_0) + \frac{E_a}{k_B \mathbf{T}}, \qquad (10)$$

where B and τ_o are the constants, independent of the temperature.

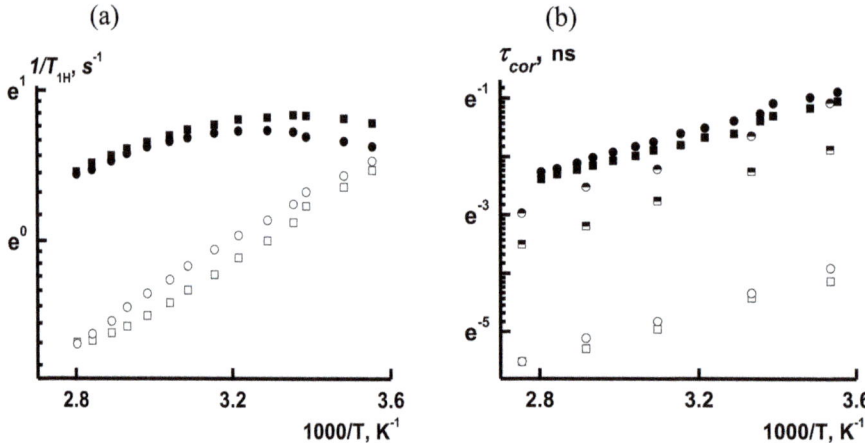

Figure 13 *Temperature dependence of the experimental spin-lattice relaxation time $1/T_{1H}$ for hydrogen atoms, corresponding to inner (solid symbols) and terminal (open symbols) CH$_2$ groups in lysine dendrimers of G = 2 (squares) and G = 4 (circles) (a). Temperature dependence of the correlation times for internal and terminal CH$_2$ groups. The results of computer simulation (open symbols (terminal groups and semi-filled symbols (internal groups)) and experimental (solid symbols, for internal groups only) for lysine dendrimers G = 2 (squares) and G = 4 (circles) (b).*

Using the equation (10) and linear dependence of $\ln(1/T_{1H})$ the value of Ea for terminal groups of dendrimers could be evaluated (Table 4). The experimental values of activation energy E_a for the terminal groups obtained using this procedure are in good agreement with simulation results. It is important to note that the activation energy of both terminal, and internal CH$_2$ groups in G = 4 dendrimer are larger then corresponding values for G = 2 dendrimer. This behavior differs from the behavior of the flexible model dendrimers (consisting of freely-jointed monomers) and NMR results for carbosilane dendrimers, where the internal correlation times are almost the same for dendrimers of different generations or for different internal subgenerations in the same dendrimer.[23–30]

Table 4 *Activation energy E_a for experimental and MD orientational correlation times τ_{cor} for terminal and internal CH$_2$ groups, shown in Fig. 2*

G	E_a, kJ/mol Terminal groups		E_a, kJ/mol Internal groups	
	NMR[a]	MD	NMR	MD
2	14.4	15.4	14.9	17.7
4	15.0	16.8	15.7	19.9

[a] *The calculation of E a was carried out from the slope of the temperature dependence of ln (1/T$_{1H}$) (see Fig. 13a) in the region where $1/T_{1H} \sim \tau_{cor}$.*

CONCLUSIONS

In this chapter we have described results of computer simulation of the polylysine dendrimers of different generations at room temperature and at different temperatures as well as NMR data for the same dendrimers. Simulations show that lysine dendrimers of generation G=1-5 have shape intermediate between plate-like and isotropic sphere and the anisotropy of shape ellipsoid decreases with G. The dendrimer size increases with generation number as $M^{0.34}$, where M is molecular weight of the dendrimer and the exponent 0.34 obtained is close to value 1/3 for a sphere with the constant density. The spacers in all lysine dendrimers are almost completely extended (up to 90% of the maximal possible extension). The angles between all short spacers in lysine dendrimers are almost fixed while angles between other spacers are more flexible. Relaxation times of spacers' length and orientation increase with the dendrimers size. Structural characteristics of lysine dendrimers do not depend on the temperature. The relaxation times of autocorrelation functions for spacer lengths (i.e. length of vector connecting neighboring branching points) and orientations increase with inverse temperature and activation energy of both processes are close to each other. The local correlation times (characteristic times of orientational mobility of CH_2 groups) of lysine dendrimers were studied by MD and NMR methods. Data obtained from MD simulation and NMR shows that the mobility of inner CH_2 groups is smaller than mobility of CH_2 terminal groups. This result is in agreement with results obtained for the flexible dendrimers both using coarse-grained and full atomic models.[23-30] At the same time, the local correlation times of internal groups are dependent on the size of the dendrimer. This behavior differs from that of flexible dendrimers simulated using both coarse grained model, consisting of freely-joint monomers, and full atomic model of carbosilane dendrimers, where the internal correlation times are practically the same for dendrimers of different generations or different internal subgenerations in the same dendrimer.[23-30] The activation energies for local correlation times of lysine dendrimers are close to activation energies for relaxation times for fluctuations of the internal spacers.

Authors acknowledge support from RFBR (grants 10-04-01156, 12-03-31243-mol-a), the Programme OHNM3 RAS and the EU Program COST TD0802. Computing resources on supercomputers "Lomonosov" and "Chebyshev" were provided by supercomputer center of Moscow State University.

References

1 E. Buhleier, W. Wehner, F.Vogtle, *Synthesis,* 1978, **2**, 155.

2 G.R. Newkome, Z.- q. Yao, G.R. Baker, V.K. Gupta, *J. Org. Chem.,* 1985 , **50**, 2003.

3 D.A. Tomalia, H. Baker, J. Dewald, M. Hall, G. Kallos, S. Martin, J. Roeck, J. Ryder, P.Smith, *Polym. J. (Tokyo, Jpn.)* 1985, **17**, 117.

4 C. Hawker, J.M.J. Frechet, *J. Chem. Soc., Chem. Commun.* 1990 , 1010.

5 R.G. Denkewalter, J. Kolc, W.J. Lukasavage, *Pat. 4 289872 USA*, 1981.

6 R.G. Denkewalter, J. Kolc, W.J. Lukasavage, *Pat. 4 410688 USA*, 1983.

7 L.Crespo, G.Sanclimens, M. Pons, E. Giralt, M. Royo, F. Albericio, *Chem. Rev.,* 2005, **105**, 1663.

8 J.P. Tam, Y. -A. Lu, J.-L.Yang, *Eur. J. Biochem.,* 2002, **269**, 923.

9 B. Klajnert, J. Janiszewska, Z. Urbanczyk-Lipkowska , M. Bryszewska, D.Shcharbin, M.Labieniec, *Int. J. Pharm.,* 2006, **309**, 208.

10 I.M. Neelov, A. Janaszewska, B. Klajnert, M. Bryszewska, N. Makova, D. Hicks, H. Pearson , G.P. Vlasov, M.Yu. Ilyash, D.S. Vasilev, N.M. Dubrovskaya, N.L. Tuma-nova, I.A. Zhuravin, A.J. Turner, N.N. Nalivaeva, *Curr. Med. Chem.*, 2013, **20,** 134.

11 Q. Yu, Y. Mu, L. Nordenskiold, J.P. Tam, *Understanding Biology Using Peptides,* Sylvie E. Blondelle (Editor), American Peptide Society, 2005.

12 S. Javor, E. Delort, T. Darbre, J.-L. Reymond, *J. Am. Chem. Soc.* 2007, **129**, 13238

13 S. Javor, J.-L. Reymond, *J. Org. Chem.* 2009, **74** , 3665.

14 B.P. Roberts, M.J. Scanlon, G.Y. Krippner, D.K. Chalmers, *Macromolecules,* 2009, **42**, 2775 .

15 B.P. Roberts, G.Y. Krippner, M.J. Scanlon, D.K. Chalmers, *Macromolecules,* 2009, **42**, 2784 .

16 G.P. Vlasov, V.I. Korolkov, G.A. Pankova, I.I. Tarasenko, A.N. Baranov, P.B. Glazkov, A.V. Kiselev, O.V.Ostapenko, E.A. Lesina, V.S. Baranov, *Bioorg. Chem.,* 2004, **30**, 15.

17 J.M.J. Frechet, D.A. Tomalia, *Dendrimers and Other Dendritic Polymers,* New York, John Wiley & Sons, 2002; S.M. Gray son, J.M.J. Frechet, *Chem. Rev.* 2001, **101**, 3819.

18 HyperChem (TM) Professional 7.5, Hypercube, Inc., 1115 NW 4th Street, Gainesville, Florida 32601, USA.

19 B. Hess, C. Kutzner, D. Spoel , E. Lindahl, *J. Chem. Theor. Comput.*, 2008, **4**, 435.

20 J.W. Ponder, D.A. Case, *Adv. Prot. Chem.*, 2003, **66,** 27.

21 B.R. Brooks, C.L. 3rd. Brooks, A.D. Jr. Mackerell, L. Nilsson, R.J. Petrella, B. Roux, Y. Won, G. Archontis, C. Bartels, S. Boresch, A. Caflisch, L. Caves, Q. Cui, A.R. Dinner, M. Feig, S. Fischer, J. Gao, M. Hodoscek, W. Im, K. Kuczera, T. Lazaridis, J. Ma, V. Ovchinnikov, E. Paci, R.W. Pastor, C.B. Post, J.Z. Pu, M. Schaefer, B. Tidor, R.M. Venable, H.L. Woodcock, X. Wu, W. Yang, D.M. York, M. Karplus, *J. Comput. Chem.,* 2009, **30**, 1545.

22 W.L. Jorgensen, J. Chandrasekhar, J. D. Madura, R. W. Impey, M. L. Klein, *J. Chem. Phys.* 1983, **79**, 926.

23 M.A. Mazo, M. Yu. Shamaev, N. K. Balabaev, A. A. Darinskii, I. M. Neelov *Phys. Chem. Phys .,* 2004 , **6** , 1285.

24 D.A. Markelov, V.V. Matveev, P. Ingman, M.N. Nikolaeva, E. Lahderanta, V.A. Shevelev, N.I. Boiko, *J. Phys. Chem. B*, 2010, **114**, 4159.

25 R. Novoa-Carballal, E. Sawen, E. Fernandez-Megia, J. Correa, R. Riguera, G.Widmalm, *Phys. Chem. Chem Phys.,* 2010, **12**, 6587.

26 D.A. Markelov, V.V. Matveev, P. Ingman, E. Lahderanta, N.I. Boiko, *J. Chem. Phys.* 2011, **135**, 124901.

27 D.A. Markelov, M.A. Mazo, N.K. Balabaev, Yu.Ya. Gotlib, *Polymer Sci. Ser. A,* 2013, **55**, 53.

28 Yu.Ya. Gotlib, D.A. Markelov, *Polymer Sci., Ser. A,* 2007, **49**, 1137.

29 D.A. Markelov, Yu.Ya. Gotlib, A.A. Darinskii, A.V. Lyulin, S.V. Lyulin, *Polymer Sci. Ser. A*, 2009, **51**, 329.

30 D.A. Markelov, S.V. Lyulin, Yu.Ya. Gotlib, A.V. Lyulin, V.V. Matveev, E. Lahderanta, A.A. Darinskii, *J.Chem.Phys*, 2009, **130**, 044907.

31 P.J.Flory, *Statistical Mechanics of Chain Molecules.*, Interscience, 1969.

32 V. N. Tsvetkov, E. Eskin, S. Ya. Frenkel, *Structure of Macromolecules in Solution,* (National Lending Library for Science and Technology, UK, Ed. C. Crane-Robinson) , 1971, **1**, 276.

CHARACTERIZATION OF DENDRIMERS AND THEIR INTERACTIONS WITH BIOMOLECULES FOR MEDICAL USE BY MEANS OF ELECTRON MAGNETIC RESONANCE

M. F. Ottaviani,[1] D. Appelhans,[2] F. Javier de la Mata,[3] S. García-Gallego,[3] A.Fattori,[1] C. Coppola,[1] M. Cangiotti,[1] L. Fiorani,[1] J. P. Majoral,[4] A. M. Caminade,[4] M. Bryszewska,[5] D. K. Smith,[6] N. Garti,[7] B. Klajnert[5]

[1] DiSTeVA, University of Urbino, Scientific Campus, Loc. Crocicchia, 61029 Urbino, Italy
[2] Leibniz Institute of Polymer Research Dresden, Hohe Str. 6, Dresden, Germany
[3] Dept. Química Inorgánica, Universidad de Alcalá, Farmacia, Alcalá de Henares, Spain.
[4] Laboratoire de Chimie de Coordination, CNRS Toulouse, France
[5] Department of General Biophysics, University of Lodz, Lodz, Poland
[6] Department of Chemistry, University of York, Heslington, York, UK
[7] Casali Inst. Applied Chemistry, The Hebrew University, Givat Ram, Jerusalem, Israel

1 INTRODUCTION

The interest to gain more fundamental knowledge about highly branched architectures combined with the high potential for applications in material science and life sciences, stimulate scientists towards strong research efforts in the expanding field of dendrimer chemistry.[1-5] The success of dendrimers is based on the availability of large molecules with unusual properties which makes them suitable for a broad range of applications. The similarities between dendrimers and globular proteins, in terms of structure and surface properties allowed dendrimers to be utilized in medical applications. Different types of dendrimers have been revealed to be successful in delivering DNA, drugs and biomolecules to target cells.

The outer shell of a dendrimer allows multiple functionalities to be added. Polyvalency provides for versatile functionalization which may produce multiple interactions with biological receptor sites, for example, in the design of antiviral therapeutic agents. Different ligands can be coupled to dendrimers to use them as transfection reagents. Functionalization of the periphery can also result in copolymers with interesting properties, such as viscosity, stability, etc.. Dendrimer properties can be easily tuned by modifying the end groups, for instance to modify the solubility in organic solvents, in CFC or in water.

Metal functionalization of the periphery has applications, for example, in catalysis. Other applications include sensing, nanoscale templates, ionic conductivity and photonic or electronic applications. Easy functionalization is also a key to enabling compatibility with other materials. The high number of reaction points can also allow dendrimers to concentrate materials to allow detection without use of amplification like MRI (Magnetic Resonance Imaging) contrast agents.

The Electron Paramagnetic Resonance (EPR) technique has been very precious to gain specific information about the dendrimer structural properties and, mainly, about the interacting ability of poly(amidoamine) (PAMAM) dendrimers towards cell membrane models, peptide and proteins, DNA and polynucleotides.[6-13] In detail, we used both the spin label and the spin probe techniques in order to characterize the dendrimers and their interactions with the biomolecular structures.

To characterize the dendrimer structure and interacting properties by means of EPR, we found it very useful to use cupric ions (Cu^{2+}).[14-21] They may enter the dendrimer structure and form complexes with the nitrogen and oxygen sites. These complexes are well identified and characterized, for their structure, geometry and mobility conditions, by means of computer aided EPR analysis. This kind of study provides interesting information about the interacting and structural properties of the dendrimer in the different regions, as a function of the chemical composition, the generation and the experimental conditions, as such as pH and ion and dendrimer concentrations.

The computer aided analysis of the EPR spectra of Cu(II)-PAMAM dendrimer complexes has already been demonstrated to be a very powerful tool to get information on the dendrimer structure and the complexation ability of different external and internal dendrimer sites.[14-17] Especially the knowledge about the location of the Cu(II) complexes within the dendritic structure is very important for the application of dendrimers as metal ion carriers in a biological environment.

In this context, in the first part of the studies presented in this report arising from collaborations in the framework of the COST action TD0802, we characterized different dendrimers by analysing the complexes formed with Cu^{2+} in water solutions in different experimental conditions.[18-21] We want to underline that we describe here the results of studies on dendrimer characterization by means of Cu(II) complexation which are already finished, but other studies are in progress on similar characterization also in collaboration with other COST members, as such as Profs. Ling Peng, Jorn Christensen, Roxana Piticescu, Jean-Pierre Majoral and Rimantas Vaisnoras

First, we selected glycodendrimers, synthesized and characterized as described by Prof. Appelhans and coworkers.[18] We aimed to characterize the Cu(II) complexation of 3rd – 5th generation PPI possessing dense maltose and maltotriose shell (Scheme 1).

The motivation of this part of our studies is to know if an extended dendritic PPI scaffold, surrounded by a dense oligosaccharide shell, is able to undergo the desired metal ion complexation in aqueous solution and if oligosaccharide shells affect internal or external metal ion complexation in the sphere of the dendrimers. This study allows a step forward in the development of dendritic metal ion carrier systems in a biological environment. In this context, the location and coordination of generation-dependent Cu(II)-dendrimer complexes were revealed by the EPR study.

Second, we studied the Cu(II) complexes with anionic carbosilane dendrimers with the aim to characterize the interacting ability of theses dendrimers towards metal ions, to be used for biomedical purposes.[19-20] Prof. De la Mata research group has already reported the synthesis and biomedical studies of anionic carbosilane dendrimers in their use as HIV-microbicides.[22] In search for a higher activity that can be provided by multivalency we have used anionic carbosilane dendrimers previously described,[22] to obtain new copper complexes that are herein characterized by EPR.[20]

Third, we performed an EPR characterization of dendrons synthesized by the group of Prof. David Smith, by both using copper ions and nitroxide radicals.[21] We characterized amine-functionalised dendrons with a cholesterol unit at the focal point which leads to self-assembly, enhanced DNA binding, and in some cases, significantly enhanced gene delivery capability.[23-24] We reported a computer aided EPR analysis of amine-functionalized dendrons with two different types of branching (G1-amide/ether and G2-ester) and with different groups at the focal point, that is a benzyl ester, or one or two cholesterol groups. We characterized the structure and interacting ability of these dendrons by means of Cu(II), which allowed analysis of the branching and peripheral groups of the dendron responsible for DNA binding, but we also analysed the aggregates formed by the dendrons using a probe, the 5-doxylstearic acid (5-DSA), able to insert into the hydrophobic domain of the aggregates formed by self-assembly of the focal point groups and report about their structure and physic-chemical properties.

The same 5-DSA probe was used to study the encapsulation of a second generation (G-2) of poly(propylene imine) dendrimer (PPI) into lamellar, diamond reverse cubic and reverse hexagonal LLCs composed of GMO (glycerol monooleate), and water (and D-α-tocopherol in the H_{II} system).[25] Such complex prospective drug delivery system was created by the group of Prof. Nissim Garti in order to enhance the performance of dendrimers as delivery agents. These LLCs based on monoglyceride were shown to form inverse water-in-oil structures such as lamellar, cubic, and reverse hexagonal which can be specifically used to solubilize dendrimers and enhance their delivery as therapeutic agent for oral and transdermal release. Comprehensive understanding of the structural properties of the LLC/dendrimer complexes is imperative for rational and successful tailoring of these potential delivery vehicles.

Similar studies are in progress on different dendrimer nanocarriers based on surfactant aggregates like vesicles and liposomes in collaboration with Profs. Garti, Demetzos, Fessas and Assimopoulou in the framework of the COST action TD0802.

The second part of this report deals on the use of EPR probes to monitor the formation of amyloid and prion fibrils, responsible of neurodegenerative diseases, and the role of different dendrimers to prevent the fibril formation.[26-27] Currently, there are not efficient treatments for the neurodegenerative diseases, as such as Alzheimer, which are eventually fatal. Therefore there is a continuous need to explore new therapeutical possibilities. Dendrimers have demonstrated to be promising materials in biomedical applications as drug carriers and transfection agents.[28-34] Especially, the interaction features of the phosphorous dendrimers synthesized by the group of Profs. Majoral and Caminade,[35] and the dense shell glycodendrimers synthesized by the group of Prof. Applehans[18] showed to be very active to prevent the formation of peptide fibrils formed by the amyloid peptide Aβ1-28 and the prion peptide PrP185-208 - both responsible for neurodegenerative disorders. These two sequences were selected because they contain the fibrilization sites and present a structural homology, which could play an important role in amyloidogenic process. The computer aided analysis of the EPR spectra was therefore used to monitor the aggregation behaviour over time in the absence and presence of phosphorous dendrimers at generation 4 and PPI dendrimers at generation 5 decorated with sugar units (maltose and maltotriose) thus providing precious information on the kinetics of aggregation and the type of interactions occurring in the system.[26-27] G4-G5 sizes are comparable with the average protein size usually present in the biomedium. These last studies aiming to use dendrimers to treat and prevent neurodegenerative diseases were performed in collaboration with Profs. Majoral, Caminade, Appelhans, Klajnert, and Bryszewska in the framework of the COST action TD0802.

2 METHOD AND RESULTS

2.1 Materials and Sample Preparation Procedures

2.1.1 Dendrimers. The dendrimers and dendrons used for the studies reported here were the following:

(a) poly(propyleneimine) (PPI) dendrimers of second (DAB-Am8), third(DABAm16), fourth (DAB-Am32) and fifth generations (DAB-Am62). The Synthesis and characterization procedure of DAB-Am8, DABAm16, DAB-Am32, and DAB-Am62 fully decorated with maltose and maltotriose units has been deeply described in ref 18. The structure is shown in Figure 1;

(b) carbosilane dendrimers decorated with anionic carboxylate and sulfonate moieties, whose synthesis has been previously described.[22] Their chemical structure and nomenclature is as follows:

G_0SulfNa : $G0(Si)-[CH_2CH_2CH_2N(CH_2CH_2SO_3Na)_2]$
G_1SulfNa : $G1(Si)-[CH_2CH_2CH_2N(CH_2CH_2SO_3Na)_2]_4$
G_2SulfNa : $G2(Si)-[CH_2CH_2CH_2N(CH_2CH_2SO_3Na)_2]_8$
G_0COONa: $G0(Si)-CH_2CH_2CH_2N(CH_2CH_2CO_2Na)_2$
G_1COONa: $G1(Si)-[CH_2CH_2CH_2N(CH_2CH_2CO_2Na)_2]_4$
G_2COONa: $G2(Si)-[CH_2CH_2CH_2N(CH_2CH_2CO_2Na)_2]_8$

(c) the dendrons we have analyzed are termed Z-G2, Chol-G1, Chol-G2 and $Chol_2$-G2 (Figure 2). The dendrons were synthesized and purified as previously reported.[23-24]
(d) Phosphorus dendrimer generation 4 (P-dendrimer G4) was synthesized as described previously.[35] Its chemical formula is as follows:

N_3P_3-[O-(C_6H_4)-CH=N-NMe-PS-(O-(C_6H_4)-CH=N-NMe-PS-(O-(C_6H_4)-CH=N-NMe-PS-(O-(C_6H_4)-CH=N-NMe-PS-(NH-CH_2-CH_2-N^+HEt_2 $Cl^-)_2)_2)_2)_2]_6$

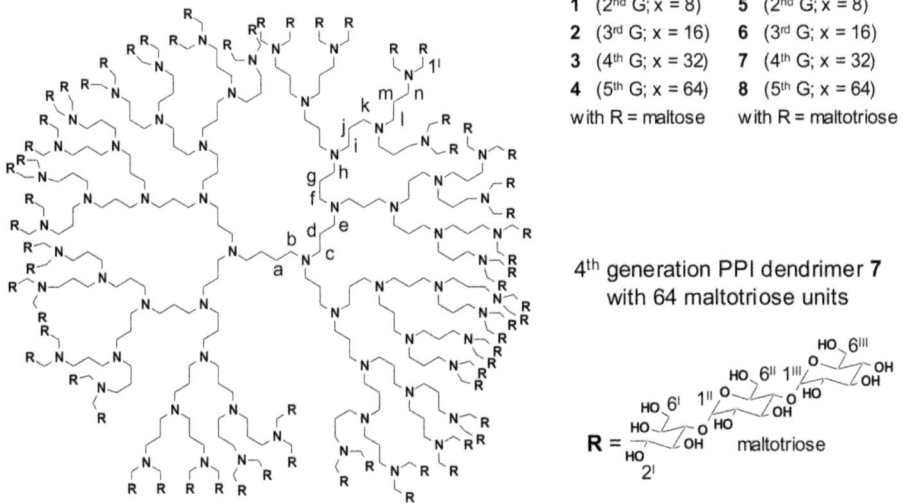

1   (2nd G; x = 8)   5   (2nd G; x = 8)
2   (3rd G; x = 16)   6   (3rd G; x = 16)
3   (4th G; x = 32)   7   (4th G; x = 32)
4   (5th G; x = 64)   8   (5th G; x = 64)
with R = maltose   with R = maltotriose

4th generation PPI dendrimer **7**
with 64 maltotriose units

R = maltotriose

Figure 1 *Structure of 4th generation PPI glycodendrimer*

2.1.2 Characterization of dendrimers by means of Cu^{2+} ions. Both dendrimers and copper nitrate hydrate ($Cu(NO_3)_2$ * $2.5H_2O$, Sigma-Aldrich, ACS reagent 98%) were dissolved in deionized water. The concentration of dendrimers was 0.1M in the external surface groups (each generation, the dendrimer concentration was multiplied by the number of surface groups), whereas the concentration of Cu(II) was varied from 0.002 to 0.1 M.

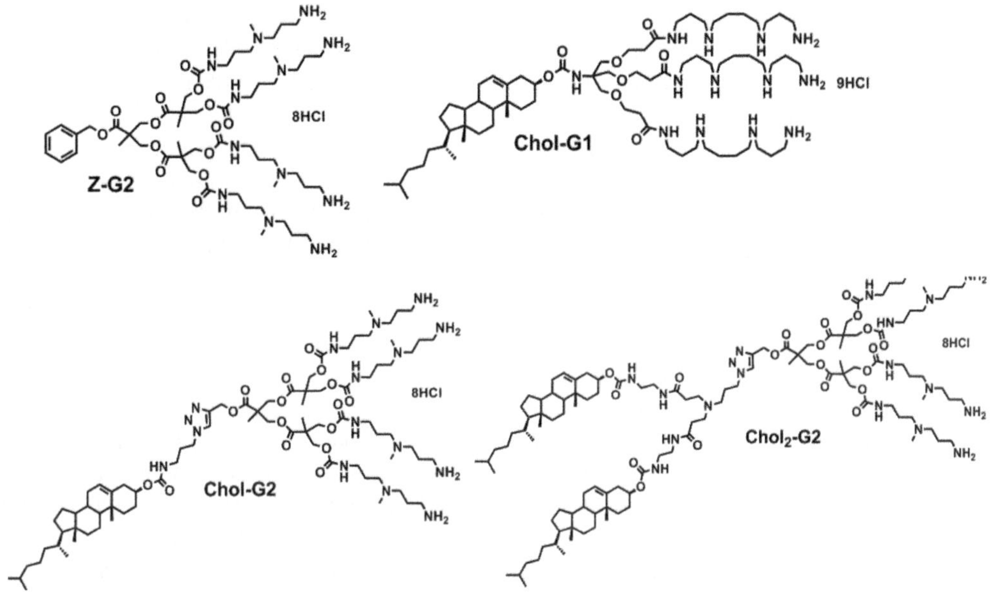

Figure 2 *Structures of self-assembling dendrons*

After different equilibration times (freshly prepared to 24 h), 100µl of the dendrimer–copper solution was inserted into an EPR tube (1 mm internal diameter). In all cases, reproducibility of the results was controlled by repeating the EPR analysis three times under identical experimental conditions for each sample.

2.1.3 Nitroxide spin probes. The nitroxide spin probe 4-octyl-dimethylammonium,2,2,6,6-tetramethyl-piperidine-1-oxyl bromide (CAT8) was kindly provided by Dr. X. Lei, Columbia University, New York., The nitroxide radicals 5-doxylstearic acid (5-DSA), 2,2,6,6-tetramethyl-piperidine-1-oxyl (Tempo), 4-hydroxy-2,2,6,6-tetramethyl-piperidine-1-oxyl (Tempol) and 4-threemethylammonium,2,2,6,6-tetramethyl-piperidine-1-oxyl bromide (CAT1) were purchased from Sigma-Aldrich and used as received., The spin probes were directly solubilized into the system to be studied at a concentration 0.1 – 0.5 mM. Before performing the EPR study we verified that the probe did not perturb the structure of the system (by varying the probe concentration and then verifying the invariance of the EPR spectrum). Since 5-DSA is not soluble in water and cannot be added to the water solutions as a solid at too low weights, a solution of 5-DSA in chloroform was prepared at a concentration of 1 mM. Then, the chloroform from 100 µL of 5-DSA solution was completely evaporated from a vial and, after that, 200 µL of the dendrimer or dendron water solution at the proper concentration was added into the vial and left to equilibrate with stirring in a cold, dark place for 1 h (longer equilibration times did not produce any difference in the results).

2.1.4 Peptide solutions. Synthetic peptides:
Aβ1–28 [DAEFRHDSGYEVHHQKLFVFFAEDVGSNK]
and PrP185-208 [KQHTVTTTTKGENFTETDVKMMER] were purchased from JPT Peptide Technology GmbH (Germany). Peptide stock solution (1 mM) was kept in 10 mM phosphate buffer pH 7.4 EPR experiments.

2.1.5 Formation of peptide fibrils in the absence and presence of dendrimers. CAT8 radical was found to be a good spin probe to monitor the formation of peptide fibrils. Other nitroxide radicals, Tempo, Tempol and CAT1 were also tested, but results are not shown since they were not informative (mainly, these radicals gave rise to very low intensity signals after fibril formation constituted by only one component). The peptides, $A\beta_{1-28}$ and $PrP_{185-208}$ solved in phosphate buffer at pH 7.4, were diluted to a final concentration of 0.5 mM (500 μM) by adding CAT8 at a concentration of 0.05 mM. Then, the aggregation was triggered by decreasing the pH to 5.5 (by titrating with diluted HCl) and adding heparin at a final concentration of 0.41 mg/mL. The aggregation process was followed both in the absence and in the presence of the dendrimers, added (before acidification and heparin addition) at concentrations 1, 10 and 100 μM for the glycodendrimer, while only the 10 μM concentration was used for the P-dendrimer.

At room temperature spectra of CAT8 in the peptide systems after acidification and heparin addition showed negligible line shape variations over time, since the paramagnetic species exchanged fast among the solution and the peptide interphase. To slow down this exchange rate, we recorded EPR spectra at 255 K by taking portions of each peptide solution (before and after acidification and heparin addition), in the absence and in the presence of the dendrimers and at subsequent times. The temperature of 255 K was selected to well differentiate in the spectra the interacting and non interacting radicals.

2.2 Method

EPR spectra were recorded by means of a EMX-Bruker spectrometer operating at X band (9.5 GHz) and interfaced with a PC (software from Bruker for handling and analysis of the EPR spectra). The temperature was controlled with a Bruker ST3000 variable-temperature assembly cooled with liquid nitrogen. The EPR spectra were recorded for the different samples as a function of temperatures (in the room temperature range, from 318 K down to 250 K; then, directly at 150 K).

2.3 Computation of EPR Spectra

2.3.1 Cu(II) Spectra. The low temperature EPR spectra were computed by using the Bruker's WIN-EPR SimFonia Software Version 1.25, and by the method reported in Ref. 36. The parameters used for the computation were the g_{ii} components (accuracy in the third decimal, on the basis of the computation itself) for the coupling between the electron spin and the magnetic field; the A_{ii} components (accuracy of about 3 %) for the coupling between the electron spin and the nuclear spin ($I_{Cu} = 3/2$) and the line widths of the x, y, and z lines. Transitions where $\Delta M_I \# 0$ were not included in the simulations. **A** and **g** were assumed to have the same principal axes, and a Gaussian lineshape was used. The values of the **g** and **A** parameters giving the best agreement with the experimental data were found by trial and error. In most cases the spectra are constituted by several components due to different coordination and complex geometries of Cu(II) in the dendrimer structure. In some cases, the subtraction between the spectra in different experimental conditions allowed to extract the signals constituting the overall spectra. In all cases we tried to get a fitting of an experimental signal by adding a maximum of two computed components, reproducing the main spectral features. However, the different components - or extracted by subtraction, or computed, - were normalized and then doubly integrated to calculate the integral area (to be used to calculate the relative intensities of the components). This means that, by both, subtraction procedure of experimental spectra and adding computed components to fit the experimental spectra, we obtained the relative percentages of the different components, with an accuracy of 3 %. We noted that simulations of observed ESR signals provide a useful means of estimating the spectral parameters but do not necessarily produce unique fits. However, we trusted the parameters which provided best fitting of a series of spectra in similar experimental conditions.

2.3.2 Nitroxide radical spectra. Computation was then performed by using Budil and Freed's program,[36] and the main parameters extracted from computation were: (a) the A_{ii} components of the hyperfine coupling tensor **A** for the coupling between the electron spin (S=1/2) and the nitrogen nuclear spin (I=1; n. of lines= 2I+1=3). The average $<A_N>=(A_{xx}+A_{yy}+A_{zz})/3$, which provides a measure of the environmental polarity of the nitroxide group; (b) the rotational diffusion mobility of the probe around the main geometrical axis (τ). An increase of this parameter indicates an increase of the local microviscosity, corresponding to an increase in the strength of interaction

2.4 Cu(II) Complexation of Glycodendrimers.

Cu(II) from water solutions localized in different sites, internally and at the periphery (externally), of glycodendrimers in water solutions. The Cu(II) coordination is affected by (i) the nature of the functional groups in the periphery (NH_2 or tertiary amino groups bearing maltose or maltotriose units), (ii) the generation (generation 2 to 5, termed G2-G5), and (iii) the Cu(II)/dendrimer ratio.[18] Different equilibration times (from freshly prepared to one day aging) did not influence the results.

The room temperature spectra are characteristic of slow motion conditions of Cu(II), since the cupric ions are trapped in the dendrimer structure. The anisotropic **g** and **A** components are already well resolved at room temperature and progressively change towards a rigid motion by decreasing the temperature. The spectral features and magnetic parameters obtained from simulation indicated two main geometries of the complexes: axial, characterized by $g_1>>g_2\geq g_3$, and rhombic, characterized by $g_1>g_2>g_3$.

Figure 3 shows: (a) an example of computation for G2-maltose (150 K) obtained by adding two axial components at different relative percentages, and (b) the differences among the spectra of G3-, G4-and G5-maltotriose due to different weights of two components, one axial and one rhombic.

The axial component (65 %) in Figure 3 for G2-maltose was attributed, on the basis of the magnetic parameters, to a $Cu-N_2O_2$ or a $Cu-NO_3$ coordination, corresponding to a square planar symmetry with a small but not negligible trigonal distortion. The less intense (35 %) component, also axial, was attributed to a $Cu-O_4$ coordination. By increasing generation, the nitrogen richer coordination increases its relative intensity (up to 80 % for G3) at the expenses of the oxygen richer coordination. These results indicate that Cu(II) ions are internalized within the dendrimer structure, and the nitrogen coordination becomes more favoured when the dendrimer structure becomes more rigid at high generation, with a larger number of nitrogen sites.

But, for glycodendrimers from G = 3 to G = 5, the spectra show two contributions from both an *axial* and a *rhombic* geometries. By increasing generation the axial component of copper decreases its relative intensity with respect to the rhombic component.

(a)   (b)

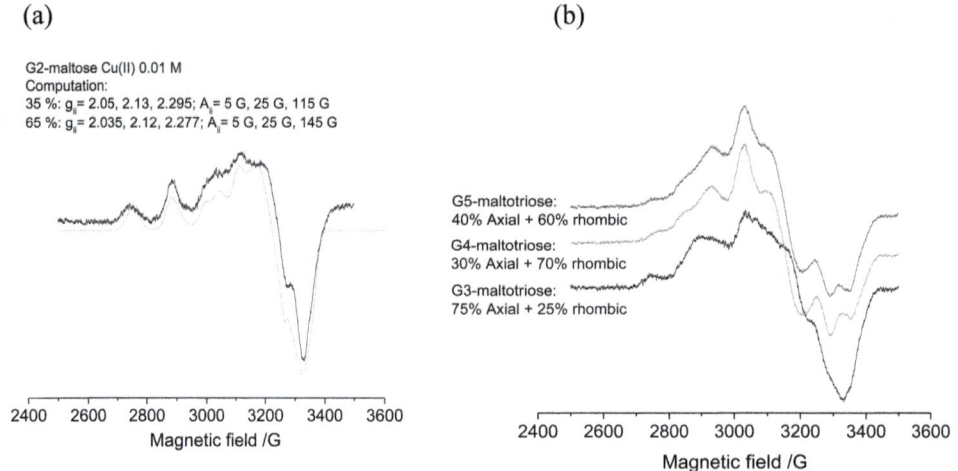

Figure 3 *(a) Example of computation for G2-maltose (150 K) obtained by adding two axial components at different relative percentages; (b) differences among the spectra of G3-, G4-and G5-maltotriose due to different weights of two components, one axial and one rhombic.*

Essentially the nitrogen complexation site for Cu(II) may be identified in the less congested area within the dendrimer, while the rhombic geometry (a distorted trigonal bipyramidal structure with a mixed ligand coordination for oxygen and nitrogen) arises from ions trapped into the dendrimer congested periphery and coordinating to both nitrogen and maltose or maltotriose OH groups . The smaller the dendrimer, the more mobile the branches and the more Cu(II) ions retains an axial symmetry where the maltose unit and water molecules can also coordinate Cu(II). The bigger the dendrimer, the larger the amount of nitrogen sites available for the axial coordination and the more congested the dendrimer periphery.

However, glycodendrimers with maltose shell show a smaller percentage of rhombic component with respect to the maltotriose ones since the constraint exerted by the sugar functions in the periphery is stronger for maltotriose compared to maltose. Furthermore, compared to maltose, the maltotriose units favour the copper-coordination with 4 nitrogen sites even at the lowest generation. This is again due to the constraint induced by the maltotriose units and the larger size and rigidity of the dendrimer structure at the lower generations.

By increasing the copper concentration, the *rhombic* component relatively decreases in intensity and the *axial* component arising from nitrogen coordination progressively broadens due to spin-spin interactions between Cu(II) in close positions. Mainly a Cu-O_4 coordination due to Cu(II) coordinating oxygen ligands was formed after saturation of the internal sites. It is interesting to note that the amino functionalized dendrimers show a resolved Cu-N_4 coordination at this Cu(II) concentration, as previously found for the amino functionalized PAMAM dendrimers.[15] This means that the sugar units lead to a lower capacity of the dendrimers to internalize the Cu(II) at the different nitrogen sites, like a structural barrier which partially impedes the localization of Cu(II) in the internal dendrimer generations.

The intensity of the broad component linearly decreases with the increase in generation since the available external-surface sites increase by increasing the dendrimer size.

2.5 Cu(II) Complexation of Carbosilane Dendrimers

The carbosilane dendrimers at generations 0, 1 and 2 showed an interesting behavior when increasing amounts of cupric ions were added.[20] Table 1 reports the main parameters obtained from the computations.

The carboxylate dendrimers give rise to two spectral components. On the basis of the magnetic parameters one indicate a location of the ions in complexation sites containing one nitrogen and 3 oxygen coordinating atoms in a square planar geometry in restricted mobility conditions. The comparison with the spectra obtained with the simple ligands,[19] and the slow motion conditions at room temperature are strongly in favour of a partial internalization of the ions into the dendrimer structure. The second component is appearing for G1 and G2 generations at Cu(II) concentrations higher than 0.0025 M, but it significantly increases in intensity with respect to the first component only at concentrations higher than 0.01 M. This component too is in slow motion conditions but the magnetic and mobility parameters indicate a weaker coordination with respect to the first component. The amount of the second component increases with the increase in generation. These results indicate that this second component arises from ions localized in the external layers (generations) of the dendrimer, where the square planar coordination of Cu(II) is more distorted also due to the branches mobility. This component increases and then decreases in intensity by increasing Cu(II) concentration (Figure 4).

Table 1 *Main parameters obtained from the computations of the EPR spectra*

Dendrimer	[Cu(II)]/M - T/K	g_{xx}	g_{yy}	g_{zz}	$<g>$	A_{xx}/G	A_{yy}/G	A_{zz}/G	$<A>$/G	τ/ns ω_{ex}/Gs
G*n*COONa	0.0025 - 298	2.015	2.022	2.225	2.086	10	20	157	63	2.35
G0COONa	0.02 - 298 (subt.0.01)	2.014	2.060	2.258	2.110	10	20	155	62	0.05
G2COONa	0.025 - 298 (subt.0.01)	2.014	2.060	2.258	2.110	10	20	155	62	1.32
G*n*COONa	0.0025 - 150	2.015	2.022	2.225	2.086	10	20	157	63	
G*n*COONa	0.025 - 150 (subt.0.01)	2.014	2.060	2.258	2.110	10	20	155	62	
G*n*COONa	0.05 - 150	2.029	2.053	2.323	2.135	5	15	136	52	
G*n*SulfNa	0.02 - 298	2.039	2.050	2.365	2.151	2	2	120	40	0.33 0.25
G*n*SulfNa	0.02 - 150	2.039	2.050	2.365	2.151	5	15	123	47	
G1SulfNa	0.015 - 150	2.012	2.027	2.236	2.092	5	5	156	55	

At Cu concentration of 0.05 M the spectrum is at quite low intensity. The parameters of computation (Table 1) are characteristic of a square planar coordination of copper with 4 oxygen sites where 2 of them probably belong to the carboxylate groups, whereas the other oxygens belong to water molecules externally to the dendrimer.

For the sulphate decorated carnbosilane dendrimers, we do not see any signal at the lowest copper contents. This effect arises from the formation of dimeric copper species which are EPR silent. This behaviour was not found in our previous study where only the external functions of these dendrimers were used as copper ligands.[19] This means that these dimeric species are formed at the dendrimer internal/external layer. At generation 1 a signal due to Cu(II) coordinating one nitrogen site is present at Cu concentrations of 0.015 M. At $[Cu^{2+}]$ = 0.02 M for all generations we found a spectrum which corresponds to copper ions mainly coordinating to water molecules and, probably, with one or two sulfonate groups at the external dendrimer surface. This means that, after saturating the dimeric coordination for all generations, at higher generation, copper ions are pushed to the external dendrimer surface to be complexed by the sulfonate groups and water. Interestingly, the increase in generation also provokes an increase in a broad component at low temperature. This means that, higher the generation, closer the external sulphonate sites where the copper ions are localizing.

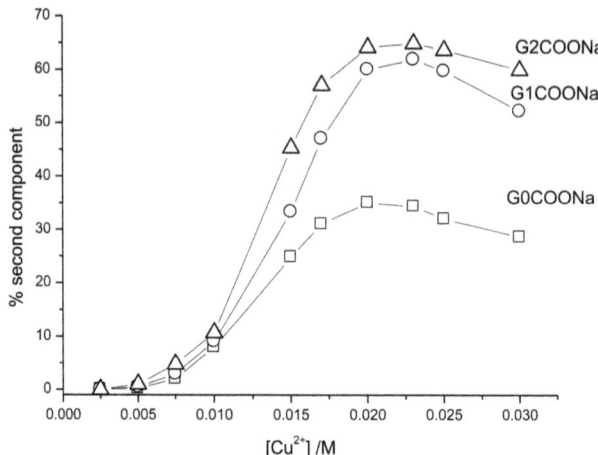

Figure 4 *Variation of the percentage of the second component as a function of Cu(II) concentration for the GnCOONa dendrimers*

2.6 Cu Complexation of Z-G2, Chol-G1, Chol-G2 and Chol$_2$-G2 Dendrons

At the lowest Cu(II) concentrations it was possible to identify two signals constituting the spectra of Cu(II) coordinating **Z-G2**, **Chol-G1**, **Chol-G2** and **Chol$_2$-G2** dendrons (structures in Figure 2).[21] These signals were termed "internal" (dendron-bound) and "external" (solvent-bound) copper, on the basis of the line shapes and the magnetic parameters extracted from computation (Table 2). The "external" component arises from Cu^{2+} ions which do not directly coordinate with dendron groups because the interacting sites are already saturated. Dendron **Z-G2** has much more 'external' copper(II) than either **Chol-G2** or **Chol$_2$-G2**. All of these dendrons only differ in the nature of the group attached at the focal point and the presence of the 1,2,3-triazole unit. We therefore suggest that the binding of copper coordination is favoured by the aggregation (micellization) of the dendrons and by the presence of 1,2,3-triazole unit and, therefore, it is favoured for **Chol-G2** and **Chol$_2$-G2** with respect to **Z-G2**.

Table 2 *Main magnetic parameters obtained from the computations of the spectra*

Dendron	g_{xx}	g_{yy}	g_{zz}	A_{xx}/G	A_{yy}/G	A_{zz}/G	$A_{zz}/x10^4 s^{-1}$
Z-G2	2.037	2.085	2.332	3	5	130	141.5
Chol-G1	2.033	2.095	2.325	3	5	132	143.3
Chol-G2	2.03	2.08	2.312	3	3	140	151.1
Chol$_2$-G2	2.03	2.08	2.312	3	3	140	151.1

On the basis of the magnetic parameters reported in the Table, the copper coordination can be assigned to Cu-NO$_3$ (for **Z-G2** and **Chol-G1**) and Cu-N$_2$O$_2$ (for **Chol-G2** and

Chol$_2$-G2) with distorted square planar coordination geometries. Nitrogen coordination only comes from unprotonated nitrogen sites, and a significant number of the amines will be protonated under the experimental conditions. The further nitrogen coordination for **Chol-G2** and **Chol$_2$-G2** with respect to **Z-G2** and **Chol-G1** may be ascribed to the presence of the triazole group, or alternatively, the self-assembly of the dendrons leading to lower degrees of protonation in the surface amine groups, and hence greater Cu(II) binding. Dendron **Z-G2** does not have a triazole and does not self-assemble and presumably predominantly binds Cu(II) via the ester groups in the dendron framework. Compound **Chol-G1** shows the least effective Cu(II) internalisation, and it is notable that this is the only dendron with a wholly different (amide/ether) 'Newkome-type' branching framework.

2.7 Following Self-assembling of Surfactant-like Dendrons

Chol-G1, **Chol-G2** and **Chol$_2$-G2** dendrons are able to self-assemble due to their surfactant nature.[23] To analyze the aggregate structure, we selected the 5-DSA probe because its surfactant nature favors insertion into micellar aggregates, with the COOH group located in the polar region and the stearic chain embedded in the hydrophobic interior.[21] In this way, 5-DSA can report on the hydrophobic focal-point-driven assembly processes, while copper ions were better for analysing interactions with the branching units and surface groups. The main parameters obtained from the computation of the spectra for the dendrons (0.05 M) containing 5-DSA at concentration 0.5 mM are reported in Table 3:

Table 3 *Main parameters obtained from the computations of the spectra*

Sample	$<A_N>$ /G (polarity)	τ /ns (microviscosity)
Water	15.75	0.08
Z-G2	15.75	0.1
Chol-G1	15.2	5.9
Chol-G2	15.2	5.9
Chol$_2$-G2	14.5	25.2

The analysis of these parameters allowed us to extract the following information:
- the probe poorly interacts with the **Z-G2** dendrons because **Z-G2** has no inherent capacity to self-assemble owing to its relatively small hydrophobic group.
- in the presence of **Chol-G1** and **Chol-G2**, the probe shows a significant decrease in mobility and polarity because 5-DSA is trapped within the hydrophobic region of **Chol-G1** and **Chol-G2** nanoscale aggregates. We have previously demonstrated that this self-assembly process is of fundamental importance in enhancing interactions of these dendrons with DNA,[37] and we therefore propose that using 5-DSA as a spin probe is an easy and rapid way of detecting self-assembly in this class of gene delivery vehicle.
- in **Chol$_2$-G2** the probe is less mobile within the aggregate and is more deeply embedded in an apolar region. Therefore, the two cholesterol groups pack the probe effectively into a disordered-low polarity region of the dendron aggregates. Pleasingly, this is in agreement with some of our recent experimental and modeling studies, which indicated that **Chol$_2$-G2** formed different aggregates to **Chol-G2**, in particular containing a larger number of dendron units and with the resulting micelles having larger diameters.[37] The ability of EPR to probe and provide insight

into these relatively subtle differences in nanoscale aggregation indicates the power of this approach for characterizing self-assembling dendron systems

2.8 Structural Behavior and Interaction of G2-PPI Dendrimer within LLC

The EPR spectra for 5-DSA probe were recorded both for the three unloaded mesophases of GMO (L_α phase, at 15 % water; Q^{224}, at 35 % water; and H_{II} phase, at 8 % VE and 20 % water) and after G2-PPI loading.[25] The microviscosity (τ) and the order parameters (S), obtained from simulation of the EPR spectra at various G2-PPI loadings are reported in Figure 5. The L_α phase is characterized by a quite fluid but partially ordered environment of the probe which is in relation with the relatively low viscosity of the L_α phase. When the water content increased, i.e; formation of the Q^{224} mesophase, both microviscosity and lipid layer order increased. In the case of H_{II} mesophase, (when VE was added to GMO and water) the EPR spectrum was very noisy that suggested a decreased solubility of the 5DSA probe into the hexagonal mesophase. However, the system is more heterogeneous, but more ordered.

When PPI-G2 is added, it interacts with water and with the hydroxyl groups of GMO in the interface and therefore it perturbs the structure. The main structural changes by increasing PPI-G2 concentration in the L_α and the Q^{224} phase are a progressive increase in order and microviscosity due to the transformation of the L_α and Q^{224} phase into H_{II} mesophase. It should be mentioned that, at 10 wt% of PPI-G2, τ and S were the lowest in the H_{II} mesophase. Thus, it can be concluded that up to this concentration PPI-G2 interacts with the GMO polar hydroxyl groups at the interface. Further solubilization causes the dendrimer to enter into the water cylinders As a consequence, at the largest PPI-G2 concentrations the H_{II} mesophase reorganized into a more ordered lipid layer.

Mainly, we verified that the introduction of PPI-G2 macromolecules led to their incorporation into the GMO hydroxyl interface (in the case of 15 and 20 wt% aq. phase) and within the water cylinder (in the case of all mesophases).

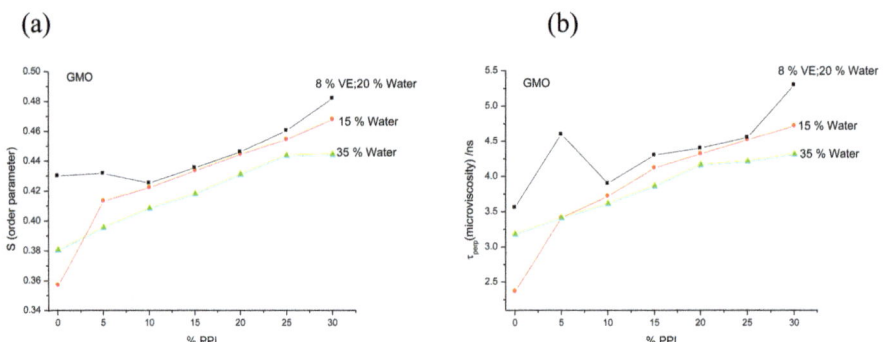

Figure 5 *(a) Order parameter (S), and (b) microviscosity (τ) obtained from simulation of the EPR spectra at various G2-PPI loadings, for the three mesophases of GMO (L_α phase, at 15 % water; Q^{224}, at 35 % water; and H_{II} phase, at 8 % VE and 20 % water)*

2.9 Dendrimers Used to Prevent and Treat Neurodegenerative Diseases

2.9.1 Interactions between phosphorous dendrimers and amyloid and prion peptides; kinetics of fibril formation:[12,13,26] The EPR spectra of the CAT8 probe in the systems containing the Aβ 1-28 and PrP 185-208 in the absence and presence of the P-dendrimer

G4 were constituted by two superimposed signals, which corresponded to a "free component" and an "interacting component" of the CAT8 probes. The interacting component due to slow moving probes is ascribed to the probes (the charged CAT group) interacting with the polar –NH-CO- groups or the termini groups of the peptides and with the peptide-dendrimer adducts. On the contrary, the free component (fast motion signal) may be ascribed to the probes at the water/peptide or dendrimer/water/peptide interphases, We analysed different parameters: (a) the relative percentages of the interacting and free components, calculated by both computation and double integration of the main EPR lines belonging to the two components; (b) the mobility parameter (A_{zz}' and/or the correlation time for motion τ), extracted by both computation and by the distance among the first and the last peaks of the interacting component; (c) the correlation time for motion τ of the free component obtained both by computation and from the height ratio between the first and the third peaks (h1/h3) of the free component; (d) the absolute intensity of the EPR signal, calculated by integration of the overall EPR signal.

Figure 6 shows examples of the variations over time of the different parameters for CAT8@peptides both in the absence and in the presence of the P-dendrimer G4.

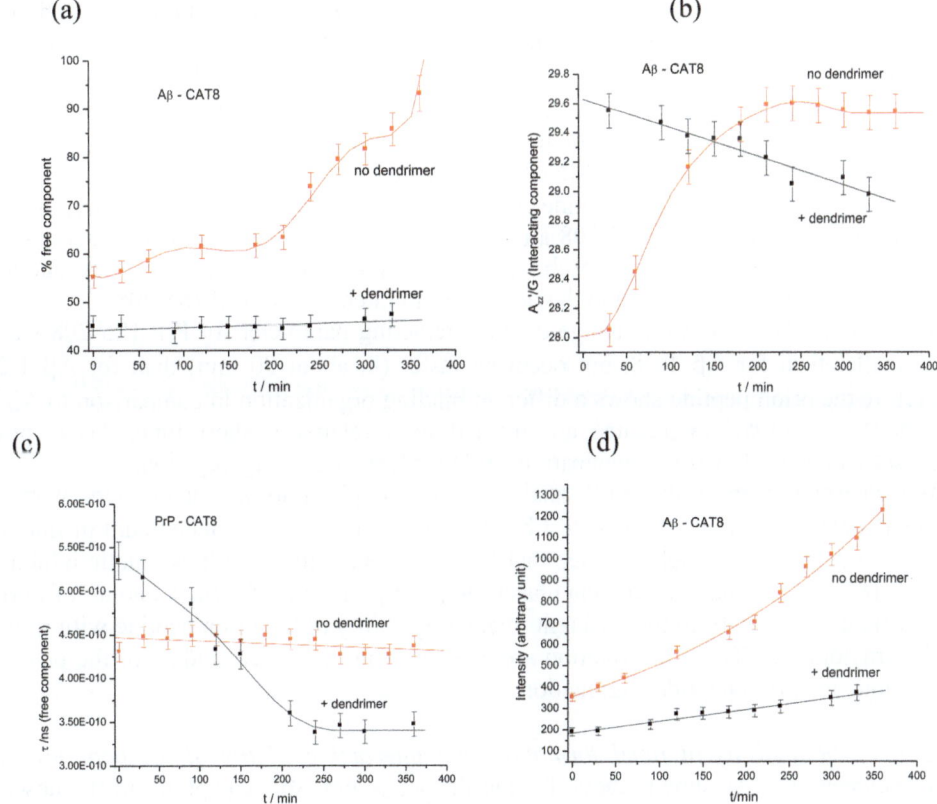

Figure 6 *Variation over time both in absence and presence of the P-dendrimer G4 of (a) the relative percentage of the free component for CAT8@Aβ 1-28; (b) the A_{zz}' parameter (corresponding to τ) of the interacting component for CAT8@Aβ 1-28; (c) τ of the free component for CAT8@PrP 185-208; (d) the absolute intensity of the EPR spectrum for CAT8@Aβ 1-28.*

Probe selfaggregation occurred at the peptide surface in solution leading to n intensity decrease of the spectra.

Aβ 1-28 without the P-dendrimer showed higher total intensity and higher percentage of the free component than in the presence of the dendrimer; this discrepancy between the absence and the presence of the dendrimer increased over time. Aβ 1-28 in the absence of the P-dendrimer preferentially host the probe in the interfacial water and a lower fraction of probes self aggregated, since the probes were better distributed at the water/Aβ 1-28 interphase. However, over time, both the intensity and the free component percentage increased, mainly after 220 min, as a consequence of Aβ 1-28 fibril formation. The peptide aggregation provoked the extrusion of the probe from the peptide surface and consequently broke down the peptide-CAT8 bond. When the fibrils are formed (after 220 min), the interacting sites available for a cooperative interactions with CAT8 are largely engaged in the peptide-peptide interactions and the probe is extracted in the fluid interphase. Conversely, in the presence of the dendrimer which interacted with Aβ 1-28, the probe remained trapped at the dendrimer/ Aβ 1-28 interphase and both the overall spectral intensity and the relative amount of the free component remained small over time.

Also the A_{zz}' value significantly increased over time for Aβ 1-28 in the absence of the dendrimer. This change may be ascribed to the progressive formation-stabilization of fibrils, which leads to a progressive trapping of the interacting probes in a restricted space. After final stabilization of the fibrils (220 min), the probe mobility did not change anymore. On the contrary, in the presence of the dendrimer, the stabilization of the Aβ 1-28/dendrimer binding led to a small increase in mobility (decrease in A_{zz}') for the interacting probe, because the dendrimer interferes in the probe-peptide binding.

Similarly as for the amyloid peptide Aβ 1-28, in the absence of the dendrimer, the free component for CAT8@ PrP 185-208 almost did not change over time, Conversely, in the presence of the P-dendrimer, the probe progressively gained freedom over time due to a competition between the probe and the dendrimer to interact with PrP 185-208.

The EPR analysis shows a change of the interacting parameter for PrP 185-208 which was smaller than for Aβ 1-28, but occurred faster (in about 90 min) than for Aβ 1-28. Therefore the prion peptide shows a different binding organization in comparison to Aβ 1-28 and less compact aggregates are formed in a relatively short time. These prion aggregates may easily work as nucleation seeds for further slow aggregation.

We clearly see from the EPR analysis that the phosphorous dendrimers work as thermodynamic inhibitors of Aβ 1-28 fibril formation because the final amount of fibrils is strongly reduced. Conversely, we see that P-dendrimers mainly work as kinetic inhibitors for PrP 185-208, by changing the lag phase and poorly changing the final amount of fibrils. This difference arises from the different interacting ability of the prion peptide with respect to the amyloid one. These information are of interest in the understanding of the pathway of amyloid and prion peptide aggregation.

2.9.2 EPR analysis of fibril formation and interacting ability of the peptides with glycodendrimers:[27] As shown above for the PrP$_{185-208}$ and Aβ$_{1-28}$ peptides in the absence and presence of the P-dendrimers, for the same peptides in the absence and presence of the glycodendrimers, the most information was obtained by comparing the parameters of computation for the various spectra in the different experimental conditions (different peptides, in the absence and presence of the different glycodendrimers, at different glycodendrimer concentrations and at subsequent equilibration times).

Figure 7 shows examples of the graphs for the variations of the different parameters (intensity, correlation time for motion, and percentage of the interacting component) over time for CAT8 in water solution with $PrP_{185-208}$ (the variation for $A\beta_{1-28}$ are similar but smaller than those for $PrP_{185-208}$) and in the absence and presence of different concentrations (1, 10, 100 mM, corresponding to a 0.1, 1, 10 dendrimer/peptide molar ratios) of PPI(G5)-dendrimers functionalized with maltose or maltotriose.

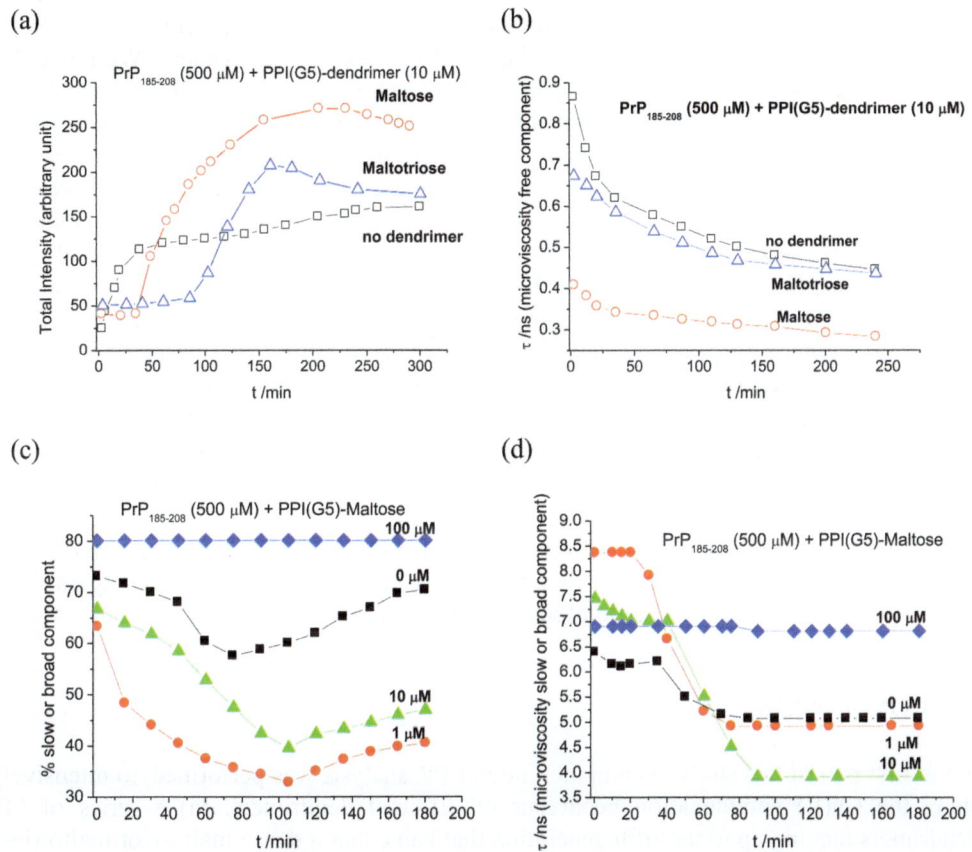

Figure 7 *Variation over time of (a) the total EPR-spectral intensity; (b) the correlation time for motion of the free component of CAT8@PrP_{185-208} in the absence and presence of PPI(G5)-dendrimers(10 mM); (c) the intensity, and (d) the correlation time for motion of the interacting component of CAT8@PrP_{185-208} in the absence and presence of PPI(G5)-maltose at different concentrations.*

For CAT8@$PrP_{185-208}$, the intensity increase is not only larger, but also delayed in the presence of the dendrimers with respect to the absence of them. In particular, the large intensity increase for PPI(G5)-Maltose starts after 30 min, while the increase for PPI(G5)-Maltotriose starts after 70 min. This means that the $PrP_{185-208}$@ PPI(G5)-Maltotriose complex needs more time for organizing and then hosting CAT8 at the interphase. We also see that the probes at the interphase (free component) gain freedom if PPI-G4-maltose is added at concentration of 10 μM. Why the peptide interacting sites are less available and the fluid region becomes more fluid over time? The most probable answer is because the peptides progressively interact with each other to form fibrils, or amorphous non-fibrillar aggregates. Such peptide-peptide interaction extrudes the CAT8 radicals from the peptide interacting sites. However, when the already formed fibrils or peptide aggregates, or clumped fibrils separate from the solution, both the interfacial and interacting CAT8 radicals follow the same destiny and disappear from the solution. Therefore, the absolute intensity of the slow-broad component decreases. However, the relative percentage of interacting nitroxide radicals with respect to the free ones increases, because the peptide fibrils or aggregates, when separating from the solution, further aggregate (probably as clumped fibrils) and the interfacial nitroxide radicals are consequently squeezed in between the fibrils, but what remains in the interfacial zone gains freedom. We noted that the above described variations of intensity, percentage and mobility hold both in the absence and in the presence of the smaller dendrimer concentrations. This indicates that small amounts of dendrimers promote peptide-fibril or peptide-aggregates formation, Furthermore, when the peptide-fibrils or aggregates are formed, promoted by the presence of the low concentrations of dendrimers, the interacting CAT8 radicals gain mobility freedom (decrease of τ) because the interacting sites of the peptides get largely involved in the peptide-peptide interactions and the CAT8 radicals gather at the few available interacting sites. At the highest dendrimer concentration (100 μM), the intensity of the interacting component progressively increases over time for all systems. Since we interpreted the maximum for the intensity and the percentage variation as indicative of the formation and subsequent separation of peptide fibrils or aggregates, therefore, at a dendrimer concentration of 100 μM, the formation-separation of $PrP_{185\text{-}208}$ and $A\beta_{1\text{-}28}$ fibrils is prevented. The $PrP_{185\text{-}208}$ + PPI(G5)-Maltotriose system shows a lower stabilization of the peptide α-helix structure.

These results provide interesting information on the mechanism of fibrilization and on the effect of the sugar-decorated PPI dendrimers in relatively large amount against the pathologies related to the formation of amyloid plaques.

3 CONCLUSION

In the first part of this study, a computer aided EPR analysis was performed to intensively study the Cu(II) complexation behaviour of different dendrimers: (a) a series of PPI dendrimers ranging up to the fifth generation that had either a dense maltose or maltotriose shell; (b) sulfonated or carboxylated carbosilane dendrimers; (c) self-assembling amine-terminated dendrons.

The Cu(II) coordination and symmetry of the generated complexes depend on the dendrimer chemical structure, the functionalization in the periphery, dendrimer generation and the ratio of the copper and dendrimer concentrations.

As generation increased, the glycodendrimers showed (a) increased nitrogen coordination in a axial symmetry, due to the increased number of nitrogen sites in the dendrimer interior, and (b) a rhombic structure which forms in the congested dendrimer periphery where the sugar units are also able to coordinate the copper ions.

At the lowest Cu(II) concentrations a $Cu\text{-}NO_3$ coordination is favored for the carbosilane dendrimers functionalized with carboxylate groups, but this partial internalization of the ions got saturated by increasing Cu(II) concentration and the ions were confined at the external surface. With the carbosilane-sulfonate dendrimers, dimeric Cu(II) complexes were found at the lowest generation, while the nitrogen coordination becomes feasible at higher generations.

Different self-assembling dendron structures had different hydrophilic coronas with different affinities for Cu(II) binding. We could determine that some of the dendrons had N_2O_2 binding sites, whilst others had NO_3 coordination modes. These could be rationalized based on the molecular structures of the dendrons involved. The self-assembling properties of these dendrons were investigated by using the 5-DSA probe. It was found that the self-assembly process depends on the number of cholesterol units which were present at the focal point of the dendron and that the spin probe can report precisely on very subtle changes.

The 5-DSA probe was also used, due to its surfactant nature, to monitor the variations of structure of drug carriers constituted by LLC upon internalization of increasing PPI-G2 concentrations. Hexagonal ordered structures become stable upon dendrimer internalization into the LLCs.

The last part of this study analyzes, by means of the CAT8 spin probe, the aggregation behavior of the amyloid peptide $A\beta_{1-28}$ and the prion peptide $PrP_{185-208}$ - both responsible for neurodegenerative disorders, in the absence and in the presence of P-dendrimer-G4 or (G5)PPI dendrimers with a dense shell of maltose and maltotriose units. The CAT8 radical well follows the progressive formation of peptide aggregates in form of fibrils by a progressive extraction of the radicals into the aggregate/water interphase. The addition of small amounts of dendrimers promotes the formation of peptide fibrils breaking them and providing a larger amount of ends that serve as sites of replications. Conversely, a high amount of dendrimers allows the peptides to well separate from each other such preventing their aggregation. EPR results also indicate that the perturbation played by PPI(G5)-Maltose are more effective onto $PrP_{185-208}$ than onto $A\beta_{1-28}$, , P-dendrimers equivalently acts to the prion and amyloid peptides, while PPI(G5)-Maltotriose is less effective in both promoting aggregation and preventing it by changing the dendrimer concentration. Our studies demonstrated that these dendrimers may be effectively used in the medical cure of prion diseases, as such as in the prevention and treatment of Alzheimer diseases.

Further studies are in progress in collaboration with several members of the COST Action TD0802: not only the co-authors of this study, but also Profs. Ling Peng, Jorn Christensen, Roxana Piticescu, Rimantas Vaisnoras, Costas Demetzos, and Andreana Assimopoulou.

References

1   A. Agarwal, A. Asthana, U. Gupta, and N.K. Jain, *J. Pharm. Pharmacol.,* 2008, **60**, 671–688.

2   U. Boas, and P.M.H. Heegaard, *Chem. Soc. Rev.*, 2004, **33**, 43–63.

3   A.W. Bosman, H.M. Janssen, and E.W. Meijer, *Chem. Rev.*, 1999, **99**, 1665–1688.

4   S.-H. Hwang, C.N. Moorefield, and G.R. Newkome, *Chem. Soc. Rev.*, 2008, **37**, 2543–2557.

5   C.C. Lee, J.A. MacKay, J.M.J. Fréchet, and F.C. Szoka, *Nat. Biotechnol.*, 2005, **23**, 1517–1526.

6   M.F. Ottaviani, P. Matteini, M. Brustolon, N.J. Turro, S. Jockusch, and D.A. Tomalia, *J. Phys. Chem. B ,* 1998, **102**, 6029-6039.

7   M.F. Ottaviani, R. Daddi, M. Brustolon, N.J. Turro, and D.A. Tomalia, *Langmuir ,* 1999, **15**, 1973-1980.

8   M.F. Ottaviani, B. Sacchi, N.J. Turro, W. Chen, S. Jockusch, and D.A. Tomalia, *Macromolecules*, 1999, **32**, 2275-2282.

9   M.F. Ottaviani, F. Furini, A. Casini, N.J. Turro, S. Jockusch, D.A. Tomalia, and L. Messori, *Macromolecules,* 2000, **33**, 7842-7851.

10   (a) M.F. Ottaviani, S. Jockush, N.J. Turro, D.A. Tomalia, and A. Barbon, *Langmuir,* 2004, **20**, 10238-10254; (b) D. Shcharbin, M. F. Ottaviani, M. Cangiotti, M.

Przybyszewska, M. Zaborski, and M. Bryszewska, *Colloids Surf B: Biointerfaces.* 2008, **63**, 27-33

11 M.F. Ottaviani, P. Favuzza, B. Sacchi, N.J. Turro, S. Jockusch, and D.A. Tomalia, *Langmuir* 2002, **18**, 2347-2357.

12 B. Klajnert, M. Cangiotti, S. Calici, J.-P. Majoral, A.-M. Caminade, J. Cladera, M. Bryszewska, M.F. Ottaviani, *Macromolec. Biosci.* 2007, **7**, 1065-1074.

13 B. Klajnert, M. Cangiotti, S. Calici, M. Ionov, J.-P. Majoral, A.-M. Caminade, J. Cladera, M. Bryszewska, M.F. Ottaviani, *New J. Chem.* 2009, **33**, 1087-1093.

14 M.F. Ottaviani, S. Bossmann, N.J. Turro, and D.A. Tomalia, *J. Am. Chem. Soc,.*1994, **116**, 661–671.

15 M.F. Ottaviani, F. Montalti, N.J. Turro, and D.A. Tomalia. *J. Phys. Chem. B*, 1997, **101**, 158–166.

16 M.F. Ottaviani, P. Favuzza, M. Bigazzi, N.J. Turro, S. Jockusch, and D.A. Tomalia, *Langmuir*, 2000, **16**, 7368–7372.

17 M.F. Ottaviani, R. Valluzzi, and L. Balogh, *Macromolecules*, 2002, **35**, 5105–5115.

18 (a) D. Appelhans, U. Oertel, R. Mazzeo, H. Komber, J. Hoffmann, S. Weidner, D. Brutschy, B. Voit and M. F.Ottaviani, *Proc. R. Soc. A*, 2010, **466**, 1489–1513. (b) D. Appelhans, Y. Zhong, H. Komber, P. Friedel, U. Oertel, U. Scheler, N. Morgner, D. Kuckling, S. Richter, J. Seidel, B. Brutschy, B. Voit, *Macromol. Biosci.*, 2007, **7**, 373–383.

19 S. Garcia-Gallego, M.J. Serramia, E. Arnaiz, L. Diaz, M.A. Munoz-Fernandez, P. Gomez-Sal, M.F. Ottaviani, R. Gomez, and F.J. de la Mata, *Eur. J. Inorg. Chem.*, 2011, **10**, 1657-1665.

20 (a) S. García-Gallego, J. Sanchez Rodríguez, J. L. Jiménez, M. Cangiotti, M. F. Ottaviani, M.A. Muñoz-Fernandez, R. Gomez, and F. J. de la Mata, *Dalton Trans.*, 2012, **41**, 6488 (b) M. Galán, J. Sánchez Rodríguez, M. Cangiotti, S. García-Gallego, J. Luis Jiménez, R. Gómez, M. F. Ottaviani, M. A. Muñoz-Fernández, and F. J. de la Mata, *Curr. Med. Chem.*, 2012, **19**, 4984-4994.

21 M.F. Ottaviani, M. Cangiotti, L. Fiorani, A. Barnard, S. P. Jones, and D.K. Smith, *New J. Chem.* 2012, **36**, 469-476.

22 (a) F.J. De la Mata R. Gómez, *Spanish Patent* ,2010, P-201030233. b) F.J. De la Mata R. Gómez, *Spanish Patent*, 2010, P-201030450. (c) B. Rasines, J. Sánchez-Nieves, M. Maiolo, M. Maly, L. Chonco, J. L. Jiménez, Mª Á. Muñoz-Fernández, F. J. de la Mata, R. Gómez, *Dalton Trans*, in press.

23 (a) M.A. Kostiainen, J.G. Hardy and D.K. Smith, *Angew. Chem. Int. Ed.* 2005, **44**, 2556–2559; (b) J.G. Hardy, M.A. Kostiainen, D.K. Smith, N.P. Gabrielson and D.W. Pack, *Bioconjugate Chem.* 2006, **17**, 172–178. (c) D.J. Welsh, S.P. Jones, D.K. Smith, *Angew. Chem. Int. Ed.* 2009, **48**, 4047-4051. (d) M.A. Kostiainen, D.K. Smith, O. Ikkala *Angew. Chem. Int. Ed.* 2007, **46**, 7600-7604. (e) M.A. Kostiainen, G.R. Szilvay, J. Lehtinen, D.K. Smith, M.B. Linder, A. Urtti and O. Ikkala *ACS Nano* 2007, **1**, 103-113. (f) S.P. Jones, N.P. Gabrielson, C.-H. Wong, H.-F. Chow, D.W. Pack, P. Posocco, M. Fermeglia, S. Pricl and D.K. Smith, *Mol. Pharm.* 2011, **8**, 416-429.

24 S. P. Jones, N. P. Gabrielson, D.W. Pack, D. K. Smith, *Chem. Commun.*, 2008, **39**, 4700-4702;

25 L. Bitan-Cherbakovsky, D. Libster, M.F. Ottaviani, .A. Aserin, N. Garti,. *J. Phys. Chem. B*, 2012, **116**, 2420-2429.

26 M.F. Ottaviani, R. Mazzeo, M. Cangiotti, L. Fiorani, J.-P. Majoral, A.M. Caminade, E. Pedziwiatr, M. Bryszewska, B. Klajnert, *Biomacromol.* 2010, **11**, 3014-3021.

27 M. F. Ottaviani, M. Cangiotti, L. Fiorani , S. Lucchi, T. Wasiak, D. Appelhans, and B. Klajnert, *Curr. Med. Chem.*, in press.

28 J.F. Kukowska-Latallo, A.U. Bielinska, J. Johnson, R. Spindler, D.A. Tomalia, J.R., Jr. Baker, *Proc. Natl. Acad. Sci. U.S.A.,* 1996, **93**, 4897-4902.

29 C. Kojima, K. Kono, K. Maruyama, and T. Takagishi, T., *Bioconjugate Chem.*, 2000, **11**, 910-917.

30 L.J. Twyman, A.E. Beezer, R. Esfand, M.J. Hardy, J.C. Mitchell, *Tetrahedron Lett.*, 1999, **40**, 1743-1746.

31 R. Esfand, and D.A. Tomalia, *Drug Discovery Today,* 2001, **6**, 427-435.

32 B.H. Zinselmeyer, S.P. Mackay, A.G. Schatzlein, and I.F. Uchegbu, *Pharm. Res.*, 2002, **19**, 960-967.

33 A.J. Hollins, M. Benboubetra, Y. Omidi, B.H. Zinselmeyer, A.G. Schatzlein, I.F. Uchegbu, S. Akhtar, *Pharm. Res.*, 2004, **21**, 458-466.

34 P.E.S. Smith, J.R. Brender, U.H.N. Durr, J. Xu, D.G. Mullen, M.M. Banaszack Holl, and A. Ramamoorthy,. *J. Am. Chem. Soc.,* 2010, **132**, 8087-8097.

35 C. Loup, M.A. Zanta, A.M. Caminade, J.P. Majoral, and B. Meunier, *Chem. Eur. J.*, 1999, 53644-53650

36 D.E. Budil, S. Lee, S. Saxena and J.H. Freed, *J. Magn. Reson. A* 1996, **120**, 155-189;

37 A. Barnard, P. Posocco, S. Pricl, M. Calderon, R. Haag, M.E. Hwang, V.W.T. Shum, D.W. Pack and D.K. Smith, *J. Am. Chem. Soc.* 2011, **133**, 20288-20300.

DENDRIMERS AS VECTORS FOR SMALL INTERFERING RNA TRANSFECTION IN THE NERVOUS SYSTEM

F. C. Pérez-Martínez[1], A.V. Ocaña[2,3], G.M. Pavan[4], A. Danani[4], and V. Ceña[2,3]

[1]NanoDrugs, S.L. Parque Científico y Tecnológico. Albacete, Spain
[2]Unidad Asociada Neurodeath. CSIC-Universidad de Castilla-La Mancha. Departamento de Ciencias Médicas. Albacete, Spain
[3]CIBERNED, Instituto de Salud Carlos III, Spain
[4]SUPSI - Laboratory of Applied Mathematics and Physics (LaMFI); Manno, Switzerland

1 INTRODUCTION

Gene therapy can be defined as an attempt to introduce functional genes into malfunctioning target cells for a therapeutic purpose. [1] However, a broader description would include both the replacement of absent or defective genes using plasmid DNA and the selective interference with signaling pathways involved in the genesis of various diseases by knocking down mRNA expression using RNA interference (RNAi) technology. [2] These latter techniques based on RNAi have great potential for drug development, but first they must overcome the key obstacle of delivering the genetic material into the affected cells. [3] Moreover, when applied *in vivo*, RNAi-based approaches are generally limited by poor penetration into the target tissue and low silencing efficiency. Small interfering RNAs (siRNAs) mimic RNAi action, and by binding to complementary mRNA sequences, promote the cleavage of these sequences and specifically inhibit the synthesis of key proteins in various signaling pathways. Not surprisingly, the use of siRNAs for the treatment of diseases that are produced by an aberrant gene expression, such as cancer and neurodegenerative diseases, constitutes a promising new therapeutic approach, and has gained wide interest. New targets for siRNA-based therapy are continuously emerging from the increasing knowledge of key molecular pathways that are critical for the development of CNS diseases.

To date, the main approach to the use of siRNA technology in postmitotic neuronal cells has relied on the use of viral vectors to deliver the genetic material to these hard-to-transfect cells. [4] However, although certain viral vectors have been shown to be useful tools for carrying genes to neurons, their potential as therapeutic agents is limited by their toxicity, immunogenicity and broad tropism as well as by the cost of large-scale formulation. Thus, the routine administration of genetic material to neurons for therapeutic purposes will inevitably involve non-viral vectors, such as therapeutic nanoparticles (NPs), due to the aforementioned drawbacks of their viral counterparts. Among non-viral vectors, dendrimers are probably the most promising NPs for successful delivery of genetic material to the central nervous system (CNS). These promising new tools constitute a relevant alternative to viral vectors, which have been shown to be useful carriers for gene delivery to CNS cells. These tools offer improved safety profiles compared to viruses, are less expensive to produce, and can be targeted to specific cell types and subpopulations. On the other hand, most of these non-viral vectors suffer from significantly lower transfection efficiencies than neurotropic viruses, which severely limits their utility in neuron-targeted delivery applications. [5] Thus, the development of therapeutic dendrimers for treating CNS diseases needs to overcome several challenges before the dendrimers can be used as a routine therapy, challenges that include better biocompatibility, blood-brain barrier (BBB) crossing, selective cellular delivery, and increased efficiency by improved endosomal escape.

Dendrimers are highly branched three-dimensional synthetic macromolecules with a well-defined structure with precise control of size and shape as well as terminal group functionality. Dendrimers have been used for numerous applications in the fields of nanotechnology, pharmaceuticals and medicinal chemistry. [6] These NPs contain three distinct domains:

(1) A central core (either a single atom or a group of atoms having two or more identical chemical functionalities).

(2) Branches emanating from the core, which are composed of repeat units with at least one branching junction whose repetition is organized in a geometric progression that results in a series of radially concentric layers.

(3) Terminal functional groups, which are located on the exterior of the NP and facilitate interactions with solvents, surfaces and other molecules.

The increasing growth of dendrimers is defined in terms of "generation number", with each generation characterized in terms of size, shape, molecular weight and number of surface functional groups. Polyamidoamine (PAMAM) dendrimers are probably the most widely studied NPs for gene or drug delivery to the brain. [7] PAMAM dendrimers are members of a class of polyamine polymers that have steadily grown in popularity in the past decade in a variety of disciplines, ranging from materials science to biomedicine. PAMAM dendrimers have demonstrated significant gene delivery ability due in part to their ability to carry nucleic acids, thanks to the amino groups at the terminal ends of the dendrimer branches. These branches are positively-charged at physiological pH and interact with the negatively-charged phosphate groups of nucleic acids. [8,9] Several research groups have tried to classically characterize selections of PAMAM dendrimers using biophysical methods to search for structural properties that correlate with transfection. The measurements of colloidal properties (size and zeta potential) as a function of the charge ratio revealed that highly transfecting dendrimer/DNA complexes had size/zeta potential values between 4 and 8. [9] However, more data is required to identify the critical parameters required to adequately predict the transfection efficiency of a given dendrimer. Moreover, further improvements in dendrimer cytotoxicity profiles, biocompatibility, and biodistribution are required to efficiently transfect CNS cells.

Advances in therapeutic drugs and medical procedures have increased life expectancy and, consequently, neoplastic and neurodegenerative diseases manifest themselves with advancing age and may involve the two main types of cells that compose the CNS: neurons and glial cells. Currently, the treatments of dysfunctions in these cell types are performed with pharmaceutical agents that generally have a selectivity that is dependent on the concentration reached in the target tissues. However, the genetic material (either siRNA or DNA) used for therapeutic purposes must be delivered to the cell cytosol where it will exert its action. In addition to its potential as a therapeutic approach, another application of genetic material delivery to CNS cells lies in understanding the role that certain proteins play in neuronal physiology and pathology. This knowledge is gained by selectively removing the target proteins to study their lack-of-function effects or, alternatively, over-expressing the proteins to explore their functions. For many years, the typical approach has consisted of generating knock-out mice that lack the target protein. [10] This is a time-consuming method, however, and the function of the removed protein can at times be replaced by another protein during development. This phenomenon is known as redundancy and leads to a lack of phenotype, making it difficult to draw conclusions from the experiments performed on these animals. A more complex approach consists of generating conditional knock-out or knock-in mice that only remove or express the protein following a specific treatment. [11] This procedure prevents the compensation of function during development, but it is very time consuming and technically difficult to achieve. Gene therapy techniques are a valuable alternative to the animal models described earlier, but the genetic material must first overcome the key obstacle of reaching the interior of the affected cells. Moreover, *in vivo* delivery of siRNA remains a crucial challenge for therapeutic success, because siRNAs on their own are not taken up by most mammalian cells in a manner that preserves their activity. Thus, the low penetration ability of siRNA through the cellular plasma membrane combined with its limited stability in blood limits the effectiveness of the systemic delivery of siRNA. Nevertheless, although gene therapy techniques such as RNAi provide a powerful strategy for modulating specific gene functions, difficulties associated with genetic material delivery to the CNS have impeded the development of efficient therapeutic applications. As mentioned earlier, dendrimers have recently emerged as promising tools for therapeutic and diagnostic applications in CNS diseases due to the presence of low permeable barriers to reach the brain. [1]

In addition to the problems described above for delivering genetic material into CNS cells, it is important to note that safe and effective dendrimers have been used for delivering genetic material to CNS cells and have shown better results than other techniques, such as electroporation, which are very inefficient in CNS cells. Dendrimers have been used in studies to deliver genetic material such as plasmid DNA, siRNA and oligonucleotides into the brain, a process that has resulted in the inhibition of undesirable gene expression and the synthesis of therapeutic proteins was recently reviewed. [1,2]

2. BLOOD BRAIN BARRIER CROSSING

Dendrimers employed as gene delivery carriers for the CNS must (1) cross one or several membrane layers (e.g., mucosa, epithelium and endothelium) before (2) being internalized in the CNS by crossing the BBB or travelling through nerve terminals. Then, (3) the dendrimers must diffuse through the cytoplasmic membrane, (4) escape from vesicular encapsulation to, ultimately, (5) target intracellular structures. Premature degradation of the dendrimer and/or the carried agent before reaching the desired intracellular target must be avoided for the dendrimer to serve as a good non-viral delivery vector. Although each step in the path that the NPs have to take to reach the cells in the CNS has its difficulties, the BBB and the endosomal escape are probably the main bottlenecks for the efficient transfection of CNS cells. [1,12] Several CNS diseases, such as neurodegenerative (Alzheimer's and Parkinson's disease), cerebrovascular and inflammatory diseases (infection and multiple sclerosis), as well as various solid brain tumors (gliomas are the most frequent primary brain tumors in humans) may lead to some loss of BBB integrity. These diseases are an on-going challenge for the use of NPs as non-viral vectors to deliver genetic material to the CNS. The described techniques for temporarily disrupting the BBB or by-passing the limited permeability of brain capillaries may provide the dendrimers with a better ability to cross the BBB. [13,14] However, all of these described techniques carry the risk of side effects such as infections, and therefore less invasive and disruptive NP administration routes are desirable.

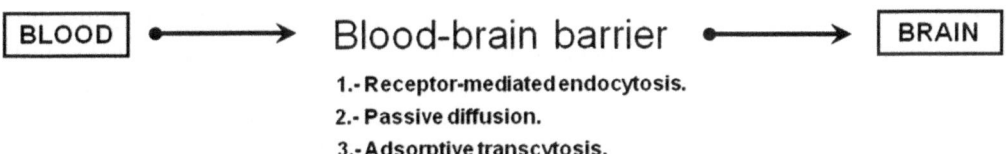

Figure 1. General mechanisms used by molecules and nanoparticles to cross the blood brain barrier.

The mechanisms used by nanoparticles to cross the BBB are indicated in Figure 1. The main mechanism used by nanocarriers to pass through the BBB is known as transcytosis. [15] Dendrimers, however, can also cross this barrier by lipid-mediated free diffusion and by receptor-mediated endocytosis. Thus, to overcome this major obstacle to CNS permeation using either passive or active transport, NPs can use specific transporters expressed on the endothelial cells of the BBB. [16] In addition, dendrimers can be functionalized with various molecules such as angiopep-2, thiamine, Tat peptides, glucose transporters, lactoferrin (Lf) and transferrin (Tf). These molecules are ligands for various receptors found on the surface of the brain endothelial cells and therefore facilitate the endocytosis of these NPs by the brain endothelial cells and the BBB crossing after intravenous administration. [1] The first study that investigated Lf as a brain-targeting ligand in the design of a PAMAM-based non-viral gene vector to the brain showed that the brain uptake and DNA transfection efficiency of Lf-modified NPs was 2.2-fold higher than that obtained using non-modified NPs *in vitro* and *in vivo*. [17] In a similar study, Lf-modified G5-PAMAM dendrimers were used as a potential non-viral gene vector to treat Parkinson's disease (PD) due to their brain-targeting and BBB-crossing ability. [18] This uptake of Lf-modified vectors was related to clathrin-mediated endocytosis (CME), caveolae-mediated endocytosis (CvME) and macropinocytosis. [19] Studies prior to the previously mentioned study investigated (*in vitro* and *in vivo*) PAMAM dendrimers conjugated to Tf via bifunctional polyethylene glycol (PEG). The results of these studies suggested that PAMAM-PEG-Tf dendrimers could be exploited as potential non-viral gene vectors. [20] PAMAM dendrimers have also been modified with angiopep through bifunctional PEG and then complexed with DNA. These dendrimers have shown great potential for application in the design of brain-targeting drug delivery systems. The angiopep-modified NPs were observed to be internalized by brain capillary endothelial cells through energy-depending endocytosis and partly through macropinocytosis.

In addition to functionalization using receptor ligands, alternative therapeutic strategies for BBB crossing have been developed. One of these strategies is based on the finding that the BBB can be easily penetrated by macrophages using a Trojan horse effect. For example, NPs were used to internalize an antiretroviral drug (indinavir) into bone-marrow-derived macrophages. These indinavir-loaded macrophages then easily reached the brain where they released the active drug. [21] In addition, other novel routes, such as intranasal administration, have raised significant interest. Several studies have shown that polymeric NPs targeting lectin receptors can use this pathway to deliver their cargo into the brain. [22]

3. CELLULAR INTERNALIZATION

The internalization pathways used by dendrimers to deliver therapeutic molecules into CNS cells include fluid-phase endocytosis (FPE) and receptor-mediated endocytosis (RME) as well as transduction, a non-endocytotic pathway for the uptake of dendrimers that occurs in many cell types and even in artificial unilamellar vesicles. Although little attention has been directed towards studying transduction, two models have been proposed to explain it: The "direct membrane penetration" model and the "inverted micelle" model, [23,24] both of which propose a three-step internalization process involving membrane interaction, membrane permeation and the release of dendrimers into the cytosol. Thus, these non-viral vectors take advantage of multiple uptake pathways simultaneously in order to become internalized in cells; however, some of these pathways lead to degradation when the uptake is higher than the efficiency of the treatment.

FPE is a non-specific mechanism used for the uptake of compounds contained in the extracellular fluid. The main characteristic of this process is its lack of selectivity. FPE results in the uptake of the extracellular fluid surrounding the cell by means of an invagination of the plasma membrane to form an endocytic vesicle. The attachment of molecules to the cell surface takes place by means of non-specific mechanisms such as electrostatic interactions, hydrogen bonding and van der Waals forces. Cationic molecules interact with the negatively charged plasmatic membrane, thereby facilitating their internalization. This process has led to the proposal that cationization may be a strategy for enhancing drug delivery to the CNS. Indeed, the most successful strategies for delivering genetic material to the CNS have involved the use of positively charged dendrimers.
On the other hand, RME takes advantage of the high affinity binding constants between the receptors and their specific ligands. Two different mechanisms have been defined, namely constitutive (class I) RME, which involves the internalization of the ligand bound to its receptor without the generation of any signal, and ligand-stimulated (class II) RME, which involves the internalization of the ligand-receptor complex following the generation of signaling molecules. CNS cells are highly differentiated and express a number of different classes of receptors, including neuropeptide, neurotrophin and neurotoxin receptors. [25] This process has led to strategies focused on brain drug delivery that take advantage of the high specificity of ligand-receptor binding. The Tf or low-density lipoprotein (LDL) receptors are among those defined as constitutive (class I) RME, whereas others, such as insulin and epidermal growth factor (EGF), are referred to as ligand-stimulated (class II) RME. Either FPE or RME can be achieved using different molecular endocytosis mechanisms that include CME, CvME and non-clathrin, non-caveolae-mediated endocytosis.

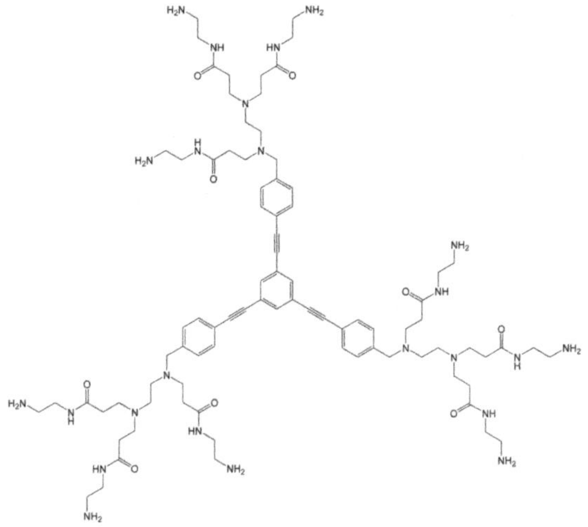

Figure 2. Chemical structure of the TRANSGEDEN dendrimer.

CME via clathrin-coated pits (CCPs) is the most fully characterized pathway for the cellular uptake of dendrimers. The CME pathway represents a common route for the cellular uptake of internalized ligands and viruses, [26,27] and for dendrimer-based genetic material delivery systems. [28] Dendrimers predominantly use this pathway for the intracellular delivery of active molecules through RME mediated by Tf, LDL and EGF receptors. [29] During CME, the membrane forms invaginations that are coated by the protein clathrin. The GTPase dynamin, along with other proteins, is mainly responsible for the detachment of CCPs from the cell membrane. CCPs also contain a high number of receptors that are involved in various interactions, such as lipid-lipid, lipid-protein and protein-protein. [30] These interactions determine the vesicle function and target. [31] CME, whether receptor-dependent or receptor-independent, is therefore very important for genetic material-loaded nanocarriers, which must release their cargo intracellularly. CME is very active in the nervous system, where it is responsible for synaptic vesicle retrieval after nerve stimulation in the retina, [32] in both central nerve termini and neuromuscular preparations following large non-physiological stimuli and after trains of action potentials within the physiological range. [33]

CvME also plays a role in the cellular uptake of various compounds. Lipid rafts have been defined as small (10-200 nm), heterogeneous, highly dynamic, sterol- and sphingolipid-enriched membrane domains that compartmentalize cellular processes. [34] The endocytic process that involves caveolae budding is defined as a clathrin-independent pathway. Ligands known to be internalized by CvME include folic acid, albumin and cholesterol. [30] The CvME pathway has received increasing attention for genetic material-delivery applications using dendrimers. [27] Folic acid (vitamin B9) appears to be an attractive target for NP-mediated nucleic acid delivery using this mechanism. Nanocarriers designed to exploit CvME may be employed to prevent degradation by lysosomal enzymes when the cargo is highly sensitive to lysosomal enzymes. Lipid rafts play important roles in neural tissue and have been shown to be involved in growth factor signaling by tyrosine kinase receptors, axonal guidance, ionic channel traffic and the recycling of receptors. [35,36,37]

Various clathrin- and caveolae-independent endocytosis pathways have only recently been described and classified. [34] Our understanding of their involvement in NP-mediated drug delivery is still at a nascent stage, although it has been suggested than this mechanism is present in the CNS. [38] Macropinocytosis is one type of non-clathrin, non-caveolae endocytic pathway that can occur in all cell types at different rates. [39] Macropinocytosis refers to the generation of large endocytic vesicles (up to 5 μm in diameter), which is associated with the formation of actin-dependent membrane ruffles. [40] This uptake mechanism shows poor selectivity and is involved in the uptake of dendrimers. [41] It is, therefore, an attractive pathway for explaining the uptake of large NPs in both glial and neuronal cells.

4. ENDOSOMAL ESCAPE

NPs internalized by endocytosis are enclosed in vesicles from which they must escape and must deliver their cargo to their targets before they encounter the degradation pathway of the lysosomal environment. This pathway is characterized by a low pH and the presence of a wide range of enzymes, including proteases, nucleases, glycosidases, lipases, phospholipases, phosphatases and sulfatases associated with the lysosomes.

Various endosome escape mechanisms, such as a possible swelling of the dendrimers resulting from an increased repulsion between the protonated groups, have been suggested. [42] Positively charged NPs, such as dendrimers, are currently major transfection agents used for the design of nanocarriers able to escape from the endosomes in neurons, although some covalent surface modifications incorporating arginines or the rabies virus glycoprotein peptide (RVG29) may improve the efficient intracellular delivery of the cargo to neural cells. [43,44] Positively charged NPs have shown remarkable transfection efficiency in various cell lines, leading to the proposal of the so-called "proton-sponge" effect. [45] According to this hypothesis, the decrease in endosomal pH results in a high protonation of NPs and consequently an osmotic swelling and subsequent vacuole disruption, which releases the dendrimers and their cargo. [45] Other strategies to improve lysosomal escape have also been proposed. NPs linking together different types of RNA as well as a promising multifunctional nanosystem known as "super pH-sensitive multifunctional polymeric micelles" have been generated. [46].

5. BIOLOGICAL ACTIONS IN CNS CELLS

Many studies exploring nanotechnology approaches for gene delivery to the brain have focused on the treatment of a variety of CNS disorders that are difficult to manage clinically using current drugs. [47] A number of groups have also encapsulated antineoplastic drugs as well as various compounds such as neuropeptides, loperamide, tubocurarine, dalargin, diminazene and a NMDA receptor antagonist in a wide variety of NPs to increase their effects when compared with the administration of the compounds in isolation (for a review see Reference 1). Moreover, new families of dendrimers have been shown to be effective in delivering genetic material to CNS cells such as astrocytes and neurons. These families include carbosilane dendrimers, [48,49] arginine-bound PAMAM dendrimers, [50] poly(l-lysine) dendrimers with silsesquioxane cubic cores, [51] nanoworms, [52] and a novel hybrid dendrimer (TRANSGEDEN) (figure 2) that combines a conjugated rigid polyphenylenevinylene (PPV) core with flexible PAMAM branches at the surface. [53,2,54] Other non-viral vectors are continuously being developed using several types of NPs such as inorganic NPs, lipid-based NPs, polymeric NPs, dendrimers and carbon-based NPs. [1]

The transfection efficiency of PAMAM-arginine dendrimers in primary neuronal cortical cultures, which are known to be quite resistant to exogenous gene transfection, has been explored. PAMAM-arginine/DNA complexes showed relatively high transfection efficiencies (35%-40%) and low cytotoxicity in primary cortical neurons, as compared with other gene carriers such as native PAMAM, cationic lipid-based NPs and polyethylenimine (PEI). [50] Efficient transfection was not limited to neurons but extended to all three glial cells (astrocytes, microglia and oligodendrocytes) present in these primary cortical cultures. [52] A more recent study has reported that PAMAM dendrimers modified with arginine allow for siRNA delivery to a primary culture of mixed cortical cells containing neurons and glia, thereby resulting in an 80% reduction in protein levels 12 h post-transfection. [50] The effects have been evaluated for another non-viral vector (carbosilane dendrimer) for the efficient delivery of siRNA to postmitotic neurons. The study analyzed the function of hypoxia-inducible factor-1 alpha (HIF1-alpha) during chemical hypoxia-mediated neurotoxicity. [49] At 18 h post-transfection, approximately 85% of the neurons contained fluorescein-labeled siRNA/dendrimer complexes. The results of this study showed that this carbosilane dendrimer can deliver specific siRNA to neurons and selectively block HIF1-alpha synthesis with similar efficiency to that achieved by viral vectors. Using this method, the authors found that this transcription factor plays a neuroprotective role during the early phase of chemical hypoxia-mediated neurotoxicity. [49] This result indicates that carbosilane dendrimers are a good alternative to viral vectors to achieve very high transfection levels in neurons *in vitro* and may be very useful for gene therapy. Other studies have used a novel hybrid dendrimer (TRANSGEDEN) as a non-viral siRNA delivery system for both cerebellar granular neurons (CGNs) and cortical neurons. [53,2,54] The TRANSGEDEN-mediated delivery of specific siRNA knocks down several genes, such as cofilin-1, beclin-1 and the enzyme SSH-1L, enabling lack-of-function studies in neurons *in vitro*. It was observed that dendriplexes formed by TRANSGEDEN and siRNAs can be incorporated into nearly 100% of neuronal cells without toxicity. Thus, TRANSGEDEN was employed to deliver a specific siRNA to rat CGNs to knock down the cofilin-1 protein. We reported that cofilin-1 removal partially protects CGNs from NMDA-mediated neuronal death. [54] Moreover, it was found that this dendrimer was very efficient in delivering siRNA to rat cortical neurons, leading to an almost complete removal of the target protein beclin-1. Silencing beclin-1 expression blocked NMDA-induced autophagy and thus potentiated NMDA-induced neuronal death, which indicates that autophagy plays a protective role during excitotoxicity and suggests that targeting autophagy might be a helpful therapeutic strategy in neurodegenerative diseases. [53] Finally, another lack-of-function study showed that only the Slingshot family of phosphatases, more specifically the enzyme SSH-1L, but not cronophin, participates in the cofilin-1 activation process during excitotoxicity. [2]

A number of studies have proposed the use of dendrimers to treat, for example, HIV-associated dementia in adults and encephalopathy in children. The authors showed that a second generation ammonium-terminated carbosilane dendrimer containing 16 positive charges (2G-NN16) was not toxic to astrocytoma cells and successfully transfected human astrocytes even after crossing an *in vitro* BBB model. The transfected siRNA reduced the replication of HIV-1 in human astrocytes. [48] In another study, generation 5 (G5)-PAMAM dendrimers efficiently delivered siRNA to U87 malignant glioma cells. [55] G5-PAMAM dendrimers have also been modified by the addition of cyclic RGD targeting peptides, maintaining the ability to complex with siRNA, although modest siRNA delivery was observed in U87 cells using either PAMAM or PAMAM-RGD conjugates. [55] In addition, the codelivery of various therapeutics has the potential to efficaciously treat human diseases via their synergetic effects. Authors have recently developed poly(l-lysine) dendrimers with silsesquioxane cubic cores (nanoglobules) to conjugate a peptide c(RGDfK) for codelivery of doxorubicin (DOX) and siRNA. [51]

A useful method for increasing transfection efficiency involves coupling either proteins or peptides to dendrimers. A number of groups have proposed the multi-functional surface modification of dendrimers with cancer targeting moieties, protective polymers and imaging agents to fabricate versatile theragnostic nanosystems that allow simultaneous cancer therapy and diagnosis. [56] Dendrimer-conjugated magnetofluorescent nanoworms have been used as a modular platform for siRNA delivery *in vivo*, with an efficient gene target knockdown and low toxicity *in vivo*. [52] Moreover, PAMAM dendrimers and Tat peptides have also been conjugated to bacterial magnetic NPs (BMPs) for the construction of an efficient and targeted gene delivery system with transmembrane ability for gene therapy of brain tumors. This study showed that modified PAMAM dendrimers might be a novel gene delivery system with potential applications in the targeted gene therapy of brain tumors. [57] The uptake of dendrimers in brain tumors has also been studied *in vivo* using G1-PAMAM through G8-PAMAM dendrimers labeled with gadolinium (Gd)-diethyl triamine penta-acetic acid, an anionic MRI contrasting agent. Xenografted RG-2 gliomas were permeable to all Gd-dendrimer generations except for Gd-G8, and it was therefore concluded that NPs ranging from 11.7 to 11.9 nm in diameter can be used as non-viral vectors in malignant gliomas. [58]

6.THE ROLE OF MOLECULAR MODELING IN UNDERSTANDING DENDRIMER-siRNA INTERACTION

Cationic dendrimers (e.g., TRANSGEDEN) can be used as vectors to deliver and release siRNA into cells mainly due to the strong binding that they can establish with nucleic acids. The nature of the interaction between their positively charged amino groups and the negatively charged P atoms present in the siRNA strands is primarily electrostatic. However, the multivalent interaction between multiple surface groups of the dendrimer with siRNA can be very complex.

Dendrimers are, in fact, far from being rigid binders for siRNA. On the other hand, they are characterized by a certain degree of flexibility that depends on structural parameters such as the scaffold architecture, the generation, the shape and size they have in solution.[59] The final conformation assumed by the dendrimer in solution can be extremely sensitive to the external conditions, especially if the solvent in which it is immerged is composed by polar molecules and charged ions, as it is the case of physiological environment. For this reason, the primary aim of molecular modeling is to allow a deep insight into the folded state of the dendrimers in solution. Several cases have been reported where atomistic simulation has provided a fundamental support to understand how complex dendritic structures looked like once immerged in solution. Moreover, considering that dendrimers properties are unavoidably related to the real folded state by the molecule in solution, molecular dynamics (MD) simulation has become in the last years a fundamental tool to understand why certain molecules behave in a certain way and the role played by the molecular structure.[60]

In general, a molecular model of the dendrimer of interest is created as composed by different residues (Figure3). As said, however, the initial drawn configuration can be far from the real solvated state of the molecule in solution. For this reason, the built model is immerged in a box containing solvent molecules (that can be water and ions depending on the experimental conditions that needs to be reproduced), and the molecular system is simulated to allow the dendrimer to reach the equilibrium configuration. This first step is necessary to have an equilibrated model that can give indication about shape, size and rigidity of the dendrimer in solution.[61]

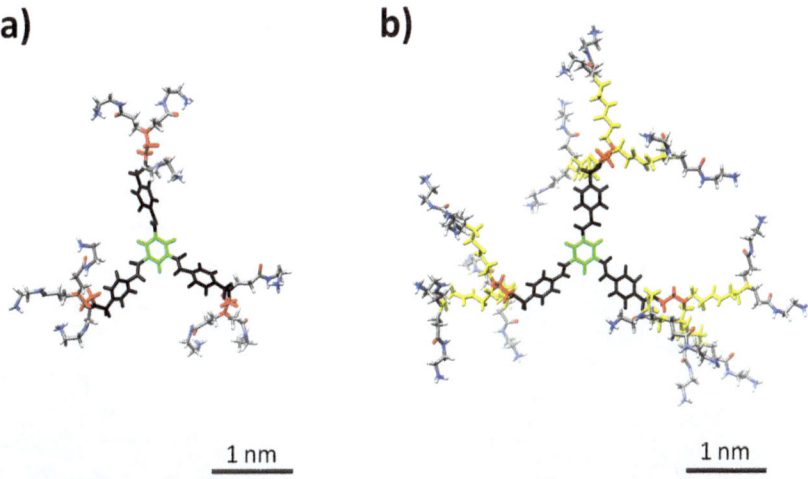

Figure 3. Molecular models for the TRANSGEDEN dendrimers – G1 (a) and G2 (b). The molecular models are built as composed by different residues. The central residue (CEN) is colored in green, the residues composing the core of the dendrirmer (COR) in black, PRE and REP residues are colored in red and yellow respectively, and the surface END groups are colored by atom (N atoms in blue, C in grey, O in red and H atoms in white).

The characterization of complex molecules as dendrimers in solution is experimentally a difficult task. Usually, information related to the average size or to the diffusion of these molecules in solution can be extracted. However, a complete characterization of dendrimers in solution is experimentally inaccessible. The single-molecule characterization provided by atomistic simulation allows to obtain information about size and shape assumed, about how much the dendrimers surface groups are backfolded or oriented toward the external environment and about the dendrimer hydration. The unique details that modeling can provide are important to understand molecular properties and to explore the interactions between the dendrimers and other molecular entities – in this case between TRANSGEDEN and siRNA.

Once an equilibrated configuration for the dendrimer in solution is achieved, this can be used as a starting point to explore the interactions between the dendrimers and different molecules including siRNA.[62] The equilibrated TRANSGEDEN is thus put in close proximity of a molecular model for siRNA and the complex is again immerged in a solvent consistent with the experimental conditions. During the MD simulation, the TRANSGEDEN-siRNAcomplex reaches the equilibrium. From the equilibrated phase of the MD trajectories it can be extracted important information about the binding between TRANSGEDEN and different siRNA molecules (figure 4).[63] MD simulations, in fact, allows to study the global affinity between a single dendrimer with the siRNA strand. Moreover, from the MD trajectories the binding interaction between TRANSGEDEN and siRNA can also be decomposed on a per-residue basis, providing indication about how much different parts of the dendrimers structure contribute to the binding.[63]

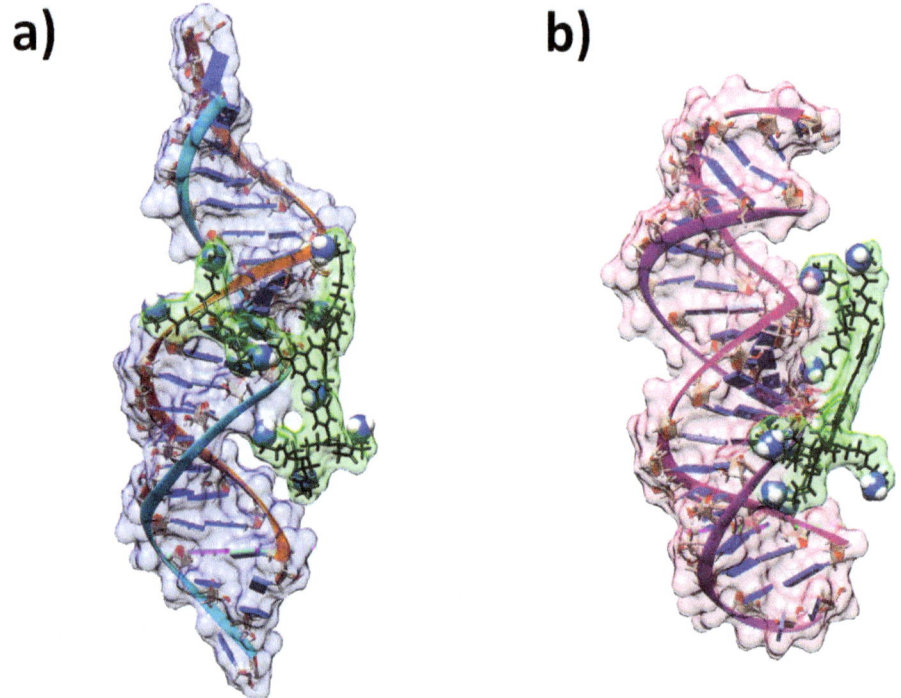

Figure 4. Equilibrated snapshot taken from the MD simulations of the TGD-G1 dendrimer in complex with GAPDH siRNA (a) and with BIRC5 siRNA (b). Within the models, the scaffold of TGD-G1 is colored in black and the primary charged amino-groups are represented as spheres and colored per atom (N atoms in blue, H atoms in white). GAPDH siRNA is represented as red and cyan strands, and its surface is colored in transparent blue. BIRC5 siRNA strands are colored in pink and purple. BIRC5 surface is colored in transparent pink and that of TGD-G1 in green.

These kind of simulations provide a unique characterization and clear structure-property relationships that cannot be achieved with the experiments. For this reason, computer simulation constitutes an ideal technique to assist and complement the experiments and to provide a complete picture of the complex molecular behavior of dendritic molecules.

In conclusion, the treatment of numerous brain diseases requires the development of non-viral vectors to deliver genetic material to the CNS. Dendrimers are promising tools for achieving this goal because of the high transfection efficiencies obtained by transfecting neurons and glial cells *in vitro* with low toxicity. However, BBB crossing and endosomal escape remain challenging for the therapeutic use of dendrimers in CNS diseases. Accordingly, several aspects of dendrimer design are relevant for good transfection efficiency, both *in vitro* and *in vivo*. These aspects include size, peripheral positive charge density and the strength of the bond between the dendrimer and the genetic material. Molecular modeling is a very useful approach to understand the complex interactions between dendrimers and other molecules including nucleic acids.

References

1. F.C. Perez-Martinez, J. Guerra, I. Posadas and V. Ceña, *Pharm.Res.*, 2011, **28**, 1843.
2. I. Posadas, F.C. Pérez-Martinez, J. Guerra, P. Sanchez-Verdu and V. Ceña, *J.Neurochem.*, 2012, **120**, 515.
3. C. Wang and Q. Zhou, *Recent Pat Drug Deliv.Formul.*, 2012, **6**, 19.
4. J.L. Dreyer, *Mol.Biotechnol.*, 2011, **47**, 169.
5. J.M. Bergen, I.K. Park, P.J. Horner and S.H. Pun, *Pharm.Res.*, 2008, **25**, 983.
6. C.C. Lee, J.A. MacKay, J.M. Frechet and F.C. Szoka, *Nat.Biotechnol.*, 2005, **23**, 1517.
7. R. Esfand and D.A. Tomalia, *Drug Discov.Today*, 2001, **6**, 427.
8. M.X. Tang, C.T. Redemann and F.C. Szoka, Jr., *Bioconjug.Chem.*, 1996, **7**, 703.
9. C.S. Braun, J.A. Vetro, D.A. Tomalia, G.S. Koe, J.G. Koe and C.R. Middaugh, *J.Pharm.Sci.*, 2005, **94**, 423.
10. R.S. Morrison, H.J. Wenzel, Y. Kinoshita, C.A. Robbins, L.A. Donehower and P.A. Schwartzkroin, *J.Neurosci.*, 1996, **16**, 1337.
11. M.A. Christophorou, D. Martin-Zanca, L. Soucek, E.R. Lawlor, L. Brown-Swigart, E.W. Verschuren and G.I. Evan, *Nat.Genet.*, 2005, **37**, 718.
12. J.S. Suk, J. Suh, K. Choy, S.K. Lai, J. Fu and J. Hanes, *Biomaterials*, 2006, **27**, 5143.
13. G. Hsich, M. Sena-Esteves and X.O. Breakefield, *Hum.Gene Ther.*, 2002, **13**, 579.
14. F. Schlachetzki, Y. Zhang, R.J. Boado and W.M. Pardridge, *Neurology*, 2004, **62**, 1275.
15. A.H. Faraji and P. Wipf, *Bioorg.Med.Chem.*, 2009, **17**, 2950.
16. A. Tsuji, *NeuroRx.*, 2005, **2**, 54.
17. R. Huang, W. Ke, Y. Liu, C. Jiang and Y. Pei, *Biomaterials*, 2008, **29**, 238.
18. R. Huang, W. Ke, Y. Liu, D. Wu, L. Feng, C. Jiang and Y. Pei, *J.Neurol.Sci.*, 2010, **290**, 123.
19. R. Huang, W. Ke, L. Han, Y. Liu, K. Shao, L. Ye, J. Lou, C. Jiang and Y. Pei, *J.Cereb.Blood Flow Metab*, 2009, **29**, 1914.

20. R.Q. Huang, Y.H. Qu, W.L. Ke, J.H. Zhu, Y.Y. Pei and C. Jiang, *FASEB J.*, 2007, **21**, 1117.

21. H. Dou, J. Morehead, C.J. Destache, J.D. Kingsley, L. Shlyakhtenko, Y. Zhou, M. Chaubal, J. Werling, J. Kipp, B.E. Rabinow and H.E. Gendelman, *Virology*, 2007, **358**, 148.

22. X. Gao, W. Tao, W. Lu, Q. Zhang, Y. Zhang, X. Jiang and S. Fu, *Biomaterials*, 2006, **27**, 3482.

23. H. Binder and G. Lindblom, *Biophys.J.*, 2003, **85**, 982.

24. D. Derossi, S. Calvet, A. Trembleau, A. Brunissen, G. Chassaing and A. Prochiantz, *J.Biol.Chem.*, 1996, **271**, 18188.

25. J.M. Bergen and S.H. Pun, *J.Gene Med.*, 2008, **10**, 187.

26. S.A. Mousavi, L. Malerod, T. Berg and R. Kjeken, *Biochem.J.*, 2004, **377**, 1.

27. M. Marsh and A. Helenius, *Cell*, 2006, **124**, 729.

28. R. Wattiaux, N. Laurent, C.S. Wattiaux-De and M. Jadot, *Adv.Drug Deliv.Rev.*, 2000, **41**, 201.

29. M. Ogris and E. Wagner, *Somat.Cell Mol.Genet.*, 2002, **27**, 85.

30. L.M. Bareford and P.W. Swaan, *Adv.Drug Deliv.Rev.*, 2007, **59**, 748.

31. M. Kirkham and R.G. Parton, *Biochim.Biophys.Acta*, 2005, **1746**, 349.

32. W.J. Jockusch, G.J. Praefcke, H.T. McMahon and L. Lagnado, *Neuron*, 2005, **46**, 869.

33. E.L. Clayton, G.J. Evans and M.A. Cousin, *J.Neurosci.*, 2008, **28**, 6627.

34. S. Mayor and R.E. Pagano, *Nat.Rev.Mol.Cell Biol.*, 2007, **8**, 603.

35. K. Bruckner, L.J. Pablo, P. Scheiffele, A. Herb, P.H. Seeburg and R. Klein, *Neuron*, 1999, **22**, 511.

36. J.R. Martens, R. Navarro-Polanco, E.A. Coppock, A. Nishiyama, L. Parshley, T.D. Grobaski and M.M. Tamkun, *J.Biol.Chem.*, 2000, **275**, 7443.

37. M. Fernandez, M.F. Segura, C. Sole, A. Colino, J.X. Comella and V. Ceña, *J.Neurochem.*, 2007, **103**, 190.

38. H. Kokubo, J.B. Helms, Y. Ohno-Iwashita, Y. Shimada, Y. Horikoshi and H. Yamaguchi, *Brain Res.*, 2003, **965**, 83.

39. S. Mukherjee, R.N. Ghosh and F.R. Maxfield, *Physiol Rev.*, 1997, **77**, 759.

40. J.A. Swanson and C. Watts, *Trends Cell Biol.*, 1995, **5**, 424.

41. O. Harush-Frenkel, E. Rozentur, S. Benita and Y. Altschuler, *Biomacromolecules.*, 2008, **9**, 435.

42. G. Creusat, A.S. Rinaldi, E. Weiss, R. Elbaghdadi, J.S. Remy, R. Mulherkar and G. Zuber, *Bioconjug.Chem.*, 2010, **21**, 994.

43. M. Lafon, *J.Neurovirol.*, 2005, **11**, 82.

44. Y. Liu, R. Huang, L. Han, W. Ke, K. Shao, L. Ye, J. Lou and C. Jiang, *Biomaterials*, 2009, **30**, 4195.

45. O. Boussif, F. Lezoualc'h, M.A. Zanta, M.D. Mergny, D. Scherman, B. Demeneix and J.P. Behr, *Proc.Natl.Acad.Sci.U.S.A*, 1995, **92**, 7297.

46. A.A. Kale and V.P. Torchilin, *J.Drug Target*, 2007, **15**, 538.

47. L.M. DeAngelis, *N.Engl.J.Med.*, 2001, **344**, 114.

48. J.L. Jimenez, M.I. Clemente, N.D. Weber, J. Sanchez, P. Ortega, F.J. de la Mata, R. Gomez, D. Garcia, L.A. Lopez-Fernandez and M.A. Munoz-Fernandez, *BioDrugs.*, 2010, **24**, 331.

49. I. Posadas, B. Lopez-Hernandez, M.I. Clemente, J.L. Jimenez, P. Ortega, M.J. de la, R. Gomez, M.A. Muñoz-Fernandez and V. Ceña, *Pharm.Res.*, 2009, **26**, 1181.

50. J.B. Kim, J.S. Choi, K. Nam, M. Lee, J.S. Park and J.K. Lee, *J.Control Release*, 2006, **114**, 110.

51. T.L. Kaneshiro and Z.R. Lu, *Biomaterials*, 2009, **30**, 5660.

52. A. Agrawal, D.H. Min, N. Singh, H. Zhu, A. Birjiniuk, M.G. von, T.J. Harris, D. Xing, S.D. Woolfenden, P.A. Sharp, A. Charest and S. Bhatia, *ACS Nano.*, 2009, **3**, 2495.
53. M.D. Perez-Carrión, F.C. Perez-Martinez, S. Merino, P. Sanchez-Verdu, J. Martinez-Hernandez, R. Lujan and V. Ceña, *J.Neurochem.*, 2012, **120**, 259.
54. A.C. Rodrigo, I. Rivilla, F.C. Perez-Martinez, S. Monteagudo, V. Ocana, J. Guerra, J.C. Garcia-Martinez, S. Merino, P. Sanchez-Verdu, V. Ceña and J. Rodriguez-Lopez, *Biomacromolecules.*, 2011, **12**, 1205.
55. C.L. Waite and C.M. Roth, *Bioconjug.Chem.*, 2009, **20**, 1908.
56. K.H. Bae, H.J. Chung and T.G. Park, *Mol.Cells*, 2011, **31**, 295.
57. L. Han, A. Zhang, H. Wang, P. Pu, X. Jiang, C. Kang and J. Chang, *Hum.Gene Ther.*, 2010, **21**, 417.
58. H. Sarin, A.S. Kanevsky, H. Wu, A.A. Sousa, C.M. Wilson, M.A. Aronova, G.L. Griffiths, R.D. Leapman and H.Q. Vo, *J.Transl.Med.*, 2009, **7**, 51.
59. D. A. Tomalia. *New J. Chem.* 2012, **36**, 264.
60. L. Albertazzi, M. Brondi, G. M. Pavan, S. S. Sato, G. Signore, B. Storti, G. M. Ratto and F. Beltram. *PLoS One* 2011, **6**, e28450.
61. G. M. Pavan, A. Barducci, L. Albertazzi and M. Parrinello. Soft Matter, DOI:10.1039/C3SM27706B.
62. M. Zheng, G.M. Pavan, N. Neeb, A.K. Schaper, A. Danani, G. Klebe, O.M. Merkel and T. Kissel. ACS Nano, 2012, **6**, 9447.
63. G.M. Pavan, S. Monteagudo, J. Guerra, B. Carrión, V. Ocaña, J. Rodriguez-Lopez, A. Danani, F.C. Perez-Martinez and V. Ceña. Curr. Med. Chem., 2012, **29**, 4929.

MULTISCALE MODELING OF DENDRIMERS AND DENDRONS FOR DRUG AND NUCLEIC ACID DELIVERY

P. Posocco,[1] E. Laurini,[1] V. Dal Col,[1] D. Marson,[1] L. Peng,[2] D.K. Smith,[3] B. Klajnert,[4] M. Bryszewska,[4] A.-M. Caminade,[5] J.P. Majoral,[5] M. Fermeglia,[1] K. Karatasos[6] and S. Pricl[1]

[1]Molecular Simulation Engineering (MOSE) Laboratory, DEA, University of Trieste, Piazzale Europa 1, 34127 Trieste, Italy
[2]Centre Interdisciplinaire de Nanoscience de Marseille, CNRS UMR 7325, 163, avenue de Luminy, 13288 Marseille, France
[3]Department of Chemistry, University of York, Heslington, York, YO10 5DD, United Kingdom
[4]Department of General Biophysics, University of Lodz, Pomorska st. 141/143, Lodz 90-236, Poland
[5]Laboratorie de Chimie de Coordination, CNRS, UPR 8241 205, route de Narbonne 31077, Toulouse, France
[6]Chemical Engineering Department, Aristotle University of Thessaloniki, University Campus, 54124, Thessaloniki, Greece

1 INTRODUCTION

Multiscale molecular simulations of drug delivery systems (DDSs) is poised to provide predictive capabilities for the rational design of targeted DDSs, including multi-functional nanoparticles such as dendrimers and dendrons as highly specialized delivery nanovectors. Realistic three-dimensional atomistic and mesoscopic models can provide a framework for understanding the fundamental physico-chemical interactions between the active principles, their nanocarriers and, ultimately, the patient physiology. The wide range of emerging nanotechnology systems for targeted delivery further increases the need for reliable *in silico* predictions.

Multiscale modeling, however, is in its infancy even for conventional drug delivery. The projection that by 2016 about 30% of pharmaceutical R&D expenditure will be on computer simulation connote that we will see more and more sophisticated molecular models developed. Due to the permutations of the confounding factors that complicate the traditional experimental (wet lab) approach, the need for multiscale computational models is even higher for the design of drug delivery systems of nanoparticles that involve multiscale processes both in the spatial and temporal dimensions. Thus, a pathway to future designs of smart delivery systems will be integration of the different elements at various levels of scales involving the physico-chemical and biological phenomena, as shown in Figure 1.

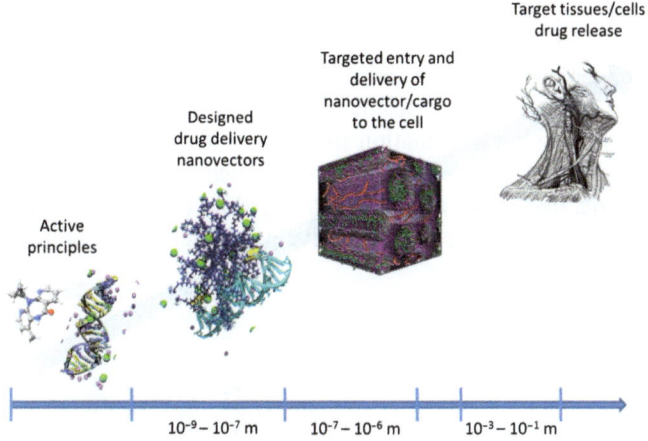

Figure 1 *The (multi)length scale of a nanovector-assisted drug delivery process.*

In recent years, the use of computer simulations as a tool for bridging between microscopic length and time scales and the macroscopic world of the laboratory has been increasing exponentially. The main reasons for this success is that, by using computational chemistry and physics, a guess at the interactions between molecules can be provided, and `exact' predictions of bulk properties can be obtained. The predictions are `exact' in the sense that they can be made as accurate as we like, subject to the limitations imposed by the available computer budget. At the same time, the hidden detail behind bulk measurements can be revealed. Simulations act as a bridge in another sense: between theory and experiment. A theory can be tested by conducting a simulation using the same model. The model can be tested by comparing with experimental results. Also, simulations can be carried out on the computer that are difficult or impossible in the laboratory (for example, working at extremes of temperature or pressure).

The actual computational modeling of biological macromolecules, mainly based on molecular dynamics (MD) simulations, commonly revolves around structure representations in atomic or near-atomic detail, with a classical description of physical interactions. In a typical MD simulation, the atomic trajectories of a system of N (e.g., 10^6) particles are generated by numerical integration of Newton's equation of motion, for a specific interatomic potential, with certain initial and boundary conditions. Such models have been quite successful in complementing experimental data with structural, dynamic, and energetic information, but involve substantial computational resources for larger systems, or when long time scales have to be considered. In particular, structure-activity calculation applications, the formation and interaction of supramolecular assemblies, and the prediction of kinetic and transport phenomena will necessarily involve extremely extensive computational resources when using models at atomic details, if they are feasible at all.

Thus, we are also in the need of developing some computational strategy to link the atomic length and time scales of MD to the macroscopic length and time scales (nanometers to micrometers and nanoseconds to microseconds): the so-called *mesoscale* phase. Only by establishing this connection from nanoscale to mesoscale it is possible to build first principles methods for describing the properties of new materials and systems for biomedical and life science applications, of which RNA/DNA delivery systems are prototypical examples.[1]

This linking through the mesoscale in which the microstructure can be described over a length scale of tens to hundred nanometers is probably the greatest challenge to develop reliable first principles method for practical material design applications. Scale integration in specific contexts in the field of (bio)macromolecular modeling can be done in different ways. Any *recipe* for passing information from one scale to another (upper) scale is based on the proper definition of many-scale modeling which considers *objects* that are relevant at that particular scale, disregards all degrees of freedom of smaller scales, and summarizes those degrees of freedom by some representative parameters (see Figure 2).[2]

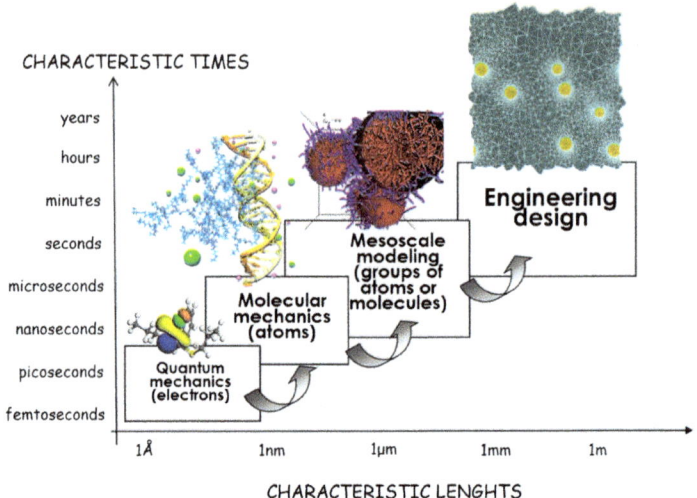

Figure 2 *The multiscale molecular modeling concept: the information obtained from simulations at a given (lower) characteristic length and time scales is used as an input for the next (upper) scale simulations.*

Under the multiscale molecular modeling perspective outlined above, the current ambitious aim of our research group is to reach the domain of nucleic acid delivery system engineering by building from fundamental principles of physics and chemistry. Hence, for fundamental predictions to play a direct role in these materials innovation and design, it is mandatory to bridge the micro-macro gap, thus establishing a tight and direct coupling between *in silico* and *in vitro/in vivo* experiments.

2   STUCTURAL CHARACTERIZATION OF DENDRONS AND DENDRIMERS

Dendrimers (or any other macromolecule) entering the systemic circulation distribute to tissues largely via the bloodstream. Therefore, the blood flow rate determines the delivery rate of macromolecules to each tissue. Dendrimers in the circulation have direct access to the capillary endothelial cells, as well as various circulating cells in the blood. These cells have the opportunity to take up the macromolecules via specific or non-specific interactions. The interaction of macromolecules with parenchymal cells in tissues can occur only when they have access through the endothelial lining.

The structure of the blood capillary walls varies greatly depending on the organ. In addition, pathological states such as inflammation could change the structure. On the basis of the morphology and continuity of the endothelial layer and the basement membrane, the capillary endothelium can be divided into continuous, fenestrated, and discontinuous endothelium. Tight junctions between endothelial cells and underlying uninterrupted basement membrane characterize the continuous endothelium, through which the passage of polymeric molecules is greatly hampered. Such type of endothelium characterizes the skeletal, cardiac, and smooth muscles, and can be found in lung, skin, and subcutaneous tissues. Dendrimeric and other polymer-based nanoparticles with diameters equal or greater than 6 nm hardly interact with parenchymal cells in these tissues, simply because of the barriers posed by the endothelium. Endothelial cells having fenestrae featuring a diaphragm - an opening 40-80 nm in diameter – form the fenestrated endothelium found in the intestinal mucosa, the endocrine and exocrine glands, and the gromerulus and peritubules of the kidney. However, the passage of macromolecules through this type of endothelium is limited by the presence of the basement membrane. The discontinuous (or sinusoidal) endothelium is found only in the liver, spleen, and bone marrow. These capillaries are characterized by endothelial gaps, intracellular junctions with a diameter up to 30-500 nm and with either no basement membrane (liver) or a discontinuous basement membrane (spleen and bone marrow). Therefore, parenchymal cells in these tissues can be accessed by macromolecules with relatively high molecular weight and, consequently, large dimensions. A similar situation (i.e., big fenestrations and enhanced vascular permeability of nanoparticle-based drug delivery systems) are also found in several solid tumours.

According to the above discussion the size and, hence, the structure of dendrimers as a function of pH is a critical issue for their utilization as drug delivery vehicles in physiological environments (pH = 7.4). Molecular simulations can provide insights into the structure and the properties of dendrimers as a function of generation by yielding, for instance out of a plethora of many others, the values of the radius of gyration R_g and the corresponding radial distribution functions of the dendrimers via fully atomistic MD simulations in explicit solvent, counterions, and ionic strength.

2.1 Dimensions and Shape of Viologen Dendrimers

Viologen-phosphorus containing dendrimers are relatively new compounds which have been seldom investigated in terms of their biological and, even less, of their structural properties.[3] These types of compounds exhibit antimicrobial properties and their behavior depends on their size, the number of viologen units and the nature of the surface groups.[3(a),4] Quite recently, Erik De Clercq and collaborators[5] proved the antiviral activity of dendrimers containing a viologen against the Human Immunodeficiency Virus (HIV), and, to a lesser extent, against other viruses such as the Herpes Simplex Virus (HSV), the Reovirus (RV), and the Respiratory Syncytial Virus (RSV).

Accordingly, we embarked in a complex computational study to determine the main structural characteristics of some representative members of the viologen-based dendrimers, and their binding to albumin.[4] In particular, we focused on two different families of new viologen dendrimers bearing phosphorus groups as additional units incorporated either at the focal point or at the periphery or both of these key structural positions of the dendritic backbone.[3] This choice of strategy was aimed by the fact that we already demonstrated the key role played by phosphorus dendrimers in biology and for biomedical applications due to several specificities.[6]

Accordingly, the two viologen-phosphorus dendrimers were built from a trifunctionalized core $P(S)(NCH_3NH_2)_3$ (**D2**, **D4**, and **D6**) or from a hexafunctionalized core $(P_3N_3)(NCH_3NH_2)_6$ (**D3**, **D5**, and **D7**), and decorated on their surface either with aldehyde groups or with phosphonate groups, the latter being well-known for their biological properties. A dendron structurally similar to **D2** but stemming from a phenyl core (**D1**) was also considered for comparison.

Scheme 1 illustrates the chemical structures of the viologen dendrimers **D1-D7**, while Figure 3 shows the MD equilibrated snapshots of **D4** and **D7** at neutral pH and in the presence of a physiological ionic strength (0.15 M) in solution.

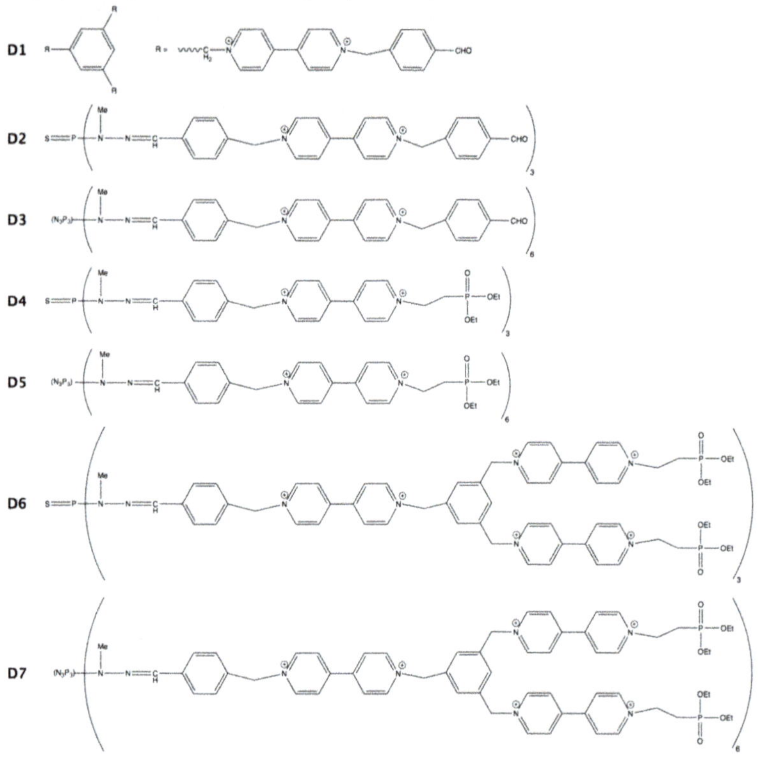

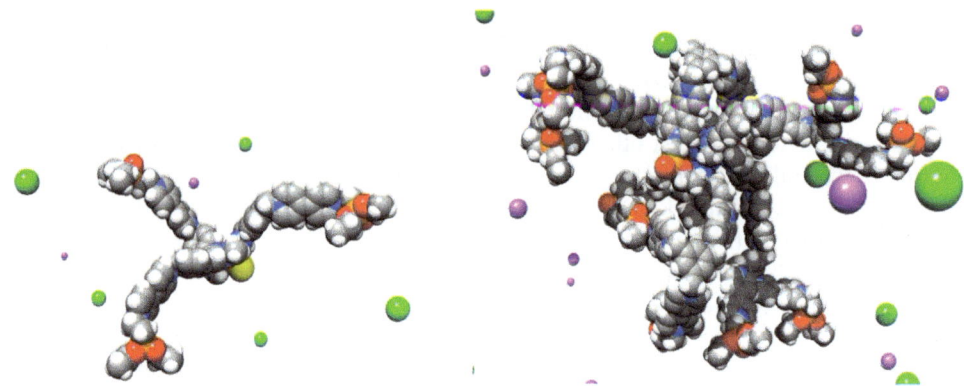

Scheme 1 *Chemical structures of the viologen dendrimers D1-D7.*

Figure 3 *Equilibrated MD snapshots of viologen-phosphorous D4 (left) and D7 (right) in solution at neutral pH and 0.15 M NaCl. The dendrimers are shown as atom-coloured spheres (grey, C; red, O; yellow, S; blue, N, orange, P, white, H). Water molecules are omitted for clarity, while some counterions are shown as green (Cl⁻) and purple (Na⁺) spheres.*

The radius of gyration R_g is a fundamental tool for the description of structural properties of dendrimeric molecules and other macromolecules as well. This quantity, related to the square root of the second invariant of the first order tensor S, takes into account the spatial distribution of the atom chain by mediating over all N molecular components. For a dendrimer, the mean-square radius of gyration is defined by:

$$R_g^2 = \frac{1}{M_w}\langle \sum_{i=1}^{N} m_i \left| r_i - R \right|^2 \rangle \tag{1}$$

where R is the centre of mass of the dendrimer, r_i and m_i are the position and mass of the ith atom, and M_w refers to the total mass of the dendrimer. The R_g values estimated by MD simulations for all viologen dendrimer generations G at pH = 7.4 and 0.15 M NaCl are listed in the fourth column of Table 1. As shown in Figure 4A, the dimensions of the viologen dendrimers linearly increase with increasing generation G.

Table 1 *Main Structural Parameters for Viologen Dendrimers D1-D7*

Dendrimer	Charge	G	R_g (Å)	Asphericity
D1	+6	0	9.25	0.078
D2	+6	0	10.76	0.063
D3	+12	0	12.32	0.020
D4	+6	0	12.19	0.081
D5	+12	0	13.07	0.023
D6	+18	1	16.59	0.069
D7	+36	1	18.82	0.026

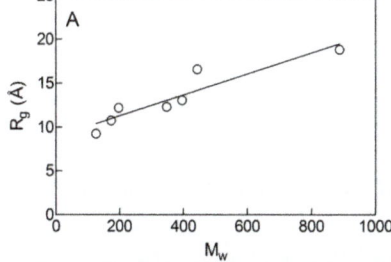
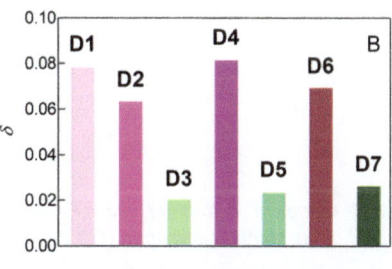

Figure 4 *(A) Plot of R_g calculated from MD simulations as a function of the viologen dendrimers molecular weight at pH = 7.4 and 0.15 M NaCl. (B) Plot of the asphericity parameter δ for all viologen dendrimers.*

While the value of R_g, yields an indication of the overall dimension of the dendrimers, it does not inform about the real shape of the molecules, that is, if the dendrimer is adopting a true spherical or, e.g., an oblong shape. To check this, MD data can be further exploited to characterize the shape of the dendrimers by calculating the molecular asphericity parameter as:

$$\delta = 1 - 3\frac{\langle I_2 \rangle}{\langle I_1^2 \rangle} \tag{2}$$

where I_1 and I_2 are the first two invariants of the radius of gyration tensor S. By definition, the asphericity parameter can take values ranging from 0 (i.e., a sphere) to 1 (a line). The fifth column of Table 1 and the graph in Figure 4B show that all viologen dendrimers tend to assume a spherical conformation; nonetheless, the dendrimers featuring the cyclotriphosphazene moiety as a core (**D3**, **D5**, and **D7**) and characterized by 6 branches all present a δ value close to 0.02 and, thus, assume a more spherical than their 3-branched trihydrazidophosphine-core or phenyl-core counterparts (**D1**, **D2**, **D4**, and **D6**). Such a behaviour can be ascribed to the presence of regularly spaced like-charges along the dendrimer branches, whose reciprocal repulsion (greater for those molecules with a higher number of ramifications) finds a global equilibrium condition in the adoption of a more regular and spherical shape.

2.2 Flexibility and Back-Folding of PAMAM-like Dendrimers

2.1.1 TEA-core PAMAM dendrimers as highly flexibly nanocarriers. Recently, Peng et al. showed that PAMAM dendrimers based on a triethanolamine (TEA) core (see Scheme 2) are effective vectors for siRNA delivery and gene silencing using both a luciferase model[7] and a functional siRNA to target the heat shock protein 27 in castrate-resistant prostate cancer.[8]

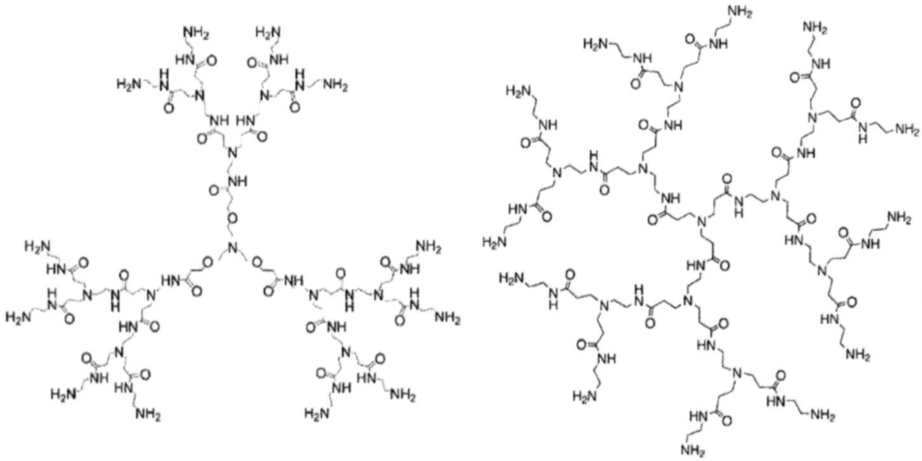

Scheme 2 *Chemical details of the TEA-core (left) and NH₃-core PAMAM dendrimers. For clarity, dendrimers of the second generation (**G₂**) are shown.*

The rationale behind the synthesis of this new dendrimer family was that the TEA-core dendrimers, having the branching units starting away from the central amine with a distance of 10 successive bonds, should feature an extended core, and are expected to be less congested in space with respect to the prototypical NH₃-core PAMAM dendrimers, for which the branches sprout directly from the small ammonia focal point. Consequently, the TEA-core dendrimers, with their branching units and terminal end groups being less densely packed than those of NH₃-core dendrimers, should be endowed with an enhanced flexibility of their arms if compared to more congested dendrimeric families and, as such, able to perform better as *e.g.*, DNA or siRNA nanocarriers. Indeed, a larger flexibility should in principle allow a nanocarrier to *i*) more effectively enwrap its genetic material and *ii*) act as a better more efficient proton sponge.

Accordingly, information on the structural diversity between TEA-core and NH₃-core based PAMAM dendrimers were obtained by applying atomistic MD simulations.[9,10] As an example, Figure 5A and 5B shows two equilibrium MD snapshots of the generation 5 dendrimers of the TEA-core (**G₅**) and the NH₃-core (**G₅'**) PAMAM dendrimers at neutral pH, respectively. The structural difference which characterizes these two macromolecules is apparent at first glance: whilst **G₅** has a more open conformation featuring uniform void spacing in its interior, the **G₅'** counterpart is more compact, with its monomer units distributed more uniformly within the entire molecule and a non-homogeneous, restricted void spacing (Figure 5A). Accordingly, the conformation of the TEA-core dendrimer **G₅** is such that the outer branches can readily move and adjust for optimizing an ultimate binding with its nucleic acid cargo. On the contrary, in the case of the NH_3-core dendrimer G_5', its more rigid and compact structure prevents this molecule for any *induced-fit* conformational readjustment and, consequently, not all terminal amine groups are available to self-orient for optimal cargo binding (see Figure 5B).

A quantitative support to this pictorial view can be obtained by considering the average radial monomer density $\rho(r)$, a quantity defined as the number of atoms whose centres of mass are located within a spherical shell of radius r and thickness Δr. Integration over r yields the total number of monomers as:

$$N(r) = 4\pi \int_0^R r^2 \rho(r) dr \qquad (3)$$

Figure 5C and 5D shows the radial monomer density profiles for the TEA-core G_5 and the NH_3-core G_5' dendrimer molecules, respectively. In each case, the plot shows the contribution to the particular generation from each of its component generations. In each case, the molecular centre of mass was taken as the origin. When considering G_5, the whole dendrimer $\rho(r)$ curve (thick continuous line in Figure 5C) shows a minimum around 10 Å away from the core, and another, smaller minimum at approximately 17 Å. These, together with the two relative maxima (located at ~ 13 and 21 Å), indicate that *i*) the core region becomes denser compared with the middle of the dendrimer, which is fairly hollow, and *ii*) the higher sub-generation monomers form a crowded layer at the dendrimer periphery. This is perfectly matching the portray of the molecule as resulting from the snapshot of the MD simulations (Figure 5A). Further, from Figure 5C we can see that this increase in density at the core stems only from the density of the inner generations. The outermost generations do not contribute to this density, but contribute mainly to the density of the outmost layers. Because of the presence of uniform, hollow spaces in the inner/middle regions of the dendrimer, a significant number of water molecules are able to penetrate to the molecular middle region, as depicted by the corresponding thick dashed curve in Figure 5C. Considering now G_5', the corresponding profile of the $\rho(r)$ curve for the whole dendrimer is pretty different (see Figure 5D). Starting form the core peak, we see a uniform decrease and then a plateau value in the monomer density all across the molecular structure, followed by a secondary peak, again at the molecular periphery. Accordingly, all sub-generations contribute substantially to the whole density curve, pointing to a more uniform monomer distribution inside the dendrimer molecule (see also Figure 5B). In harmony with this evidences, water does not show a pronounced maximum in any specific region of the molecule but is also uniformly distributed within the molecular interior (thick dashed curve in Figure 5D).

2.1.2 Back-folding of PAMAM dendrimers. A further, peculiar feature of dendrimeric structures which may affect their performance as nanocarriers is the high degree of back-folding. The usual schematic diagrams found in the literature for dendrimers, particularly the 2D representations, convey the idea that the terminal groups are located at the periphery of the molecule. However, actual MD simulations reveal the presence of a substantial back-folding of the end groups toward the dendrimer core.[10,11] To quantify this aspect, the radial distribution functions for terminal nitrogen atoms for various generations of the "gold standard" diethylenediamine (DEA) PAMAMs are reported in Figure 6A and 6B.

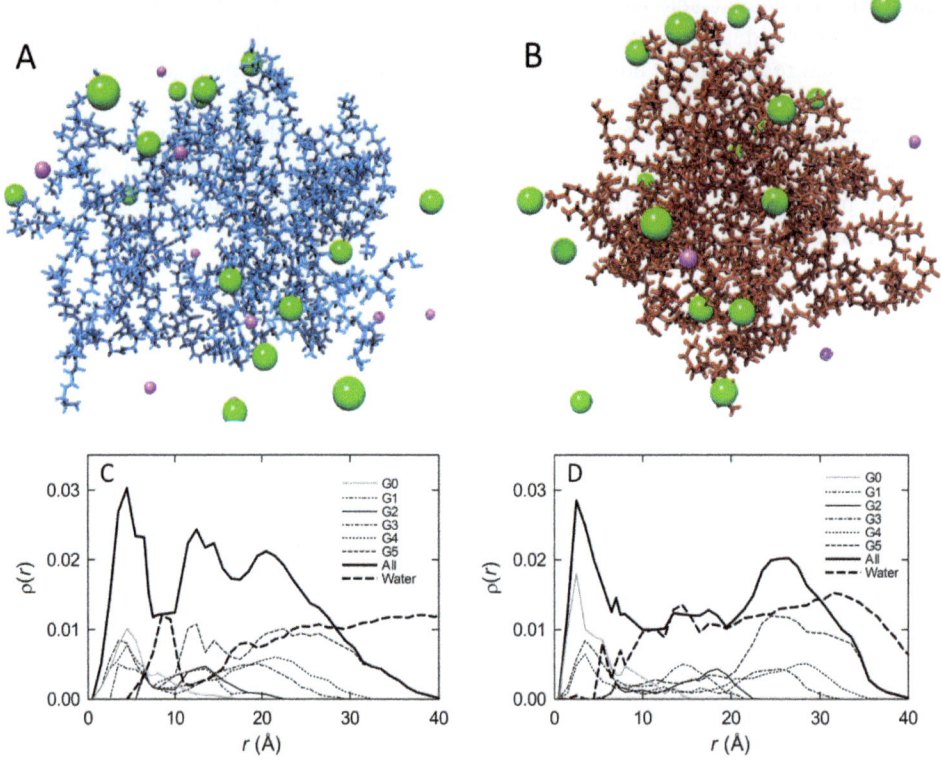

Figure 5 *Top panels: snapshots of typical equilibrium configurations of G5 (A) and G5' (B) dendrimers at pH = 7.4 and 0.15 M NaCl. Dendrimers are shown as coloured sticks, while some counterions are portrayed as green (Cl⁻) and purple (Na⁺) spheres. Water is not shown for clarity. Bottom panels: radial monomer density profiles for TEA-core dendrimer G_5 (C) and NH₃-core dendrimer G_5' (D).*

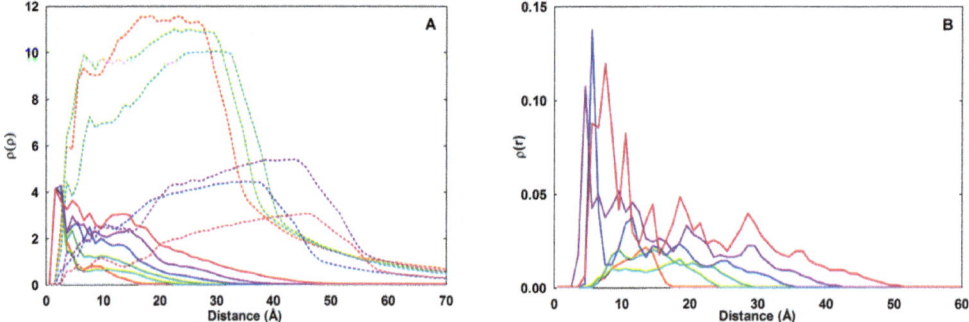

Figure 6 *(A) Radial density distributions for PAMAM generations G_1 to G_6 (continuous lines) and water (broken lines) at pH = 7.4. (B) Radial density distributions for terminal nitrogen atoms of PAMAM generations G_1 to G_6 at pH = 7.4. Colour legend: red, G_1; light green, G_2; dark green, G_3; blue, G_4; purple, G_5; dark red, G_6. Adapted from PAMAM dendrimers for siRNA delivery: computational and experimental insights, Pavan, G.M.; Posocco, P.; Tagliabue, A.; Maly, M.; Malek, A.; Danani, A.; Ragg, E.; Catapano, C.V.; Pricl, S. Chemistry Eur. J. 16(26), Copyright © [2010], John Wiley & Sons, http://onlinelibrary.wiley.com/doi/10.1002/chem.200903258/pdf.*

These distributions reveal that the dendrimer end groups are sufficiently flexible to interpenetrate nearly the whole molecule. In particular, the end groups of higher generations come even close to the core of the molecule, and the extent of back-folding increases with increasing dendrimer generation G. This effect is more evident at neutral pH; higher generations show pronounced peaks near the core of the molecule and, for smaller generations, the back-folding pervades the entire molecular architecture. Obviously, the presence of a substantial back-folding is detrimental to nucleic acid binding, as less protonated terminal groups are available on the dendrimer surface; accordingly, the overall dendrimer surface charge is diminished, the corresponding ionic interactions with the genetic material is lower, and the nucleic acid cargo might be lost along the way to the target cell under the action of drag forces in the blood stream or the uptake of plasma proteins. On the other hand, a too strong interaction between the nanovector and its cargo can turn out to be unfavourable in a later stage of the delivery process, that is during cargo release in the cell cytoplasm: a tight electrostatic bond between the two molecular entities may disfavour the nucleic acid detachment from its vector, thus making the genetic material unavailable for further, therapeutic action.

3 BINDING OF DENDRON/DENDRIMERS TO NUCLEC ACIDS

The ability of a nanocarrier to generate a stable complex with its nucleic acid payload is a background postulate for its usefulness in gene delivery. This property can be experimentally explored and quantified through the use of many disparate techniques, ranging from the standard Ethidium Bromide (EthBr) displacement fluorescence spectroscopy assay to the more sophisticate and quantitative isothermal titration calorimetry (ITC) or differential scanning calorimetry (DSC). Multiscale molecular simulations, however, not only can yield the same information in a less expensive way (both from time and money standpoint), but may offer a reliable molecular rationale to explain the generation, structural, ionic strength, and other chemico-physical properties and mechanisms determining the dependence of the affinity of a given dendrimer/dendron carrier to its nucleic acid cargo.[1,9-12]

Thus, in a recent study we demonstrated that the structurally flexible TEA-core poly(amidoamine) (PAMAM) dendrimers are excellent nonviral vectors for siRNA delivery both *in vitro* and *in vivo*.[8,9,13] Of particular interest, the generation 7 dendrimer (G_7) can mediate efficient siRNA delivery and produce potent gene silencing of the heat shock protein 27 (Hsp27) leading to effective anticancer activity in a castration-resistant prostate cancer model.[8] Unfortunately, however, the large-scale synthesis of the good quality TEA-core dendrimer G_7 is particularly challenging. This is due to the seemingly easy but rather time-consuming and meticulous control of the reaction conditions as well as the tedious procedures of purifying the resulting, high generation PAMAM dendrimers. Accordingly, the possibility of developing low generation dendrimers for the effective delivery of siRNA therapeutics constitutes *per se* a challenging but worthwhile goal.

Recently, Behr et al. discovered that siRNAs with short complementary A_n/T_n (n = 5 - 8) 3′ overhangs, named " sticky " siRNA could dramatically increase gene silencing efficiency when using polyethylenimine (PEI) as the delivery vector.[14] Given these premises, since the large-scale synthesis of good quality, high generation dendrimers is particularly challenging, we reasoned that, resorting to sticky siRNAs, it could be possible to achieve the same gene efficiency by exploiting lower generation dendrimers as nanovectors.

Indeed, we verified that TEA-core PAMAM dendrimers of generation 5 are able to deliver sticky siRNAs bearing complementary A_n/T_n with (n = 5 or 7) 3'overhangs efficiently to a prostate cancer model both in vitro and, most notably, in vivo, and produce potent gene silencing of the heat shock protein 27, leading to a notable anticancer effect.[15]

We further checked whether, in addition to the hypothesized formation of gene-like longer double strand RNA molecules, the two complementary A_n/T_n (n = 5 or 7) overhangs of the sticky siRNAs might also behave as a sort of protruding molecular arms, allowing the siRNA molecule to enwrap the spherical, low generation dendrimers with higher binding affinity compared with a conventional siRNA which has two short T_2/T_2 overhangs.

Therefore, we studied the complex formation of G_5 with different siRNA molecules (conventional siRNA with T_2/T_2 overhangs, and sticky siRNAs with either A_5/T_5 or A_7/T_7 overhangs) by atomistic MD techniques.[15] The *in silico* predicted affinities of each sticky siRNA and the G_5 dendrimer, as quantified by the corresponding free energy of binding ΔG_{bind}, reveal that the ΔG_{bind} values obtained for G_5 and the sticky siRNAs with A_5/T_5 or A_7/T_7 overhangs are lower (i.e., more negative and, hence, more favourable) than those calculated for G_5 and the conventional siRNA with T_2/T_2 overhangs (Table 3), which indicates that the binding affinity of G_5 for sticky siRNAs is higher than that of G_5 for conventional siRNA. Based on these results, we hypothesized that, in addition to the possible formation of gene-like longer double strand RNA molecules, stronger binding to dendrimer of sticky siRNAs over conventional siRNAs might also contribute to the enhanced delivery activity of G_5.

Table 2 *Free energy of binding between a TEA-core PAMAM dendrimer of generation 5 (G_5) and a siRNA with T_2/T_2, A_5/T_5, and A_7/T_7 overhangs (conventional siRNA and sticky siRNAs), respectively. Adapted with permission from Liu, X.; Liu, C.; Laurini, E.; Posocco, P.; Pricl, S.; Qu, F.; Rocchi, P.; Peng, L. Efficient delivery of sticky siRNA and potent gene silencing in a prostate cancer model using a generation 5 triethanolamine-core PAMAM dendrimer. Mol. Pharm., 2012, 9, 470-481. Copyright {2012} American Chemical Society.*

System	ΔH_{bind} (kcal/mol)	$-T\Delta S_{bind}$ (kcal/mol)	ΔG_{bind} (kcal/mol)
G_5/siRNA (T_2/T_2 overhangs)	-571.1 ± 2.6	254.3 ± 4.3	-316.8 ± 5.0
G_5/sticky siRNA (A_5/T_5 overhangs)	-637.40 ± 2.8	250.0 ± 4.1	-387.4 ± 5.0
G_5/sticky siRNA (A_7/T_7 overhangs)	-690.2 ± 4.7	267.3 ± 5.3	-422.9 ± 7.1

4   SOLVATION OF DENDRIMER/NUCLEIC ACID COMPLEXES

Soft colloids and macromolecules with flexible structures and void pervading their entire complex molecular structure are necessarily hydrated not only in their outer shell. Indeed, ions and water can penetrate along the tortuous pathways of holes and channels of the macromolecular entity, eventually reaching down to the inner core. Upon binding of a dendrimer to a nucleic acid, water plays even more determining roles. First, it creates a bridge between the carrier and the DNA/RNA, by maintaining an hydration layer and ensuring the instauration of a hydrogen bond network between the carrier and the nucleic acid, critical to their complex formation and stability. More important, perhaps, is the role of overall solubilization. Water and the solution navigating salts must pervade the entire system to guarantee uniform hydration and dispersion of the loaded nanoparticles, avoiding their aggregation and collapse.

Mesoscale simulations offer the possibility to predict and study this type of behaviour; in fact, a typical result of a mesoscale simulation is the morphology and the structure of matter at nanoscale level at the desired environmental conditions.[2,9] Let us then consider Figure 7, where the nanoscale morphology of a DNA/G_6 complexes of TEA-core dendrimer (see §2.2.1 and §3) is presented. As it can be seen from this Figure, the TEA dendrimers are able to complex the DNA strands efficiently and homogeneously, with the DNA chains well enwrapped in the systems and the absence of DNA bundles at the nanoscopic level. Further, the water density maps at the mesoscopic level not only support the lower-scale (i.e., atomistic MD) results discussed above of a higher degree of hydration but also confirm the uniform water molecule distribution within the nucleic acid/TEA-core PAMAM dendrimer.

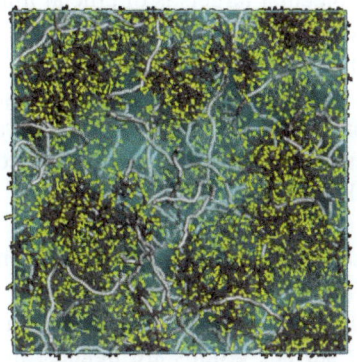 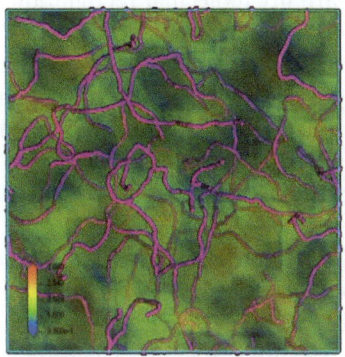

Figure 7 *(Left) Mesoscale morphologies of the assembled systems between TEA-core dendrimers G_6 and DNA. The dendrimers are represented as dark grey and yellow sticks while the DNA is shown as light grey sticks. Water is portrayed as a light grey field. (Right) DNA chains and water molecules distribution within the architectures of the TEA-core DNA/G_6 nanoscopic assembly. In this case, water is represented as a coloured density field: according to the scale reported in the lower left corners of the panels, blue density values are black, while high density values are white. Adapted with permission form Liu, X.X.; Wu, J.; Yammine, M.; Zhou, J.; Posocco, P.; Viel, S.; Liu, C.; Ziarelli, F.; Fermeglia, M.; Pricl, S.; Victorero, G.; Nguyen, C.; Erbacher, P.; Behr, J.P.; Peng, L. Structurally flexible triethanolamine core PAMAM dendrimers are effective nanovectors for DNA transfection in vitro and in vivo to the mouse thymus. Bioconjug. Chem., 2011, 22(12), 2461-2473. Copyright {2011} American Chemical Society.*

From a structure-activity relationship (SAR) standpoint, the enhanced swelling capacities of the TEA-core dendrimers at low pH values may result in a higher buffering capacity which, in turn, can be beneficial to endosomal escape of the nucleic acid cargo via the proton sponge effect. At the cellular level, in fact, inadequate cytosolic access is one major challenge that must be overcome if nanovector/DNA(RNA) systems are to become effective in vivo therapeutics. The increased swelling and, possibly, the increased proton sponge effect of more flexible and open structure dendrimers such as the TEA-core PAMAMs undoubtedly concur to enhance the capacity of these nanovectors and their cargoes to enter the endosome, adsorb protons, swell and cause an influx of negative (e.g., Cl⁻) counterions which, in turn, creates an osmotic effect ultimately leading to water uptake. This escalation of events are purported to cause endosome membrane destabilization and rupture, with subsequent release of the nanodelivery complex in the cellular cytosol. Thus, should the proton sponge effect be the operative mechanism underlying endosome escape of the nanovector and release of it payload, then flexibility, softness, and conformational freedom are all key molecular parameters in a dendrimer-based nanocarrier.

5   DENDRIMERS AND DENDRONS AS MULTIVALENT NANOVECTORS

Multivalent systems are widely found in nature, and especially in biology: adhesion of viruses or bacteria to cells' surface, cell to cell adhesion, and cell to polyvalent molecule interactions. A good example of multivalency resides in the defence process of the immune system involving bacteria, antibodies, and macrophages. Antibodies have the ability to recognize non-self entities, such as bacteria, upon polyvalent binding with antigens, or other proteins, located at their surface. It is noteworthy that weak ligand-receptor interactions can be made much stronger simply by the simultaneous bonding of these ligands to these multiple receptors.

High-affinity molecular recognition of biomolecular targets is of crucial importance in the development of synthetic systems capable of intervening in biological pathways; multivalent recognition is a key principle in enhancing binding strength and hence developing systems with potential biomedical applications. Experimental studies and mathematical models have demonstrated that once the first ligand in a multivalent array has bound to the target, the binding of a second ligand is usually a cooperative, entropically less disfavoured process, with a local concentration effect also enhancing binding.

Dendrimers and dendrons are inherent multivalent ligands that can present multiple recognition elements from a central scaffold. The scaffold plays a crucial role because it moulds the final architecture in term of shape, orientation of recognition elements, flexibility, size and valency. When the multiple surface groups are ligands, the dendritic scaffolding can be considered to act as a kind of nanoscaffolding, organizing the ligand array. As such, dendritic systems have been widely exploited for their potential applications in multivalent biological recognition. ,

Self-assembly is an incredibly powerful concept in modern molecular science. The ability of carefully designed building blocks to spontaneously assemble into complex nanostructures underpins developments in a wide range of technologies, from materials science to molecular biology. Self-assembly is a supramolecular approach which relies on complementary noncovalent interactions, such as electrostatic and van der Waals forces, hydrogen bonds, coordination interactions and solvophobic effects. In self-assembled structures, these temporal intermolecular forces connect to the molecular scale building blocks in a reversible, controllable, and specific way. Of particular value are the possibilities offered by self-assembly to generate nanoscale complexity with relatively little synthetic input. Furthermore, the ability of self-assembled superstructures to behave as more than the sum of their individual parts, and exhibit completely new types of behaviour, is of special interest and appealing in (bio)nanotechnology.

There are a number of different ways in which dendrimers or dendrons can be assembled in solution; perhaps the most efficient approach is the one that gives rise to well-defined (i.e., monodisperse) assemblies of dendritic building blocks. The supermolecular structures generated using this approach are generally based on well-established, specific intermolecular interactions; consequently, each assembly contains a defined number of dendritic building blocks. Such supermolecular dendrimeric structures have an equivalent degree of structural definition to a traditional covalent dendrimer; however, they are held together by reversible, nonbonded interactions. Given the relative simplicity of using self-assembly as a noncovalent synthetic tool, this approach is relatively cost-effective, and its potential for genuine future applications is therefore significantly enhanced.

Surface-active amphiphilic molecules are well-known to assemble into discrete structures such as micelles and vesicles in water solution. Amphiphilic dendritic systems are not exception to this rule, and a range of dendrimers with surfactant-like assembly properties have been reported. Indeed, when mixed with water, the apolar and polar regions of these Janus-type molecules will attempt to phase separate via self-assembly into structures such as micelles. Importantly, only in some cases does the aggregation process give rise to true micellar structures: this occurs at molecular concentrations C greater than the so-called critical micellar concentration (CMC), which is one of the key parameter in self-assembly. When C > CMC, aggregates with a variety of different, non-micellar structures – often ill-defined – are formed. In other words, CMC defines the thermodynamic stability of the micelles. The latter is a very critical property in drug-delivery applications of micelles because intravenous injection of micellar solutions are associated with extreme dilutions by circulating blood (usually about 25-fold dilution at bolus injection or a much higher dilution at infusion). If the concentration of a micelle forming molecule in the circulation drops below the CMC, the micelles may be prematurely destroyed, resulting in the release of their cargo into the bloodstream before it reaches its target. This, in turn, will not only result in a poor therapeutic regime but, perhaps more importantly, could be dangerous because off-target and other unwanted side effects might (and likely will) originate. On the other hand, amphiphilic compound concentration cannot be increased above some critical values that correspond to the onset of micellar aggregation and precipitation, provoked by the interpenetration of the hydrophilic micellar coronas.

5.1 Aggregation of Amphiphilic Dendrons in Solution

Under the perspective outlined above, Smith's group recently synthesized a series of dendrons with a variety of lipophilic units at their focal points and tested these molecules for DNA binding and cell transfection capacities, revealing a set of stimulating evidences: not only all modified dendrons were able to tightly bind DNA and efficiently transfect cells, but for the first time and with the aid of multiscale molecular modeling a structure-activity relationship (SAR) could be formulated between the DNA binding affinity and the overall surface charge σ_m of the micellar assemblies but, perhaps more importantly, the SAR could be extended to cellular gene delivery, as σ_m plays a fundamental role in controlling the extent of the endosomal escape.[1(c)]

Thus, state-of-the-art multiscale simulation techniques were employed to monitor the dendrons self-assembly processes and to gain an insight into the types of aggregates eventually formed. First of all, the simulations revealed that all hydrophobically modified dendrons of generation 1 were able to form spherical supermolecular structures (see Figure 8) with diameters D_m in the range of 3 - 5 nm (see Table 3 and Scheme 3).

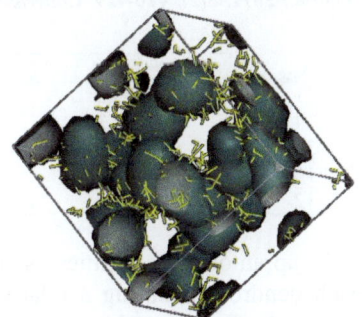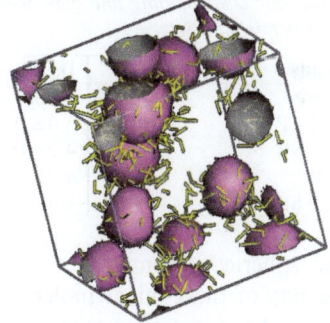

Figure 8 *Mesoscale modeling of amphiphilic dendrons showing aggregation into spherical micellar objects. In all pictures, the yellow sticks represent the dendron head groups while sea green and purple spheres are adopted to portray the various hydrophobic regions. Water and counterions are omitted for clarity. Adapted with permission from Jones, S.P.; Gabrielson, N.P.; Wong, C.H.; Chow, H.F.; Pack, D.W.; Posocco, P.; Fermeglia, M.; Pricl, S.; Smith, D.K. Hydrophobically modified dendrons: developing structure-activity relationships for DNA binding and gene transfection. Mol. Pharm., **2011**, 8(2), 416-429. Copyright {2012} American Chemical Society.*

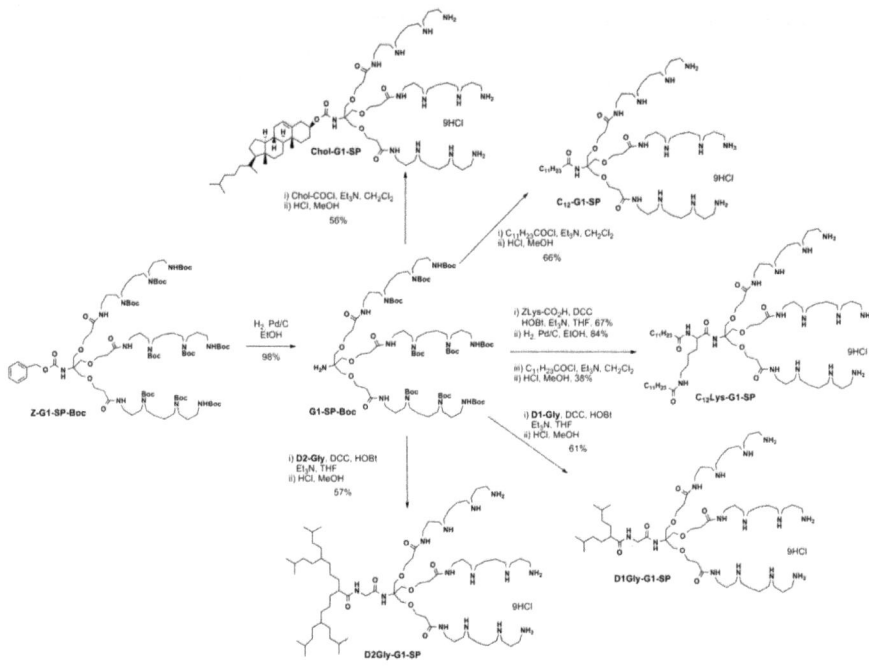

Scheme 3 *Chemical structures of the first generation dendron-based nanovectors with different hydrophobic groups at the focal point. Adapted with permission from Jones, S.P.; Gabrielson, N.P.; Wong, C.H.; Chow, H.F.; Pack, D.W.; Posocco, P.; Fermeglia, M.; Pricl, S.; Smith, D.K. Hydrophobically modified dendrons: developing structure-activity relationships for DNA binding and gene transfection. Mol. Pharm., 2011, 8(2), 416-429. Copyright {2012} American Chemical Society.*

Table 3 *Values of the micellar diameter D_m (nm), aggregation number N_{agg}, and micelle surface charge density σ_m (e/nm^2) for different amphiphilic dendrons as obtained from mesoscale simulations. Adapted with permission from Jones, S.P.; Gabrielson, N.P.; Wong, C.H.; Chow, H.F.; Pack, D.W.; Posocco, P.; Fermeglia, M.; Pricl, S.; Smith, D.K. Hydrophobically modified dendrons: developing structure-activity relationships for DNA binding and gene transfection. Mol. Pharm., 2011, 8(2), 416-429. Copyright {2012} American Chemical Society.*

Compounds	D_m	N_{agg}	σ_m
Chol-G1-SP	3.4 ± 0.1	21	5.2
C_{12}Lys-G1-SP	4.0 ± 0.2	24	4.3
D2Gly-G1-SP	4.9 ± 0.2	32	3.8
C_{12}-G1-SP	4.0 ± 0.1	16	2.8
D1Gly-G1-SP	4.0 ± 0.2	12	2.1

The spherical geometry of the self-assembled supramolecular entities is a direct consequence of the conical molecular shape of each dendron, featuring a relative large cationic head and a comparatively small lipophilic part. In fact, assembly geometries for amphiphilic molecules is dictated by the proportions of their polar and apolar domains, aptly described by the so-called packing parameter $P = v_h/a_0l_c$,[16] in which v_h is the volume of the densely packed hydrophobic segment, a_0 is the effective cross-sectional area of the hydrophilic group, and l_c is the chain length of the hydrophobic moiety normal to the interface. Based on simple geometric considerations of micellar core volume *vs.* surface area, it is easy to show that $P < 1/3$ is characteristic of spherical micelles, $1/3 < P < 1/2$ characterizes self-assembly of cylindrical shape, $1/2 < P < 1$ corresponds to vesicles, flat lamellae are formed at $P = 1$ and, lastly, inverted micelles are expected for $P > 1$.

By coupling basic molecular modeling concepts to the dimensional micellar parameters estimated by mesoscopic simulations we were able to calculate the corresponding value of packing parameter P for all modified dendrons under hydrated conditions, which in all cases fell between 0.24 and 0.32, in agreement with the corresponding spherical morphologies predicted by our mesoscopic simulations.

5.2 Aggregation of Amphiphilic Dendrons in the Presence of a Nucleic Acid

Mesoscale simulations of the same dendron micelles carried out in the presence of DNA neatly showed that, in all cases, the overall systems consist of parts of free, unfolded, single-chain DNA that connect micelles on which a partial amount of DNA has been adsorbed (see Figure 9). In other words, all dendron/DNA complexes present a typical beads-on-a-string structure, made of dendron micelles connected by a DNA thread. Importantly, this predicted morphology is supported by detailed AFM studies between G4 PAMAM dendrimers and DNA – indicative that these self-assemblies of dendrons can be considered to be somewhat like covalently bound higher generation spherical dendrimers. These structures are also somewhat reminiscent of the structure of open chromatin, which consists of an array of nucleosome core particles, separated from each other by up to 80 base pairs of linker DNA. However, in clear contrast to the periodic structure of open chromatin, the dendron micelles appear to be distributed in a non-periodic, more irregular way.

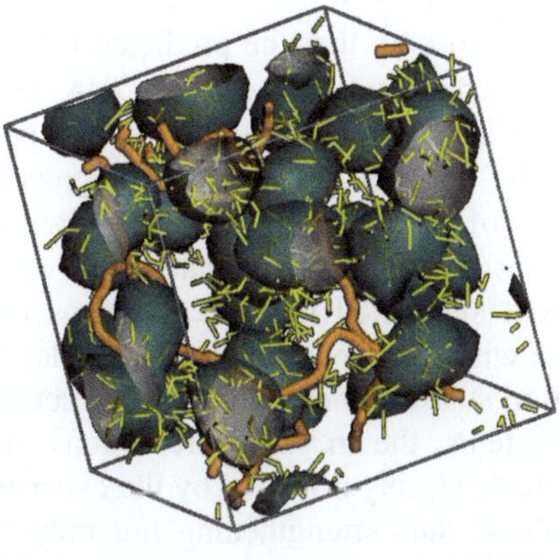

Figure 9 *Mesoscale modeling of the interaction of DNA with an amphiphilic dendron. In this Figure, yellow sticks represent dendron head groups, while coloured spheres are adopted to represent the hydrophobic region of the micelles. Water is omitted for clarity. DNA molecules are depicted as orange sticks. Adapted with permission from Jones, S.P.; Gabrielson, N.P.; Wong, C.H.; Chow, H.F.; Pack, D.W.; Posocco, P.; Fermeglia, M.; Pricl, S.; Smith, D.K. Hydrophobically modified dendrons: developing structure-activity relationships for DNA binding and gene transfection. Mol Pharm., 2011, 8(2), 416-429. Copyright {2012} American Chemical Society.*

5.3 Critical Micellar Concentration of amphiphilic dendrons

According to the classical laws of thermodynamics, the free energy of micellization ΔG_{mic} – i.e., the driving force that might eventually lead the amphiphilic molecules to spontaneously aggregate in water – can be expressed in the simple form $\Delta G_{mic} = -RT\ln K_m$, where K_m is the equilibrium constant between the aggregated and free forms of the given amphiphile in the aqueous environment. For conditions near or above the CMC, it can be shown that the above expression for ΔG_{mic} can be approximated to the form $\Delta G_{mic} =$

RTln(CMC). Accordingly, once either ΔG_{mic} or CMC is known, the other parameter can be easily estimated through this simple, fundamental relationship.

Following the theory originally proposed by Tanford and subsequently modified by other authors, and using the information available from our multiscale simulations, we were able to calculate the values of ΔG_{mic} and the corresponding CMCs for the five modified dendrons of Table 3. Interestingly, ΔG_{mic} at room temperature has large, negative values, indicating that micellisation is a spontaneous and highly favourable process for all amphiphilic dendrons, although ΔG_{mic} decreases on going from Chol-G1-SP to D_1Gly-G1-SP (in the order: -87.56 kcal/mol and 0.021 μM; -80.42 kcal/mol and 0.089 μM; -77.97 kcal/mol and 0.15 μM; -55.92 kcal/mol and 12.5 μM; -49.29 kcal/mol and 47.6 μM, respectively). Since the head group architecture is the same in all amphiphiles, the main differential contribution to ΔG_{mic} must originate from differences in the size and structure of the hydrophobic component.

Typically, micellar aggregates have CMCs of the order of 10^{-3}-10^{-5} M, while lower CMCs, even down to the nanomolar range can be found for amphiphiles that form either membranes or cylindrical aggregates. Amphiphiles showing low CMCs tend to have relatively large hydrophobic segments, and this normally results in an assembly shape with a lower curvature. However, our series of modified dendrons combine a large hydrophobic portion with a very large head group, resulting in a roughly conical amphiphile. The size of the hydrophobic segment is responsible for the low CMCs, while the large size of the head group results in the spherical geometry of the assembly.

It is of particular interest to note that the predicted CMC values for C_{12}-G1-SP and D_1Gly-G1-SP lie above the concentrations of the DNA binding assays (i.e. low μm concentrations) – as such, it is possible that the relatively poor DNA binding ability of these compounds reflects the fact that they are not aggregated under the experimental conditions as a consequence of their relatively small hydrophobic segments. Although a word of caution is due about the fact that the calculated values of ΔG_{mic} and CMC are obtained using validated but simplified theoretical approaches, the trends exhibited by these parameters are in line with the experimental data. Indeed, we were able to carry out full experimental aggregation studies on a closely related set of hydrophobically modified dendrons, and for these systems, the in silico predictions of micelle diameters, charge densities and CMC values were closely mirrored by the experimental results, both in terms of trends and absolute values, thus strengthening not only the reliability of the entire computational procedure applied but, perhaps more importantly, validating its predictive capacity.

Figure 10 graphically recaps the major finding of the study summarized and discussed above in terms of a graphical perspective of the qualitative relationship between the main properties of the self-assembled dendron systems investigated and their performance as gene delivery nanovectors.

6   CONCLUSIONS

In conclusion, the extensive series of examples illustrated and discussed above - taken from our own experience in the field - emphasizes the role and potentiality of multiscale molecular modeling in the pre- and post-development of nanodevices for gene delivery. Accurate and reliable molecular modeling can be performed more easily than experiments. In silico evaluation can take into account the molecular specificity of the problem and dramatically reduce the time and cost required to formulate a new device and therapeutic intervention, and eventually translate it into the clinical setting. In nanomedicine, the need for accurate multiscale molecular modeling is even more pressing. Despite its rapid growth and extraordinary potential, the field is still in its infancy, is highly interdisciplinary, and aims at solving problems of extraordinary and unprecedented complexity. With such a scenario, multiscale molecular modeling could afford a substantial contribution in dictating the success of nanomedicine and make the difference between several years of unfruitful research and the development of new, revolutionary therapeutic strategies readily available to the public.

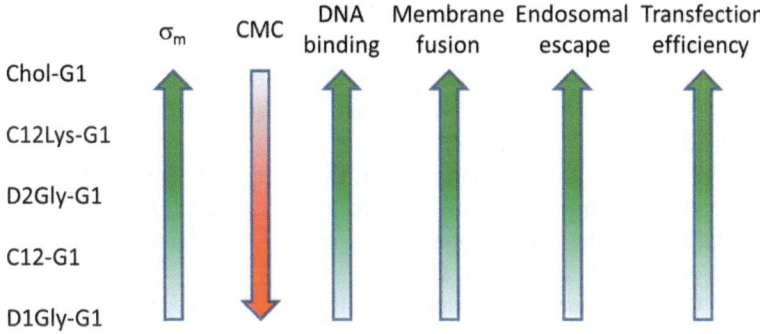

Figure 10 *Qualitative structure-activity relationship (SAR) of the main properties of the self-assembled dendron systems and their performance as gene delivery nanovectors. The green colour denotes a positive effect while the red colour a negative one. The direction of the arrow head indicates an increase (upward direction) or a decrease (downward direction) of the relevant property/performance.*

References

1 (a) P. Posocco, E. Laurini, V. Dal Col, D. Marson, K. Karatasos and S. Pricl, *Curr. Med. Chem.* 2012, **19**, 5062.; (b) A. Barnard, P. Posocco, S. Pricl, M. Calderon, R. Haag, M.E. Hwang, V.W. Shum, D.W. Pack and D. K. Smith, *J. Am. Chem. Soc.* 2011, **133**, 20288; (c) S.P. Jones; N.P. Gabrielson, C.H. Wong, H.F. Chow, D.W. Pack, P. Posocco, M. Fermeglia, S. Pricl and Smith, D.K., *Mol. Pharm.* 2011, **8**, 416; (d) P. Posocco, S. Pricl, S. P. Jones, A. Barnard and D. K. Smith, *Chem. Sci.* 2010, **1**, 393, and reference therein.

2 (a) P. Posocco, C. Gentilini, S. Bidoggia, A. Pace, P. Franchi, M. Lucarini, M. Fermeglia, S. Pricl and L. Paquato, *ACS Nano* 2012, **6**, 7243; (b) R. Toth, F. Santese, S.P. Pereira, D.R. Nieto, S. Pricl, M. Fermeglia and P. Posocco, *J. Mater. Chem.* 2012, **22**, 5398; (c) P. Posocco, M. Fermeglia and S. Pricl, *J. Mater. Chem.* 2010, **20**, 7742, and references therein.

3 (a) K. Ciepluch, N. Katir, A. El Kadib, A. Felczak, K. Zawadzka, M. Weber, B. Klajnert, K. Lisowska, A.M. Caminade, M. Bousmina, M. Bryszewska and J.-P. Majoral, *Mol. Pharm.* 2012, **9**, 458; (b) K. Milowska, J. Grochowina, N. Katir, A. El Kadib, J.-P. Majoral, M. Bryszewska and T. Gabryelak, *J. Lumin.* 2012, article asap http://dx.doi.org/10.1016/j.jlumin.2012.08.060.

4 D. Marson, P. Posocco, E. Laurini, M. Fermeglia, K. Ciepluch, B. Klajnert, M. Bryszewska, N. Katir, A. El Kadib, A.-M. Caminade, J.-P. Majoral and S. Pricl, manuscript in preparation.

5 S. Asaftei and E. De Clercq, *J. Med. Chem.* 2010, 53, 3480.

6 A.-M. Caminade, C.-O, Turrin and J.-P. Majoral, *New J. Chem.* 2010, **34**, 1512.

7   J. H. Zhou, J. Y. Wu, N. Hafdi, J.-P. Behr, P. Erbacher and L. Peng, *Chem. Commun.* 2006, 2362.

8   X. Liu, P. Rocchi, F. Q. Qu, S. Q. Zheng, Z. C. Liang, M. Gleave, J. Iovanna and L. Peng, *ChemMedChem* 2009, **4**, 1302.

9   X. Liu, J. Wu, M. Yammine, J. Zhou, P. Posocco, S. Viel, C. Liu, F. Ziarelli, M. Fermeglia, S. Pricl, G. Victorero, C. Nguyen, P. Erbacher, J.P. Behr and L. Peng, *Bioconjug. Chem.* 2011, **22**, 2461.

10   K. Karatasos, P. Posocco, E. Laurini and S. Pricl, *Macromol. Biosci.* 2012, **12**, 225.

11   G.M. Pavan, P. Posocco, A. Tagliabue, M. Maly, A. Malek, A. Danani, E. Ragg, C.V. Catapano and S. Pricl, *Chemistry Eur. J.* 2010, **16**, 7781.

12   (a) S.P. Jones, G.M. Pavan, A. Danani, S. Pricl and D.K. Smith, *Chemistry Eur. J.* 2010, **16**, 4519; (b) G.M. Pavan, A. Danani, S. Pricl and D.K. Smith, *J. Am. Chem. Soc.* 2009, **131**, 9686.

13   J. Zhou, C.P. Neff, X. Liu, J. Zhang, H. Li, D.D. Smith, P. Swiderski, T. Aboellail, Y. Huang, Q. Du, Z. Liang, L. Peng, R. Akkina and J.J. Rossi, *Mol. Ther.* 2011, **19**, 2228.

14   A.L. Bolcato-Bellemin, M.E. Bonnet, G. Creusat, P. Erbacher and J.P. Behr, *Proc. Natl. Acad. Sci. U.S.A.* 2007, **104**, 16050.

15   X. Liu, C. Liu, E. Laurini, P. Posocco, S. Pricl, F. Qu, P. Rocchi and L. Peng, *Mol Pharm.* 2012, **9**, 470.

16   (a) J.N. Israelachvili, D.J. Mitchell and B.W. Ninham, *Biochim. Biophys. Acta, Biomembr.* 1977, **470**, 185; b) J.N. Israelachvili, D.J. Mitchell and B.W. Ninham. *J. Chem. Soc., Faraday Trans. II* 1976, **72**, 1525.

POLY(AMINOESTER) DENDRIMERS: DESIGN, SYNTHESIS AND CHARACTERIZATION

G. Quélever,[1] C. Bouillon,[1] P. Moreno,[1] A. Tintaru,[2] L. Charles,[2] S. Pricl[3,4] and L. Peng[1]

[1] Aix Marseille Université, Centre Interdisciplinaire de Nanoscience de Marseille, CINaM CNRS UMR 7325, 163, avenue de Luminy, F-13288, Marseille Cedex 9, France
[2] Aix Marseille Université, Institut de Chimie Radicalaire, CNRS UMR 7273, F-13397, Marseille Cedex 20, France
[3] Molecular Simulation Engineering (MOSE) Laboratory, Department of Engineering and Architecture (DEA), University of Trieste, Via Valerio 10, 34127 Trieste, Italy
[4] National Interuniversity Consortium for Material Science and Technology (INSTM), Research Unit MOSE-DEA, University of Trieste, Italy

1 INTRODUCTION

Dendrimers have attracted particular attention for their potential as drug delivery vehicles showing high drug payload confined within a nanosized volume.[1-7] Among the various families of dendrimers studied for drug delivery applications, poly(aminoester) dendrimers (Figure 1), also referred to as poly(amino)ester or poly(esteramine) dendrimers in the literature, are particularly appealling thanks to their multiple advantageous structural features.[8] Firstly, they contain labile ester groups, and thus are expected to be biodegradable *via* ester hydrolysis, under acidic or basic conditions or in the presence of enzymes such as esterases. Small molecules encapsulated within these dendrimers are expected to be easily released by cleavage of the ester bonds. The resulting fragments can also be conveniently cleared from the body, thus reducing any eventual toxicity related to dendrimer accumulation or repeated use. Secondly, the amine functionalities can serve as a buffer to neutralize the acids produced during the ester hydrolysis, generating a benign and

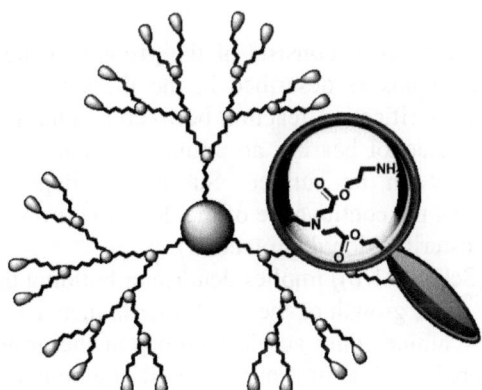

Figure 1 *Poly(aminoester) dendrimers*

non-aggressive environment throughout the cellular metabolism of the dendrimer. Moreover, the presence of a large number of ester and amine functionalities within the dendritic scaffold may help the formation of hydrogen bonds and electrostatic interactions with cargo drug molecules. This would favour the encapsulation of active particles and improve their solubility and delivery properties. Finally, the peripheral ester or amine groups can be chemically modified into various other functionalities in order to meet the special needs for diverse drug delivery requirements.

Despite these advantages over other families of dendrimers, only a few examples of poly(aminoester) dendrimers have been reported so far.[8] Consequently, their applications in drug delivery have rarely been disclosed, mainly because of their complicated synthesis and the limited synthetic methods available for their preparation. Indeed, the synthesis of poly(aminoester) dendrimers is not as trivial as one could expect. The reason is essentially the simultaneous presence of both ester and amine functionalities. Esters are sensitive to both acidic and basic conditions, and can also easily react with nucleophilic functionalities and readily undergo various derivatizations even under mild conditions. Concerning the amines, they can easily form zwitterions or H-bonds with carboxylic acids in the reaction medium. The reactivity of the carboxylic acids is hence reduced for the coupling reaction for ester formation. Another liability of the large number of both primary and tertiary amines is that amines can impart high polarity and water solubility to the dendrimers, which complicate later separation and purification procedures. Consequently, the reliable synthesis of high quality poly(aminoester) dendrimers constitutes a considerable challenge for synthetic chemists.

In this chapter, we will first present a brief overview on the synthesis of poly(aminoester) dendrimers, and then report a novel strategy recently developed by us within this COST action. The synthetic method is based on an iterative 4-step synthesis *via* the formation of active cyanomethyl ester intermediates offering high product yields and easy purification of the synthesized dendrimers. All dendrimers produced by this method have been examined by mass spectrometry in order to identify possible structural defects. Also computer modelling was applied to characterize these dendrimers in terms of their potential biological applications.

2 STRATEGIES FOR SYNTHESIZING POLY(AMINOESTER) DENDRIMERS

The very first synthesis of poly(aminoester) dendrimers was reported in 2002 by Sha *et al.*[9] Since then, several strategies have been developed to construct poly(aminoester) dendrimers. These strategies are schematically presented in Scheme 1, and will be briefly highlighted below.[8]

The first strategy (Scheme 1(a)) consists of the growth of the dendrimer through the direct formation of ester bonds as described in the literature.[10-13] The key step of this synthetic pathway is the esterification reaction between a central entity having peripheral carboxylic acids, and an alcohol bearing an amine function at the branching point and protected carboxylic acids on its surface. Subsequent deprotection of the terminal carboxylic functions allows the continuance of the dendritic growth process by iteration of the two main steps (i.e., esterification/deprotection).

The second strategy (Scheme 1(b)) implies dendrimer building through functionalization of peripheral amines.[14-19] The growth of the dendrimer is then achieved through a Michael addition process of these amines onto acrylate groups at the growing unit. Nevertheless, difficulties are encountered in obtaining pure desired compounds due to the presence of various double bonds available for Michael addition as peripheral groups on the growing units.

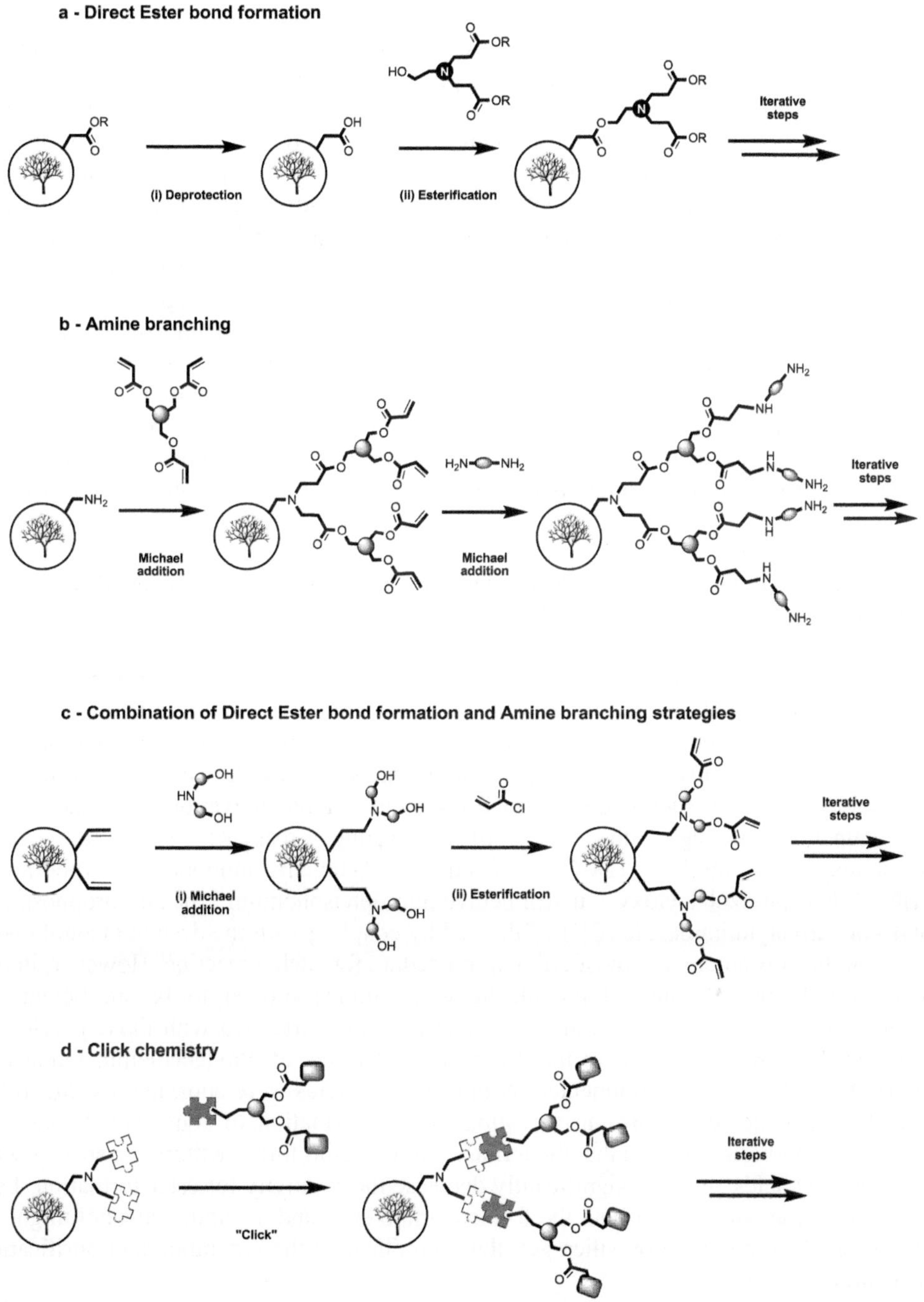

a - Direct Ester bond formation

b - Amine branching

c - Combination of Direct Ester bond formation and Amine branching strategies

d - Click chemistry

Scheme 1 *Strategies for the synthesis of poly(aminoester) dendrimers via (**a**) direct ester bond formation, (**b**) amine branching, (**c**) combined ester bond formation and amine branching and (**d**) "click" chemistry*

The third strategy (Scheme 1(c)) results from combining the two previously described approaches, namely, direct ester formation and amine branching. One of the two key steps involves the introduction of the ester functions through a reaction between a hydroxy functionalized moiety and an acryloyl acid derivative. During the second main step, the resulting acryloyl end groups are submitted to a Michael addition in the presence of amino growing units. This strategy has been successfully employed by Sha *et al.* in the synthesis of the very first poly(aminoester) dendrimers previously mentioned.[9]

Very recently, a fourth strategy based on "click" chemistry has been reported (Scheme 1(d)). Since "click" reactions often lead to high-yield production under mild conditions and within short reaction periods, their potential in synthesizing dendritic macromolecules is attracting increasing amounts of attention. Among the so-designated reactions, the Cu(I) catalysed azide-alkyne cycloaddition is the most popular and has been successfully exploited for the synthesis of poly(aminoester) dendrimers.[20] Similarly, thiol-ene[18] and thiol-yne[21] "click" coupling reactions have also been employed for such purposes.

It is noteworthy that all these strategies are based on the principle of the divergent approach,[22] the growing dendrimer being constructed from its centre towards the periphery. To our knowledge, no example of convergent synthesis[23] or of a combination of the divergent and convergent approaches[24] has been reported to date. We have recently reviewed the current status of the synthesis of various poly(aminoester) dendrimers.[8] Readers are encouraged to refer to this review and the references therein for detailed information.

3 SYNTHESIS OF POLY(AMINOESTER) DENDRIMERS VIA CYANOMETHYL ACTIVATED ESTER INTERMEDIATES

When we started our synthesis of poly(aminoester) dendrimers, we focused particularly on the first strategy (Scheme 1(a)) because of the seemingly simple coupling reactions between properly selected carboxylic acids and alcohols as growing units. Formation of an ester bond is a frequently required reaction in organic synthesis. A wide range of methods is available to perform such coupling reactions. Conventional activation of the carboxylic acid function through the use of activating reagents such as N,N'-dicyclohexylcarbodiimide (DCC), N-ethyl-N'-3-dimethylaminopropyl)carbodiimide (EDC), benzotriazol-1-yloxy tris(dimethylamino)phosphonium hexafluorophosphate (BOP) or carbonyldiimidazole (CDI), followed by coupling with the desired alcohol under mild conditions is among the most efficient procedure for such a reaction. However, in our hands and despite all our efforts, all these conditions proved to be inefficient for synthesizing poly(aminoester) dendrimers. These results correlated with those previously described by Buschhaus *et al.* in the preparation of esters of ethylenediaminetetraacetic acid (EDTA).[11] Indeed, as commented by the authors, yields were poor, mainly due to the difficulty encountered performing the simultaneous formation of four ester bonds. An additional hypothesis could be that the tertiary amines could form zwitterionic species with the carboxylic acids and thus significantly decrease the reactivity for ester formation. Last but not least, the polarities of both the formed amino ester and the amino alcohol might be very close when migrating on silica gel, thus complicating the separation and purification procedures.

In order to overcome all these difficulties, we therefore challenged ourselves to develop an original strategy based on the formation of a cyanomethyl ester intermediate which involves a four-step synthetic sequence (Scheme 2).[25] The first step of this novel synthetic strategy involves the deprotection of peripheral *tert*-butyl esters to generate carboxylic acid functionalities. The second step consists in the conversion of these acid functions into their corresponding cyanomethyl esters by reaction with chloroacetonitrile. During the third step, the cyanomethyl activated esters are transesterified by treatment with an excess of the selected amino alcohol in the presence of 1,8-diazabicyclo[5.4.0]undec-7-ene (DBU). It is noteworthy that the use of DBU has been found to be essential since no reaction occurs in its absence or when it is replaced by weaker bases such as triethylamine or 4-(dimethylamino)pyridine (DMAP). Finally, the scavenging of the excess of alcohol by treating the crude product mixture with benzoic anhydride and DMAP quantitatively converts the alcohol into its less polar benzoate derivative. The purification procedure was hence simple and could be easily achieved using column chromatography, delivering the desired poly(aminoester) dendrimer in pure form.

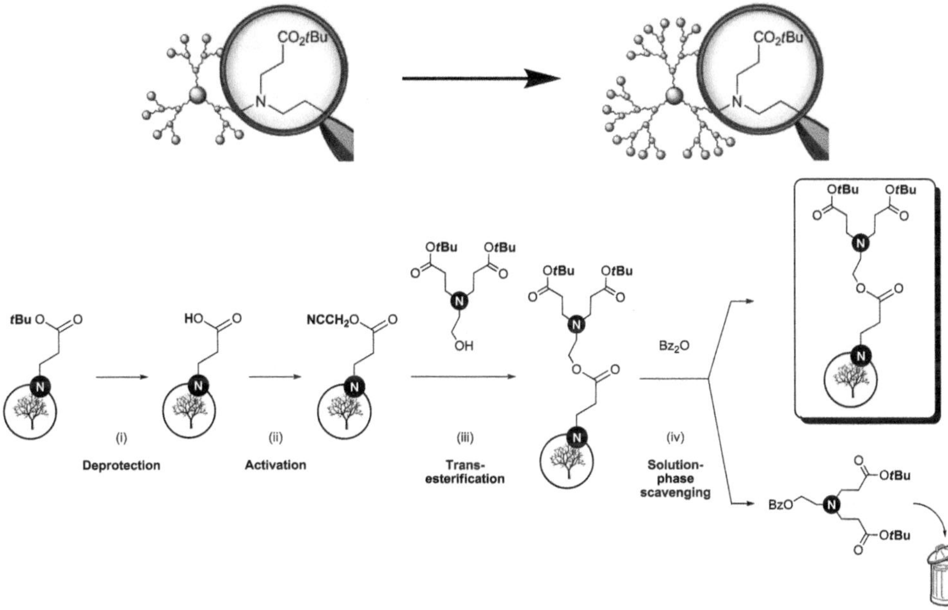

Scheme 2 *4-step cyanomethyl activated ester strategy*[25]

This strategy proved to be particularly efficient for the synthesis of various esters containing tertiary amine functionalities either in the acid or alcohol moieties[25] where, as previously mentioned, conventional conditions were found to be inefficient. This synthetic scheme has also been successfully applied to the divergent synthesis of poly(aminoester) dendrimers functionalized with peripheral *tert*-butyl esters with good to excellent yields (Scheme 3).[26] While it was difficult to achieve high generation dendrimers using this strategy, we were able to synthesize poly(aminoester) dendrimers up to generation 3 (Scheme 3). We are currently focusing our efforts on developing novel strategies permitting the construction of higher generations of poly(aminoester) dendrimers.

4 MASS SPECTROMETRIC CHARACTERIZATION AND STRUCTURAL DEFECTS

Dendrimers are polyfunctionalized macromolecules of rapidly increasing size and molecular weight when generation goes up. When synthesized through a divergent approach, dendrimers are built step by step with an increasing number of reactions to be conducted simultaneously at high generations. With such requirements, deemed perfection of high dendrimer generations can be subjected to caution. Statistically, as mentioned by Meijer, structural defects are therefore a reality.[27] These anomalies are synthetic defect but can also result from the intrinsic reactivity of the molecule itself, such as the intra- and intermolecular transamidation reactions observed in PAMAM dendrimers.[28] These defects concern not only to PAMAM but also to other families of dendrimers.[29] Fortunately, while

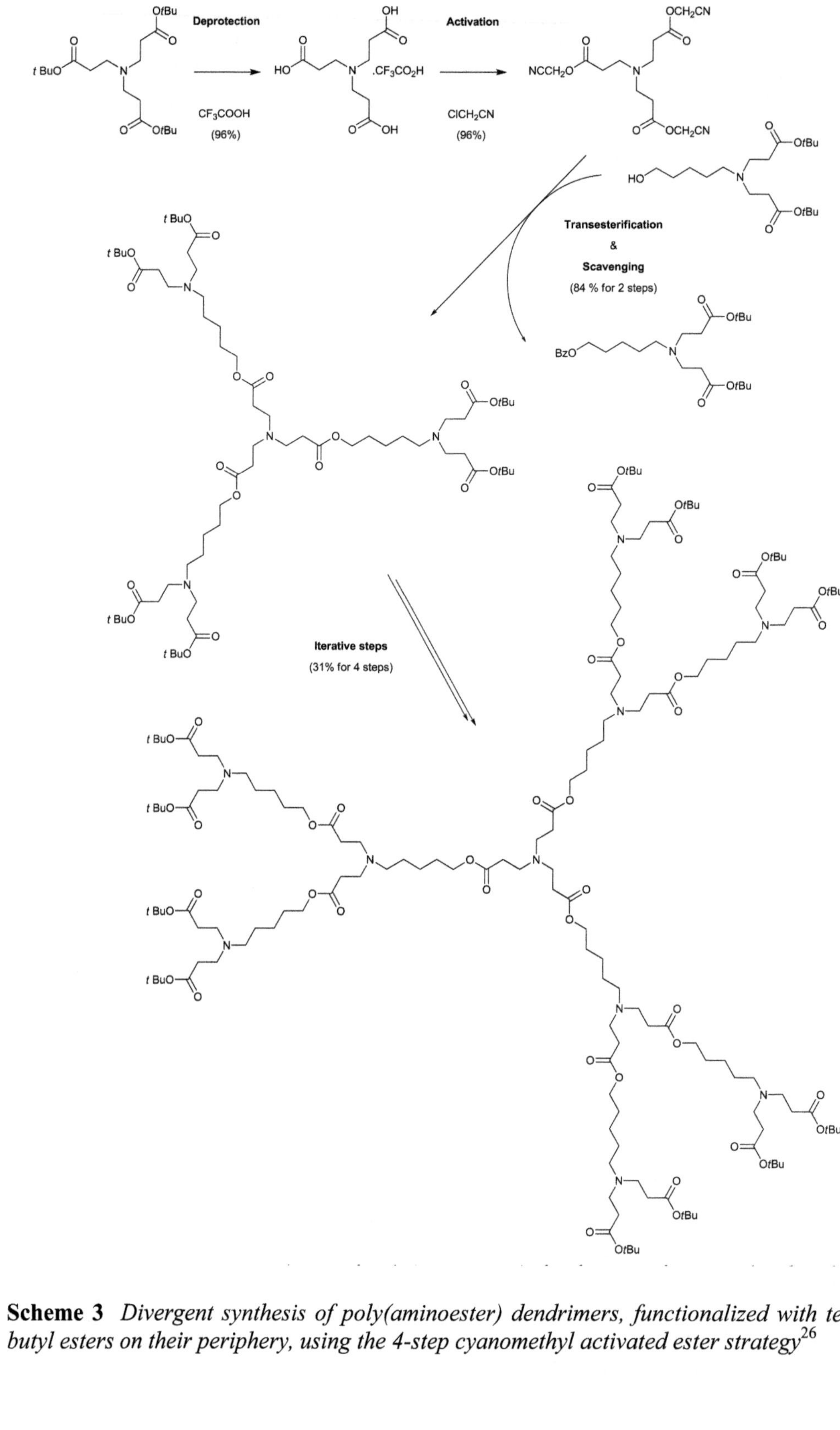

Scheme 3 *Divergent synthesis of poly(aminoester) dendrimers, functionalized with tert-butyl esters on their periphery, using the 4-step cyanomethyl activated ester strategy*[26]

these anomalies are most often not detectable by nuclear magnetic resonance NMR, they can be readily detected and characterized as traces using mass spectrometric techniques.

In order to characterize our synthesized dendrimers and to analyse such eventual undesirable imperfections, we developed an analytical methodology based on tandem mass spectrometry. Mass spectrometry (MS) associated with electrospray ionization (ESI) or matrix-assisted laser desorption/ionization is a method of choice for the characterization of dendrimers. The information obtained through the use of these techniques can shed light on structural defects since the imperfect molecules differ from the ideal structure by a known amount in mass. Further deviations can be identified by collision-induced dissociation (CID)[30] or by post-source decay (PSD).[30c, 30d, 31]

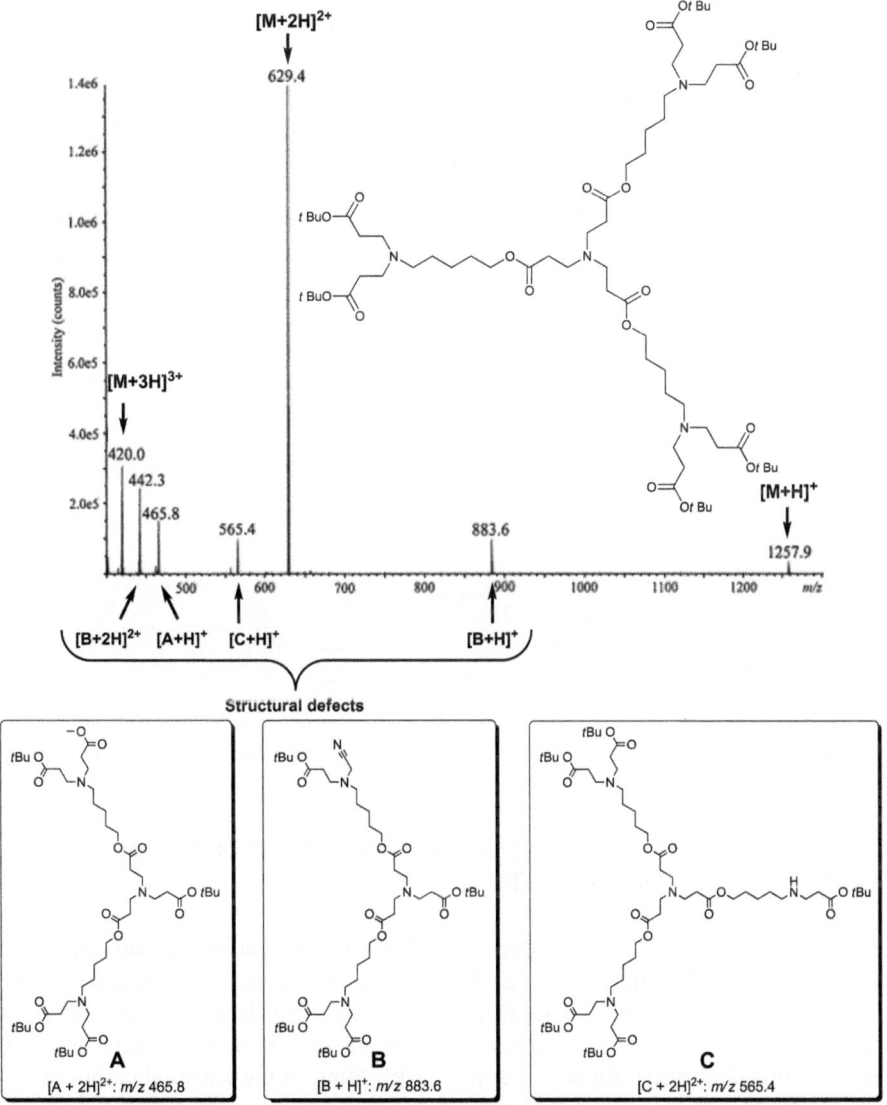

Figure 2 *MS spectrum of generation 1 tert-butyl ester terminated poly(aminoester) dendrimer synthesized through the active cyanomethyl ester 4-step strategy, and its structural defects.[32, 33]* **M** *refers to the perfect dendrimer molecule, and* **A**, **B**, *and* **C** *to dendrimers with defects*

Thanks to this powerful analytical tool, our synthesized poly(aminoester) dendrimers were precisely characterized (Figure 2) and their fragmentation behaviour was established by studying the CID of their protonated forms. The high level of symmetry of the ions in the perfect dendrimer, and the occurrence of sequential neutral losses upon its activation permitted establishing a reference CID behaviour. Based on this, any deviation observed during MS/MS of any dendritic precursor ions allowed an unambiguous characterization of the defective part and its localization within the molecules. Using this approach, we uncovered some defective structures in our dendrimer samples (Figure 2).[32] These defects were identified as originating from our synthetic strategy. For example, lack of a whole branch in impurities **A** and **B** could be explained by the subquantitative success of (i) the deprotection reaction (step 1 in Scheme 3), (ii) activation of carboxylic functions (step 2 in Scheme 3), or (iii) the transesterification reaction (step 3 in Scheme 3). The defective moiety in **C** might suggest the presence of an impurity in the amino alcohol used in the transesterification step. Concerning the cyanomethyl side-arm structural defect in **B**, we can hypothesize that during the activation step, some internal tertiary amines were quaternized in the presence of chloroacetonitrile (Scheme 4). The resulting quaternary ammonium species would have been further engaged in a retro-Michael reaction with the loss of an acryloyl arm. Fortunately, as mentioned previously and as indicated by the much higher relative contribution of $[M+nH]^{n+}$ ions to the whole MS signal, these defects were only observed as traces in the ESI-MS spectrum.

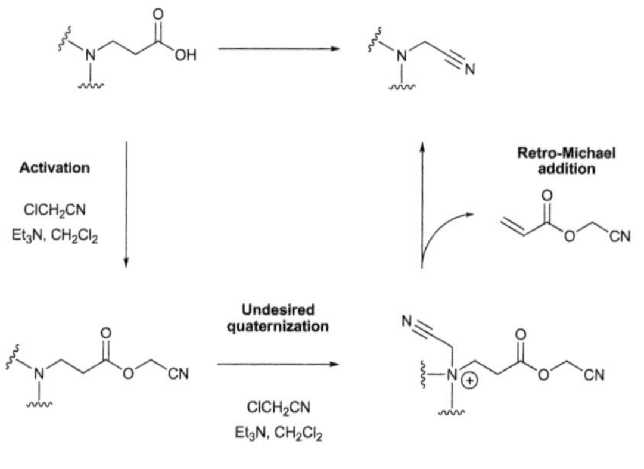

Scheme 4 *Possible mechanism to hypothesize the cyanomethyl side-arm structural defect observed in **B** in Figure 2*

5 PRELIMINARY MOLECULAR MODELING CHARACTERIZATION OF POLY(AMINOESTER) DENDRIMERS

Preliminary all-atom molecular dynamics (MD) studies performed on the two early generations of the poly(aminoester) dendrimers are shown in Figure 3. Interestingly, the first generation maintains an open conformation throughout the entire MD trajectory (see Figure 3(a)), with the arm stretched out into the solvent. In spite of this, the very high flexibility of this dendrimer allows for some backfolding of the terminal carboxylic groups toward the dendrimer core, as detected by the corresponding radial distribution function (see black curves in Figure 4). The overall regular and almost spherical symmetry of the first generation dendrimer is testified by the corresponding values of the aspect ratios of the principal moments of inertia. Indeed, none of the three molecular dimensions prevails over the other, and the three I_i/I_j values are very close to unity ($I_x/I_z = 1.08$; $I_y/I_x = 0.98$;

I_z/I_y = 0.96). As expected, for the second generation dendrimer a more compact conformation is detected along the corresponding MD trajectory (see Figure 3(b)), characterized by the presence of some of the –COOH terminal groups pointing towards the inner part of the molecule itself (see red lines in Figure 4). With respect to its lower generation counterpart, this dendrimer is significantly less symmetrical, as testified by the corresponding values of aspect ratios of the principal moments of inertia: I_x/I_z = 1.31; I_y/I_x = 0.93; I_z/I_y = 0.79.

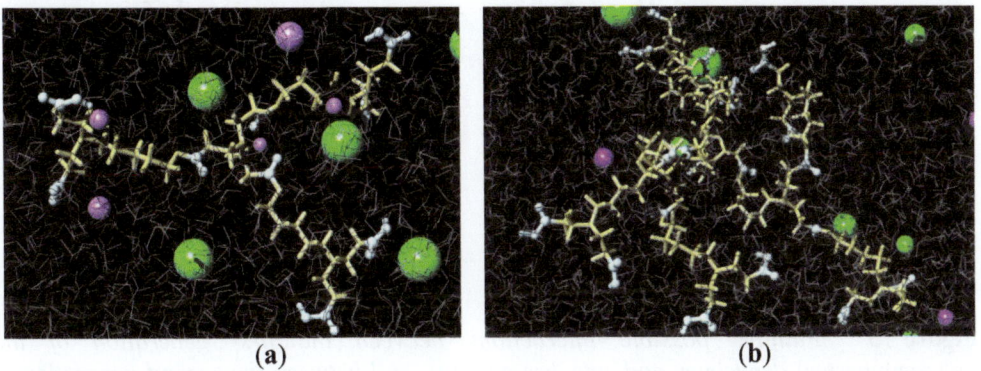

(a)   (b)

Figure 3 *Equilibrated MD snapshots of the first (a) and second (b) generation of the poly(aminoester) dendrimers. All simulations were performed in water in the presence of 0.15 M NaCl to a mimic physiological ionic strength. The dendrimer molecules are portrayed as sand-coloured sticks, with the internal C=O groups and the terminal –COOH groups highlighted as light blue sticks-and-balls. Water molecules are shown as grey lines. Some counter ions are shown as purple (Na$^+$) and green (Cl$^-$) spheres*

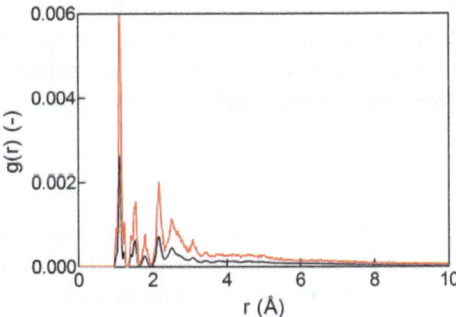

Figure 4 *Radial distribution functions (RDFs) from the center-of-mass of the poly(aminoester) dendrimers. Black lines, first generation; red lines, second generation*

The calculated average value of the hydrodynamic radius R_h was 1.08 nm for the first generation and 1.49 nm for the second generation dendrimers. Interestingly, these two values are close to the 1.18 nm and 1.47 nm determined for the ethylenediamine (EDA) core and terminal NH$_2$ groups of the gold standard PAMAM dendrimers.[34] Another, interesting structural aspect of these two dendritic molecules concerns their molecular surface area (MSA), also known as *addressable area* (AA). According to Chiba *et al.*,[35] who established that a given dendrimer might exhibit a specifically higher affinity towards a protein with interfacial area comparable to its AA, the AA value of 1046 Å^2 calculated for the first generation of the poly(aminoester) dendrimer suggests that this molecule might have a high binding affinity for cytochrome c, which has a interfacial area of 1100 Å^2 (See Figure 5(a)). Along the same lines, the second generation of these dendrimers, with an AA of 2437 A^2, might be a tight binder of chymotrypsin, which has an interfacial area of 2400 Å^2 (see Figure 5(b)).

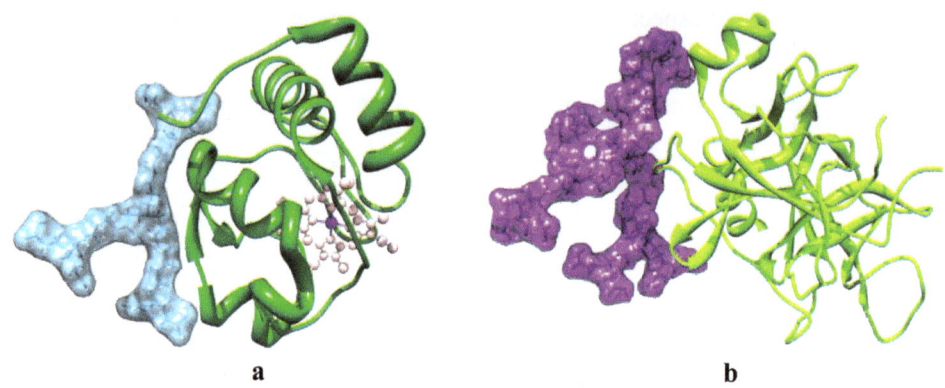

a   b

Figure 5 *Putative possible interactions between the first generation of the poly(aminoester) dendrimer and cytochrome c (**a**), and between the second generation of the poly(aminoester) and chymotrypsin (**b**). The dendrimers are emphasized by highlighting their van der Waals surface while the proteins are shown as forest green and chartreuse ribbons, respectively. The heme group of cytochrome c is also represented by in stick-and-ball representation*

Protein-protein interactions play an essential role in many biological systems. When such interactions occur in an undesirable or uncontrolled fashion, disease is often a result. Macromolecular systems capable of interrupting these unwanted interactions may represent viable and realistic therapeutic agents. In this perspective, these low generation poly(aminoester) dendrimers could be exploited in a size selective binding mechanism at aimed at inhibiting of protein-protein aggregation.[34, 35]

6 CONCLUSION

Over the last few decades, dendrimers have received increasing amounts of interest. Thanks to their well-defined architecture, these macromolecules are powerful tools for use in a wide range of applications in the field of nanomedicine. We have been particularly interested in structurally flexible and amphiphilic poly(amidoamine) dendrimers and we have already demonstrated their efficiency as vectors for nucleic acid delivery.[36, 37] As part of the COST program, we have been engaged in synthesizing another family of biodegradable dendrimers, poly(aminoester) dendrimers.[8] To Confront the difficulties encountered during the synthesis of such molecules, we have developed an original synthetic strategy based on the formation of active cyanomethyl ester intermediates with the iteration of 4 consecutive steps of deprotection, activation, transesterification and scavenging. Using this method, we were able to synthesize various small generation dendrimers.[26] At present, we are working actively towards developing novel strategies for the synthesis of higher generations of poly(aminoester) dendrimers. For this purpose, we are putting our faith in "click" chemistry which we believe is one of the most promising approaches available to construct various poly(aminoester) dendrimers.

Acknowledgement

We acknowledge financial support from the international ERA-Net EURONANOMED European Research project DENANORNA, Association Française contre les Myopathies, Canceropôle PACA, French Ministry of Education and CNRS. This work was carried out under the auspice of European COST Action TD0802 "Dendrimers in Biomedical Applications".

References

1 D. A. Tomalia, A. M. Naylor and W. A. Goddard, *Angew. Chem. Int. Ed. Engl.*, 1990, **29**, 138.
2 J. M. J. Fréchet and D. A. Tomalia, in *Dendrimers and other dendritic polymers*, ed. Wiley, Amsterdam, The Netherlands, 2001.
3 G. R. Newkome, C. N. Moorefield and F. Vögtle, in *Dendrimers and dendrons: Concepts, synthesis, applications*, ed. Wiley, Weinheim, Germany, 2001.
4 D. A. Tomalia and J. M. J. Fréchet, *J. Polym. Sci. Pol. Chem.*, 2002, **40**, 2719.
5 J. M. J. Fréchet, *J. Polym. Sci. Pol. Chem.*, 2003, **41**, 3713.
6 F. Vögtle, G. Richardt and N. Werner, in *Dendrimer chemistry: Concepts, synthesis, properties, applications*, ed. Wiley, Weinheim, Germany, 2009.
7 M. A. Mintzer and M. W. Grinstaff, *Chem. Soc. Rev.*, 2011, **40**, 173.
8 Y. Wang, G. Quéléver and L. Peng, *Curr. Med. Chem.*, 2012, **19**, 5011.
9 Y. W. Sha, L. Shen and X. Y. Hong, *Tetrahedron Lett.*, 2002, **43**, 9417.
10 J. Kawakami, T. Mizuguchi and S. Ito, *Anal. Sci.*, 2006, **22**, 1383.
11 B. Buschhaus, F. Hampel, S. Grimme and A. Hirsch, *Chem. Eur. J.*, 2005, **11**, 3530.
12 D. Soto-Castro, J. A. Cruz-Morales, M. T. R. Apan and P. Guadarrama, *Molecules*, 2010, **15**, 8082.
13 T. R. Krishna and N. Jayaraman, *J. Org. Chem.*, 2003, **68**, 9694.
14 D. M. Xu, K. D. Zhang and X. L. Zhu, *Tetrahedron Lett.*, 2005, **46**, 2503.
15 D. M. Xu, K. D. Zhang, C. H. Ning and X. L. Zhu, *J. Appl. Polym. Sci.*, 2005, **97**, 60.
16 D. M. Xu, Z. L. Zhao, A. F. Wang, K. D. Zhang and X. L. Zhu, *J. Appl. Polym. Sci.*, 2008, **107**, 2578.
17 D. M. Xu, K. D. Zhang and W. J. Wu, *J. Appl. Polym. Sci.*, 2005, **98**, 341.
18 D. R. Swanson, B. Huang, H. G. Abdelhady and D. A. Tomalia, *New J. Chem.*, 2007, **31**, 1368.
19 X. P. Ma, J. B. Tang, Y. Q. Shen, M. H. Fan, H. D. Tang and M. Radosz, *J. Am. Chem. Soc.*, 2009, **131**, 14795.
20 M. Li, L. Q. Xu, L. Wang, Y. P. Wu, J. Li, K.-G. Neoh and E.-T. Kang, *Polym. Chem.*, 2011, **2**, 1312.
21 R. J. Amir, L. Albertazzi, J. Willis, A. Khan, T. Kang, C. J. Hawker, *Angew. Chem. Int. Ed.*, 2011, **50**, 3425.
22 (a) D. A. Tomalia, H. Baker, J. Dewald, M. Hall, G. Kallos, S. Martin, J. Roeck, J. Ryder and P. Smith, *Polymer J.*, 1985, **17**, 117; (b) D. A. Tomalia, H. Baker, J. Dewald, M. Hall, G. Kallos, S. Martin, J. Roeck, J. Ryder and P. Smith, *Macromolecules*, 1986, **19**, 2466.
23 (a) C. J. Hawker and J. M. J. Fréchet, *J. Am. Chem. Soc.*, 1990, **112**, 7638; (b) C. J. Hawker and J. M. J. Fréchet, *J. Chem. Soc., Chem. Commun.*, 1990, 1010.
24 K. L. Wooley, C. J. Hawker and J. M. J. Fréchet, *J. Am. Chem. Soc.*, 1991, **113**, 4252.
25 C. Bouillon, G. Quéléver and L. Peng, *Tetrahedron Lett.*, 2009, **50**, 4346.

26 C. Bouillon, A. Tintaru, V. Monnier, L. Charles, G. Quéléver and L. Peng, *J. Org. Chem.*, 2010, **75**, 8685.

27 A. W. Bosman, H. M. Janssen and E. W. Meijer, *Chem. Rev.*, 1999, **99**, 1665.

28 R. Giordanengo, M. Mazarin, J. Wu, L. Peng and L. Charles, *Int. J. Mass Spectrom.*, 2007, **266**, 62 and references therein.

29 For an example, see: J. C. Hummelen, J. L. J. van Dongen and E. W. Meijer, *Chem. Eur. J.*, 1997, **3**, 1489.

30 (a) J. W. Weener, J. L. J. van Dongen and E. W. Meijer, *J. Am. Chem. Soc.*, 1999, **121**, 10346; (b) S. A. McLuckey, K. G. Asano, T. G. Schaaff and J. L. Stephenson, *Int. J. Mass Spectrom.*, 2000, **195**, 419; (c) A. Adhiya and C. Wesdemiotis, *Int. J. Mass Spectrom.*, 2002, **214**, 75; (d) M. He and S.A. McLuckey, *Rapid Commun. Mass Spectrom.*, 2004, **18**, 960; (e) C. L. Mazzitelli and J. S. Brodbelt, *J. Am. Soc. Mass Spectrom.*, 2006, **17**, 676; (f) R. Giordanengo, M. Mazarin, J. Y. Wu, L. Peng and L. Charles, *Int. J. Mass Spectrom.*, 2007, **266**, 62.

31 J. Subbi, R. Aguraiuja, R. Tanner, V. Allikmaa and M. Lopp, *Eur. Polym. J.*, 2005, **41**, 2552.

32 A. Tintaru, C. Chendo, V. Monnier, C. Bouillon, G. Quéléver, L. Peng and L. Charles, *Int. J. Mass Spectrom.*, 2011, **308**, 56.

33 A. Tintaru., V. Monnier, C. Bouillon, R. Giordanengo, G. Quéléver, L. Peng and L. Charles, *Rapid Commun. Mass Spectrom.*, 2010, **24**, 2207.

34 J. Giri, M. S. Diallo, A. J. Simpson, Y. Liu, W. A. Goddard III, R. Kumar and G. C. Woods, *ACS Nano*, 2011, **5**, 3456.

35 F. Chiba, T.-C. Hu, L. J. Twyman and M. Wagstaff, *Chem. Comm.*, 2008, **36**, 4351.

36 (a) J. H. Zhou, J. Y. Wu, N. Hafdi, J.-P. Behr, P. Erbacher and L. Peng, *Chem. Commun.*, 2006, 2362; (b) X. Liu, P. Rocchi, F. Qu, S. Zheng, Z. Liang, M. Cleave, J. Iovanna and L. Peng, *ChemMedChem*, 2009, **4**, 1302; (c) J. Zhou, P. Neff, X. Liu, J. Zhang, H. Li, D. D. Smith, P. Swiderski, Y. Huang, Q. Du, Z. Liang, L. Peng, R. Akkina and J. Rossi, *Mol. Ther.*, 2011, **19**, 2228; (d) X. Liu, J. Wu, M. Yamine, J. Zhou, P. Posocco, S. Viel, C. Liu, F. Ziarrelli, M. Fermeglia, S. Pricl, G. Vicotrero, C. Nguyen, P. Erbacher, J.-P. Behr and L. Peng, *Bioconjugate Chem.*, 2011, **22**, 2461; (e) M.-F. Lang, S. Yang, C. Zhao, G. Sun, K. Murai, X. Wu, J. Wang, H. Gao, C. E. Brown, X. Liu, J. Zhou, L. Peng, J. J. Rossi and Y. Shi, *PLoS ONE*, 2012, **7**, e36248; (f) X. Liu, C. Liu, E. Laurini, P. Posocco, S. Pricl, F. Qu, P. Rocchi and L. Peng, *Mol. Pharmaceut.*, 2012, **9**, 470.

37 T. Yu, X. Liu, A.-L. Bolcato-Bellemin, Y. Wang, C. Liu, P. Erbacher, F. Qu, P. Rocchi, J.-P. Behr and L. Peng, *Angew. Chem. Int. Ed.*, 2012, **51**, 8478.

FROM MULTIVALENT DENDRONS TO SELF-ASSSEMBLED MULTIVALENT DENDRIMERS: A COMBINED EXPERIMENTAL AND THEORETICAL APPROACH

David K. Smith[1,*] and Sabrina Pricl[2]

[1] Department of Chemistry, University of York, Heslington, York, YO10 5DD, UK
[2] Molecular Simulations Engineering (MOSE) Laboratory, Department of Engineering and Architecture (DEA), University of Trieste, Piazzale Europa 1, 34127 Trieste, Italy

1 INTRODUCTION TO DENDRIMERS AND MULTIVALENCY

Dendrimers are well-defined nanoscale branched molecules.[1] Unlike many nanostructures, dendrimers can be made using a wide range of different synthetic methodologies, and as a consequence, many different biologically active units can be incorporated, giving them the capacity to transform a number of areas of nanomedicine.[2] One of the most interesting regions of the dendritic architecture is occupied by the peripheral surface groups, which constitute a multivalent nanoscale array, and can therefore form high-affinity interactions with a variety of biological targets.

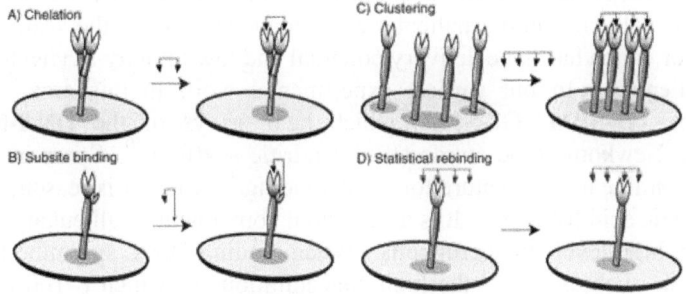

Figure 1 *Mechanisms of Multivalency in Host-Guest Binding*

Multivalency describes the simultaneous interaction of multiple binding groups on one molecule with the complementary receptors on another and is widely employed by biological systems which employ high-affinity binding in very competitive aqueous environments.[3] In multivalent interactions the binding of the second ligand is favoured as a consequence of being 'intramolecular' in nature (Fig. 1).[4] The average free energy of interaction between one ligand and receptor in a multivalent system can either be greater than, equal to or less than the free energy in the analogous monovalent interaction, referred to as positively cooperative (synergistic), non-cooperative (additive) or negatively cooperative (interfering), respectively. Positively cooperative multivalent binding is very rare,[5] but multivalency does not require positive cooperativity – the key aspect is whether the multivalent system has higher affinity for its target than the monovalent analogue.

Whitesides and co-workers defined a binding enhancement factor, a ratio of multivalent to monovalent binding, to capture this enhancement in overall affinity.[3a] Given the importance of multivalency in biological systems, and the ability of multivalent interactions to adhere synthetic nanoscale surfaces to one another, it has become a primary tool for chemists working in the fields of biomolecular recognition and nanotechnology and is an ideal approach for exploitation by dendrimer chemists.

This article provides an overview of collaborative work carried out in the Smith (experimental) and Pricl (theoretical) research groups to probe and understand multivalency effects in dendritic systems. In particular, as our research evolved, we developed a novel approach to organising dendritic multivalent arrays of ligands – self-assembled multivalency.[6] Our research has been motivated by understanding and manipulating the interactions between dendritic molecules and a variety of biological targets, such as DNA, heparin and integrin proteins. As such, this research has potential applications in areas of nanomedicine as varied as gene therapy, post-surgical treatment of patients, tumour targeting and tissue engineering. Although our research has potential applications, this article will primarily focus on how our combined approach has led to new fundamental insights into multivalency. This article gives an overview of key results and their significance, leading to design principles for the future, and providing intriguing hints as to how such systems may be applied in the future of nanomedicine.

2 MULTIVALENT DENDRONS

2.1 Dendrons for DNA Binding – New Paradigms in Multivalency

High generation spherical dendrimers are well-known to bind DNA and deliver it into cells.[7] Such systems have potential applications in gene therapy, in which therapeutic DNA would be delivered into a patient's cells, however, so far, the search for a suitable non-viral vector which has gene delivery potential and low toxicity *in vivo* has remained an unsolved challenge.[8] In our earliest experimental work in this area,[9] we developed dendrons (e.g., **G1-SPM**, **G2-SPM**) which held arrays of the DNA-binding ligand spermine on a Newkome-type amide-ether dendritic scaffold.[10] Spermine is a naturally occurring tetra-amine used in nature for DNA binding,[11] where it is reasoned to play a role in helping nucleic acid folding.[12] It is an essential component of all eukaryotic cells and is present at very high levels in sperm cells. When binding DNA, spermine has to compete with counterions such as Na^+,[13] the high concentrations of which (>100 mM) mean that relatively large quantities of spermine are required to effectively bind DNA. We therefore considered that a multivalent array of spermine ligands may be better able to compete with electrolyte and potentially yield useful DNA binding systems and/or delivery vehicles.

By using a combination of gel electrophoresis and an Ethidium Bromide (EthBr) assay[14] we demonstrated that our dendritic systems **G1-SPM** and **G2-SPM** (Fig. 2) could achieve high-affinity DNA binding (Table 1). The EthBr displacement assay allowed us to gain a comparative quantitative estimate of the binding strengths. In this experiment EthBr was bound to calf thymus DNA and then the concentration of dendron required to reduce the fluorescence intensity of EthBr by 50% through competitive binding, was determined. These concentrations (C_{50} values) represent the binding of the dendron to DNA – the lower the value, the more effective the binding. The data can also be presented as charge excess (CE_{50}) values, where CE_{50} represents the charge excess of cationic dendron to anionic DNA needed to displace 50% of the EthBr. Dendron **G2-SPM**, with nine surface spermine ligands, had a C_{50} value of 30 nM – a significantly lower concentration than monovalent

G0-SPM, which was in the micromolar range. Furthermore, we found that the binding of **G2-SPM** to DNA, unlike **G1-SPM**, was remarkably independent of salt concentration.

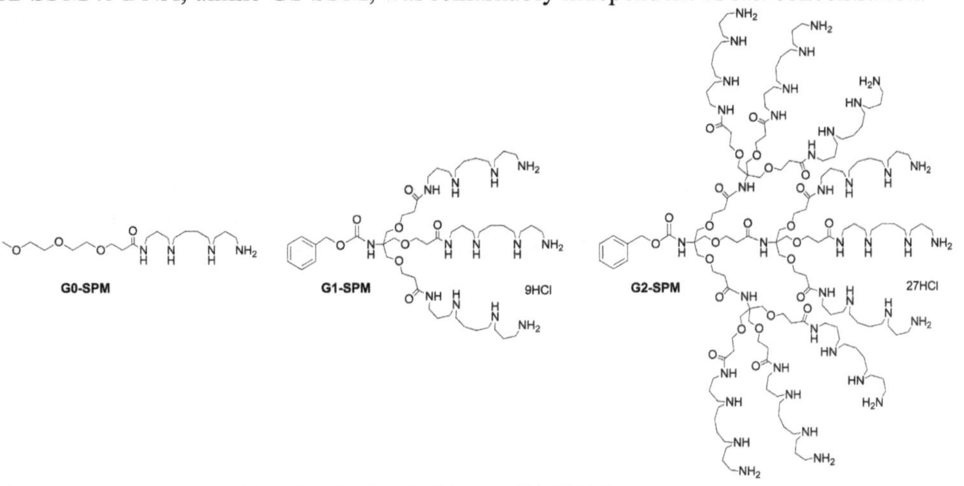

Figure 2 *Structures of G0-SPM, G1-SPM and G2-SPM*

Table 1 *Experimental and Theoretical Data for the binding of Gn-SPM to DNA.*

Dendron	Charge	[NaCl] (mM)	Experimental			Theoretical	
			C_{50} (nM)[a]	CE_{50}[b]	CE_{50} ratio[c]	ΔG_{bind} (kcalmol^{-1})[d]	$\Delta\Delta G_{bind}$[e]
G1-SPM	+9	9.4	76	0.68	3.97	-61.7	+1.3
G1-SPM	+9	150	300	2.7		-60.4	
G2-SPM	+27	9.4	30	0.81	0.94	-196.2	0.0
G2-SPM	+27	150	28	0.76		-196.2	

[a] C_{50} represents the concentration of dendron required to displace 50% of the EthBr ([DNA Base] = 1 μM, [EthBr] = 1.26 μM). [b] CE_{50} represents the charge excess (ratio of protonatable nitrogen atoms on the dendron to deprotonatable phosphate groups on the DNA) at which 50% of EthBr is displaced. [c] CE_{50} ratio = CE_{50} (150 mM NaCl) / CE_{50} (9.4 mM NaCl), and represents how much th binding decreases on the addition of salt. [d] ΔG_{bind} is determined by molecular dynamics methods for the binding of dendrons **G1** and **G2** to DNA. [e] $\Delta\Delta G_{bind} = \Delta G_{bind}$ (150 mM NaCl) – ΔG_{bind} (9 4 mM NaCl).

At the start of our collaboration, we wanted to understand the origins of this remarkable salt-independent multivalency – such an observation had not previously been reported. We employed atomistic molecular dynamics (MD) methods to evaluate the global binding affinities of **G1-SPM** and **G2-SPM** with a 21-mer base-paired model DNA at both 9.4 and 150 mM NaCl.[15] We employed the MM/PBSA simulation scheme[16] in a solvent box,[17] to generate binding energies ΔG_{bind} (Table 1). It was immediately apparent that the binding model for **G1-SPM** exhibited pronounced salt dependency. This $\Delta\Delta G_{bind}$ of 1.3 kcal mol^{-1} on addition of salt reflects a weakening in binding by approximately an order of magnitude – a significant change. Conversely, modelling indicated that the overall binding affinity of **G2-SPM** to DNA was not affected by NaCl. As such, these MD calculations supported the experimental data.

In order to understand the origin of these effects, we focused attention on the 1:1 binding models (Fig. 3) and considered them as an assembly of residues – monitoring the interaction between each part of the dendron structure and DNA. Considering energetic values for each residue within the dendron, it was clear that the spermine ligands were, as expected, responsible for binding DNA due to electrostatic interaction between protonated amines and anionic phosphates. We modelled the effect of increasing salt concentration on the interaction of each residue with DNA. For **G1-SPM** one of the spermine ligands was very seriously disturbed (in energetic terms) by salt, and effectively prevented from binding to DNA – hence the salt-induced decrease in binding affinity. For **G2-SPM**, however, although some SPM ligands were adversely affected by the increase in NaCl concentration, some of the other units then bound DNA significantly more strongly. Modelling suggested that as NaCl concentration increases, some SPM residues 'sacrifice' their own interaction with DNA and act as a kind of barrier, protecting the remaining residues from the surrounding medium (a 'screening' effect) and allowing their interaction with DNA to be optimised and strengthened. This means that increasing NaCl concentration had minimal impact on the overall strength of the complex.

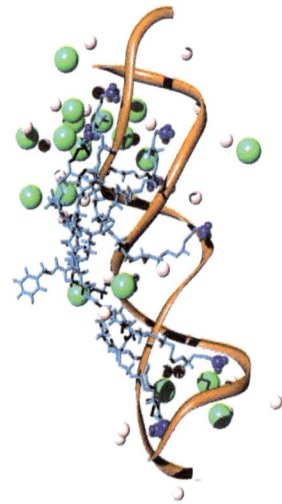

Figure 3 *Molecular Dynamics modelling of **G2-SPM** bound to the DNA double helix*

By combining experimental work and theoretical modelling, we were therefore able to suggest a new paradigm in multivalency – i.e., although some ligands may not bind to the target, they can still play an active role in enhancing the binding of the remainder of the dendron. It is sometimes argued that multivalent ligands are more effective if they are highly pre-organised (and hence rigid),[3] but this work clearly indicated that a degree of flexibility in the multivalent display of ligating groups can be highly beneficial.

2.2 Effect of Surface Groups – Thermodynamic Insights into Multivalency

In order to probe multivalency in more detail, we made an experimental study of surface ligand structure on DNA binding, to determine whether spermine was particularly preferred, or whether other amines on a dendron surface would operate in similar ways.

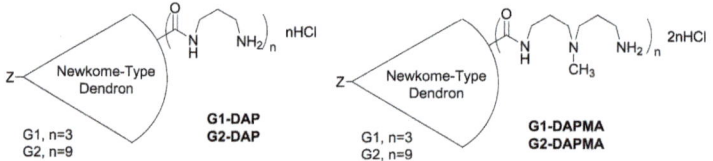

Figure 4 *Newkome-type dendrons displaying different cationic ligands on the surface*

We therefore synthesised **G2-DAPMA** and **G2-DAP** (Fig. 4).[18] The ability of these systems to bind DNA was probed using the EthBr displacement assay, which indicated that, as expected, the **G2** systems are significantly better DNA binders than their **G1** analogues – a clear simple multivalency effect (Table 2). However, dendrons **G1-SPM** and **G2-SPM** were by far the most effective DNA binders in terms of the CE_{50} parameter – which reflects the relative ability to bind anionic DNA per cationic charge. Spermine was clearly the optimal ligand for DNA binding – outperforming **DAPMA** and **DAP** by one and three orders of magnitude, respectively. The data clearly demonstrated that it is not just higher charge which gives spermine ligands their overall advantage – spermine is optimized for minor groove DNA binding,[11] whereas the synthetic amines are not.

Table 2 *Experimental and Theoretical Data for the binding of dendrons with different surface ligands to DNA.*

Dendron	Charge	Experimental		Theoretical			
		$C_{50}{}^a$	$CE_{50}{}^b$	$\Delta G_{bind}{}^c$	ΔG_{bind}/charge^d	ΔH_{bind}	$-T\Delta S_{bind}$
G1-DAP	+3	367	550	-16.7	-5.6	-49.9	+33.2
G2-DAP	+9	n/a	n/a	-49.6	-5.5	-109.9	+60.2
G1-DAPMA	+6	10.7	32	-33.8	-5.6	-68.9	+35.1
G2-DAPMA	+18	0.567	5.1	-126.3	-7.0	-227.3	+101.0
G1-SPM	+9	0.600^e	2.7	-60.4	-6.7	-106.3	+45.9
G2-SPM	+27	0.056^e	0.76	-196.2	-7.3	-310.2	+114.0

^{a} C_{50} represents the concentration of dendron required to displace 50% of the EthBr ([DNA Base] = 2 μM, [EthBr] = 2.52 μM). ^{b} CE_{50} represents the charge excess (ratio of protonatable nitrogen atoms on the dendron to deprotonatable phosphate groups on the DNA) at which 50% of EthBr is displaced. ^{c} ΔG_{bind} is determined by molecular dynamics methods for the binding of dendrons to DNA. ^{d} ΔG_{bind}/charge represents the free energy per positively charged nitrogen. ^{e} These values are different to those in Table 1 because the assay conditions had doubled the concentration of DNA and EthBr for this study.

We modelled the binding using MD methods and found that in general terms as the charge of the dendron increases, so does its ability to bind DNA.[18] However, the relationship between total charge and binding affinity is not linear. For example, dendrons **G2-DAP** and **G1-SPM** both have total charges of +9, but **G1-SPM** has a more favourable ΔG_{bind} value than **G2-DAP**. This indicates that ligand structure plays an important role in optimising the individual charge-charge interactions – multivalency is not simply a function of total charge. Modelling agreed with the experimental observation that each charge is most effectively used when the surface groups are **SPM** (i.e. ΔG_{bind}/charge is ca. -7.0 kcalmol^{-1} per charge), whereas those dendrons with **DAP** surface groups are the least effective (only ca. -5.5 kcalmol^{-1} per charge). In general, each charge contributes ca. -12.0 kcalmol^{-1} to the value of ΔH_{bind}, reflecting the simple electrostatic interactions between dendron and DNA. However, the entropies (ΔS_{bind}) are highly variable. For example, **G2-DAP** and **G1-SPM** have identical charges (+9), and similar ΔH_{bind} values, but the binding of **G2-DAP** to DNA is entropically much more disfavoured than **G1-SPM**. Evidently more degrees of freedom are lost when **G2-DAP** binds DNA than **G1-SPM**. This entropic difference underpins the difference in ΔG_{bind}. It is clearly better to have individual amines grouped together into three spermine units, than spread onto the termini of nine separate flexible branches – the immobilisation of which is much more entropically challenging.

When we sub-divided the dendron into individual residues, we found that **G2-DAPMA** and **G2-SPM** optimise the interaction of selected surface ligands with DNA, and still achieve high affinity binding. Conversely, **G2-DAP** attempts to optimize the interaction of as many of the individual point surface charges as possible with DNA, which has significant entropic cost. This entropic difference helps explain why the dendrons with polyvalent surface amines (**SPM** and **DAPMA**) are experimentally so much more effective than those with individual surface amines (**DAP**) and clearly demonstrates the importance of charge organisation in multivalent electrostatic binding.

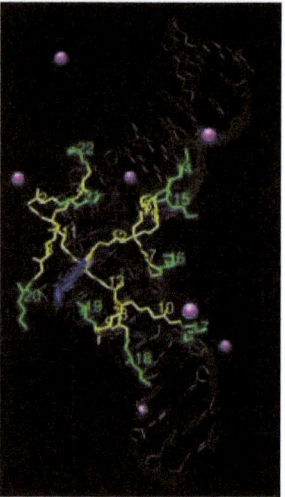

Figure 5 *G2-DAPMA binding to DNA*.

Interestingly, we noted experimentally that the best systems for gene delivery, had **DAPMA** ligands, even though this was not the best DNA binder. Modelling indicated that for **DAPMA**, the interaction between the tertiary amine and the DNA caused back-folding, which in turn led to significant distortion of the DNA double helix (Fig. 5). We suggested this may help explain the enhanced gene delivery – DNA compaction is an important step in transfection. However, further experimental evidence to support this is still required.

2.3 Degradable Multivalent Arrays – 'On-Off' Multivalency

One of the inherent problems with applying multivalent systems in nanomedicine is that they have high affinity for their biological binding partner. This can cause serious problems if the structure persists in the cell for any length of time, as it can interact with a number of targets *in vivo*. For example, it has been shown that when PAMAM dendrimers are used for gene delivery, remnant dendrimers can be found bound to cellular components some time after transfection.[19] As such, there is considerable interest in the development of degradable vectors.[20] Such an approach would be particularly powerful with a multivalent array – as it degrades, the number of ligands decreases, and the binding affinity will diminish – i.e., a high-affinity delivery vehicle degrades into non-binding fragments.

In early work, we developed an experimental system which underwent UV-triggered degradation as a consequence of having a UV-cleavable linker between the surface ligands and the spermine surface groups.[21] On UV irradiation (350 nm), the dendron-DNA complex disassembled as a consequence of dendron degradation. However, this approach is impractical for use *in vivo*. Kostinainen and co-workers developed systems which employed reversible disulfide bond formation to achieve chemically/enzymatically mediated cleavage,[22] while we turned our attention to the development of DNA binding dendrons which were hydrolytically degradable.

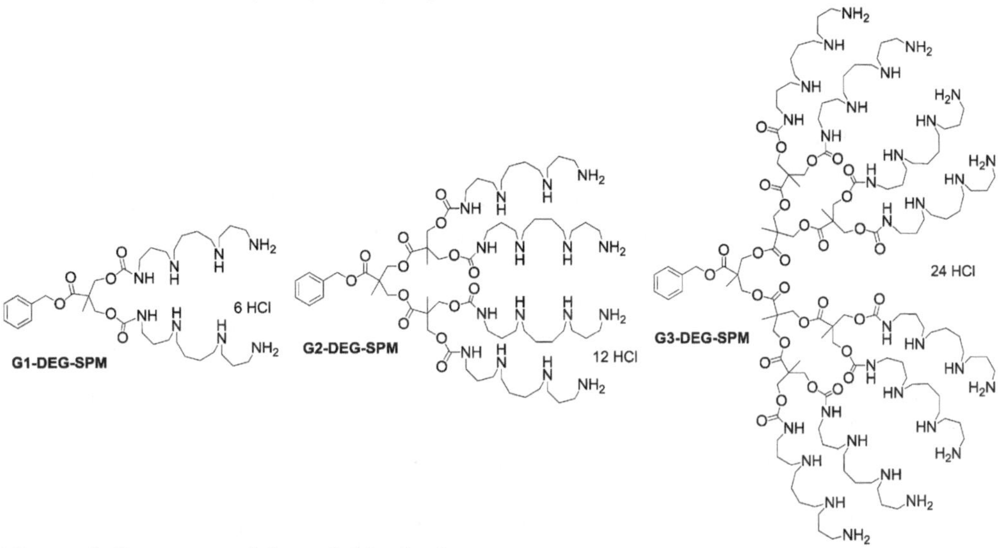

Figure 6 *Structures of degradable dendrons*

We made use of the ester-carbamate dendron synthesis originally disclosed by Fréchet and co-workers,[23] based on the hyperbranched polymer structures developed by Hult and co-workers.[24] Fréchet and co-workers demonstrated that this kind of dendron scaffold degraded over a number of days. We therefore synthesised compounds **G1-DEG-SPM**, **G2-DEG-SPM** and **G3-DEG-SPM** (Fig. 6) to determine their ability to bind DNA, and assess their potential to degrade under bio-relevant conditions.[25] These dendrons are based on a two-fold branching motif. The third generation system contains eight surface groups, whereas the Newkome based dendron, with three-fold branching points has nine surface ligands at the second generation. The DNA binding ability increased with dendritic generation. First generation **G1-DEG-SPM** binds at micromolar levels (13.8 μM), whilst for **G3-DEG-SPM**, only low nanomolar amounts of the dendron were required (78 nM). Normalising the data to yield the effective concentration per spermine unit demonstrated multivalency, with the largest enhancement on going from **G1-DEG-SPM** to **G2-DEG-SPM** (15-fold) with a smaller improvement on going to **G3-DEG-SPM** (3-fold).

We probed stability under physiologically relevant conditions. Fréchet and co-workers had previously reported that this dendrons framework can degrade on standing in aqueous solution.[23] In particular, they reported that at pH 7.4, both ester and carbamate hydrolysis occurred over a time period of days. We incubated **G3-DEG-SPM** at pH 7.4 and at various times monitored its ability to bind DNA. After incubation, **G3-DEG-SPM** was no longer able to effectively displace EthBr from its complex with DNA. This is a consequence of the dendron being degraded – switching off the multivalency. Control **G2-SPM**, without a degradable framework, retained its ability to bind DNA. In this way, we introduced the concept of temporary 'on-off' multivalency as a unique approach through which it is possible to gain the benefits of high-affinity binding to biological targets, with slow degradation of the dendron under biological conditions helping avoid longer term negative effects of high-affinity recognition once the desired bio-intervention is complete.

3 FROM MULTIVALENT DENDRONS TO SELF-ASSEMBLED MULTIVALENT DENDRIMER ARRAYS

All of our studies described above were performed with individual low generation dendrons. This gave excellent insights into fundamental multivalency effects, but in general, their ability to carry out gene delivery was limited.[26] It is well-known that higher generation cationic dendrimers have greater capacity to buffer the endosome within the cell, facilitating cellular entry.[27] However, the synthesis of higher generations is synthetically challenging – the surface groups become more numerous, making complete divergent reaction difficult, whilst the focal point becomes sterically hindered and unreactive. In order to achieve larger multivalent nanoscale arrays, we decided to develop an alternative strategy. One advantage of using dendrons rather than spherical dendrimers as synthetic building blocks is that the focal point remains available for further functionalisation. We therefore chose to attach a self-assembling unit at the focal point of the dendron – in particular, hydrophobic units which aggregate in biologically-relevant aqueous conditions. In this way, we reasoned we could use simple, spontaneous self-assembly to multiply up the small multivalent array on each individual dendron into a larger multivalent nanoscale assembly. We argued this might introduce new aspects to multivalent binding and provide us with an additional level of control over interactions. We refer to this approach as 'self-assembled multivalency'[6] – the resulting structures can be thought of as self-assembled dendrimers (Fig. 7).[28]

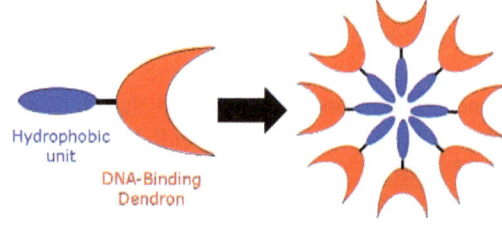

Figure 7 *Schematic illustration of self-assembled dendrimer formation*

There are a number of advantages to this self-assembly approach to multivalent dendrimer arrays: (i) spontaneous assembly/easy to make, (ii) well-defined low-molecular-weight building blocks suitable for clinical approval, (iii) easily tunable ligands, (iv) tunable nanostructure morphologies, (v) ability to assemble different active components into a single nanostructure, (vi) reversible and addressable assemblies.

Self-assembled dendrimers have been of interest since the pioneering work of Zimmerman and co-workers who used arrays of hydrogen bonds to hold together multiple dendritic building blocks in organised nanoscale architectures,[29] and a wide variety of non-covalent interactions have since been exploited for the assembly of supramolecular dendrimers.[30] In a key study, dendrons with a hydrophobic polymer grafted at the focal point were shown to self-assemble into giant micelles, with low critical micelle concentrations, by Meijer and co-workers.[31]

There has also been increasing interest in the use of self-assembled multivalency to achieve high-affinity binding, and we recently drew this together in a key review.[6] Early pioneers of this approach were Whitesides and co-workers, who used self-assembly to generate arrays of sialic acid which could bind with enhanced affinity to hemagglutinin.[32] A number of researchers have assembled systems which express RGD peptides in order to yield enhanced interactions with cell surfaces.[33] The groups of Florence,[34] Hammond[35]

Diederich,[36] Haag[37] and Peng,[38] have all explored self-assembling dendrons for applications in gene delivery. Once again, in our studies we had a focus on using a combined experimental and theoretical approach to gain new fundamental insight.

4 SELF-ASSEMBLED MULTIVALENCY

4.1 Self-Assembled Multivalency – Charge Density and Multivalent Binding

We explored the effect of a hydrophobic unit at the dendron focal point on the binding affinity of DNA to surface ligands and synthesised a family of modified compounds **HYD-G1-SPM** (Fig. 8).[39] In each case, the DNA binding ligand array is identical, therefore any difference in binding must arise from differences in how the hydrophobic unit multiplies up the ligands into a self-assembled multivalent array. As the data in Table 3 indicate, modifying the hydrophobic unit exerted a dramatic effect on the affinity of the dendrons for DNA, even though this group is not itself directly responsible for binding DNA.

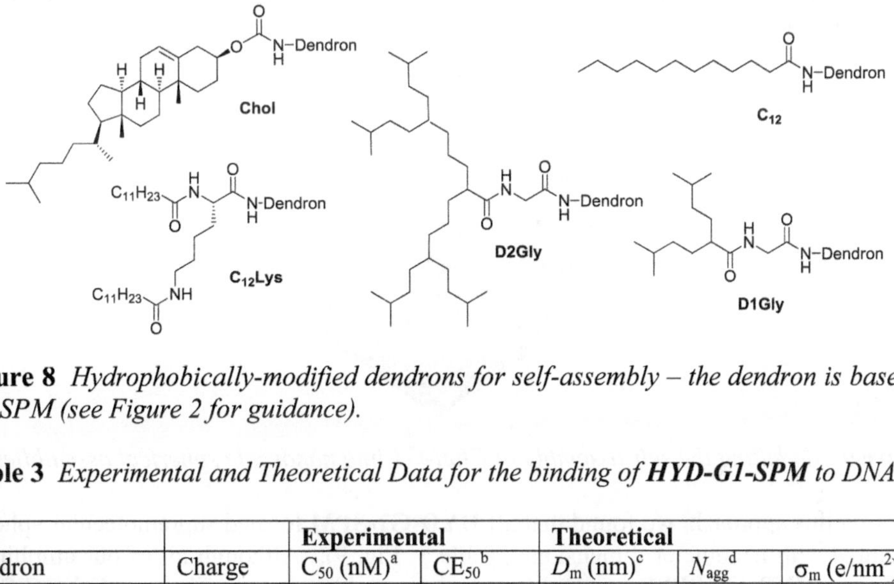

Figure 8 *Hydrophobically-modified dendrons for self-assembly – the dendron is based on G1-SPM (see Figure 2 for guidance).*

Table 3 *Experimental and Theoretical Data for the binding of **HYD-G1-SPM** to DNA*

Dendron	Charge	Experimental		Theoretical		
		C_{50} (nM)[a]	CE_{50}[b]	D_m (nm)[c]	N_{agg}[d]	σ_m (e/nm²)[e]
D1Gly-G1-SPM	+9	955	4.3	4.0	12	2.1
C$_{12}$-G1-SPM	+9	733	3.3	4.0	16	2.8
G1-SPM	+9	600	2.7	n/a	n/a	n/a
D2Gly-G1-SPM	+9	400	1.8	4.9	32	3.8
C$_{12}$Lys-G1-SPM	+9	189	0.85	4.0	24	4.3
Chol-G1-SPM	+9	122	0.55	3.4	21	5.2

[a] C_{50} represents the concentration of dendron required to displace 50% of the EthBr ([DNA Base] = 2 µM, [EthBr] = 2.52 µM). [b] CE_{50} represents the charge excess (ratio of protonatable nitrogen atoms on the dendron to deprotonatable phosphate groups on the DNA) at which 50% of EthBr is displaced. [c] D_m represents the micellar diameter. [d] N_{agg} represents the number of dendrons per self-assembled nanostructure. [e] σ_m is the surface charge density of the self-assemblies.

Dendrons **Chol-G1-SPM** and **C$_{12}$Lys-SPM** had the lowest CE_{50} values of 0.55 and 0.85 respectively, indicating very effective DNA binding – some of the best ever reported, and significantly better than previously observed even for our second generation spermine arrays, which have many more spermine units per dendron (Table 1).[9] Compound **D2Gly-**

SPM was somewhat better than **G1-SPM** having a CE_{50} value of 1.8. On the other hand, compounds **C$_{12}$-G1-SPM** and **D1Gly-G1-SPM** had higher CE_{50} values of 3.3 and 4.3 respectively, indicating they have lower affinities for DNA than **G1-SPM**.

In an attempt to rationalise these observations and better understand the structure-activity effects, we employed mesoscale modeling. Many interesting problems in soft matter science occur at length and time-scales between the atomistic scale and the macroscopic continuum – this is true of the self-assemblies proposed for these dendrons. Such problems cannot be addressed by atomic-level molecular dynamics. Rather, one needs to take recourse to computational techniques at the intermediate scale. Over the last few years, different approaches have been developed to address problems at this mesoscale level, which could be broadly classified as particle-based or density-based. We decided to use a particle-based method called Dissipative Particle Dynamics (DPD),[40] in which groups of atoms are coarse-grained into a bead, substantially reducing the number of particles to be simulated. Further, rather than interact through Lennard-Jones forces, the beads feel a simple soft pair-wise conservative potential which embodies the essential chemistry of the system. This force is of short range, and has a simple analytical form, resulting in fast computation per time step and, hence, providing the opportunity to expand the simulation from nanoseconds to real time periods.

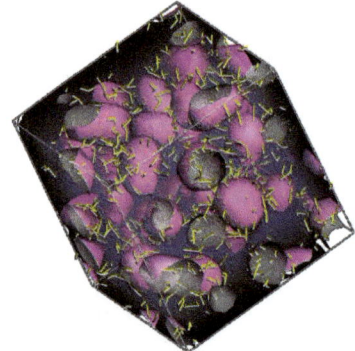

Figure 9 *Modelling the self-assembly of **Chol-G1** into nanoscale spherical assemblies*

Using this approach, we found that all **HYD-G1-SPM** formed supramolecular spherical structures with nanometer dimensions (Table 3, Fig. 9). Although all of our amphiphilic dendrons (**HYD-G1-SPM**) are predicted to assemble in a similar way, the different architectures of the hydrophobic portion result in differently sized micelles (D_m) and/or different numbers of dendrons per micelle (N_{agg}), and, hence, different micellar surface charge densities (σ_m). This key parameter shed light on the very different abilities of the dendrons to bind DNA. Pleasingly, the experimentally verified CE_{50} values directly correlated with the calculated σ_m values. The best DNA binder, **Chol-G1-SPM**, assembles into much smaller micelles than **C$_{12}$Lys-G1-SPM** and **D2Gly-G1-SPM** due to the less sterically demanding nature of cholesterol leading to more effective packing. As such, even though the nanostructures formed by **Chol-G1-SPM** contain fewer dendrons and have less total positive charge than the others, their smaller size means they have a higher surface charge density, and are therefore much more effective DNA binders. We confirmed these proposals using detailed experimental approaches on related degradable dendron structures (see Section 4.4). This study clearly demonstrated how the hydrophobic unit controls the packing within the nanoscale assembly, which in turn controls the effective surface charge density, and the affinity of the aggregates for polyanionic DNA. Self-assembly-induced control of charge density is a new concept in multivalency.

4.2 Self-Assembled Multivalency – Inverting Dendritic Effects

We then moved on to consider the performance of second generation hydrophobically-modified dendrons **Chol-G2-SPM** and **C$_{12}$-G2-SPM**.[41] Unlike the **G1** system, there were minimal differences between the CE$_{50}$ values observed for **Chol-G2-SPM** (CE$_{50}$ = 1.4) and **C$_{12}$-G2-SPM** (CE$_{50}$ = 1.7). For these **G2** compounds, the hydrophilic dendron is much larger than for **G1**, and dominates the molecular shape. As such, these second generation dendrons have less potential to self-assemble in a surfactant-like manner. We propose that the nine spermine surface groups, which contain 27 amines, dominate DNA binding, and the focal point group exerts less influence on binding.

Notably, **Chol-G2-SPM** is a less effective binder than **Chol-G1-SPM** even though taken individually, the former compound has many more spermine groups. Mesoscale modeling was used to provide insight into this counter-intuitive observation. Both **Chol-G1-SPM** and **Chol-G2-SPM** were predicted to form spherical micelles with average diameters of 3.4 and 3.8 nm, respectively. However, when these aggregates were considered in more detail, there was a significant difference between them. The **G1** system assembles into a much more highly charged aggregate than the **G2** analogue. This may seem counterintuitive, because **Chol-G2-SPM** has 27 amine groups, whereas **Chol-G1-SPM** only has 9. However, the greater relative degree of hydrophobicity in **Chol-G1-SPM** means self-assembly is significantly more effective, meaning it assembles into a more effectively packed aggregate with a dense-packed positively charged surface (Fig. 10). The simulated surface charge density (σ_m) for **Chol-G1-SPM** was 5.3 e/nm^2, whilst for **Chol-G2-SPM** it was only σ_m = 4.2 e/nm^2.

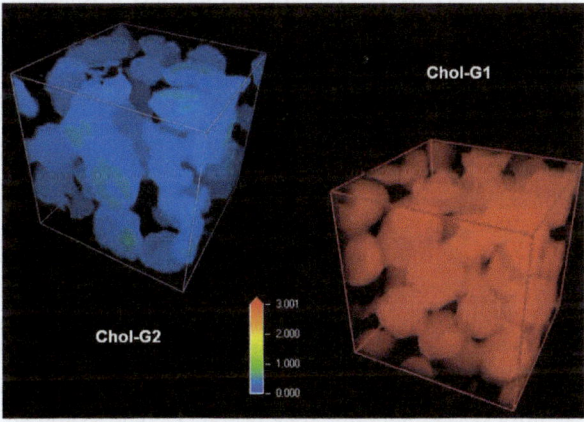

Figure 10 *Cationic surface charge densities of **Chol-G1-SPM** and **Chol-G2-SPM** leading to a self-assembly-mediated inverted dendritic effect – less is more*

The surprising observation, that a lower generation dendron can be more effective in terms of DNA binding reinforced our new hypothesis about multivalent electrostatic interactions, in which self-assembly controls the surface charge of the aggregate, and hence the relative affinities of these systems for DNA. In this sense, 'less is more', and the smaller dendron is actually better able to bind DNA once the multivalency is expressed on the nanoscale.

4.3 Self-Assembled Multivalency – Controlling Morphology

An interesting aspect of using self-assembly to create nanoscale structures is that the morphologies can be diverse and tunable. Israelachvili developed a series of rules to predict the way in which amphiphilic systems would self-assemble into different nanostructures.[42] His simple analysis is based on dividing the structure of the amphiphile into hydrophilic and hydrophobic parts and determining their relative sizes. As the hydrophobic group becomes larger relative to the hydrophilic one (as represented by the packing parameter, P) the geometry preferred for the self-assembly changes from a spherical micelle, to a cylindrical (rod-like) micelle, to a bilayer-type assembly, and ultimately to an inverted (inside-out) micelle (in an appropriate solvent). This is a simple consequence of the amount of space required by the hydrophobic group.

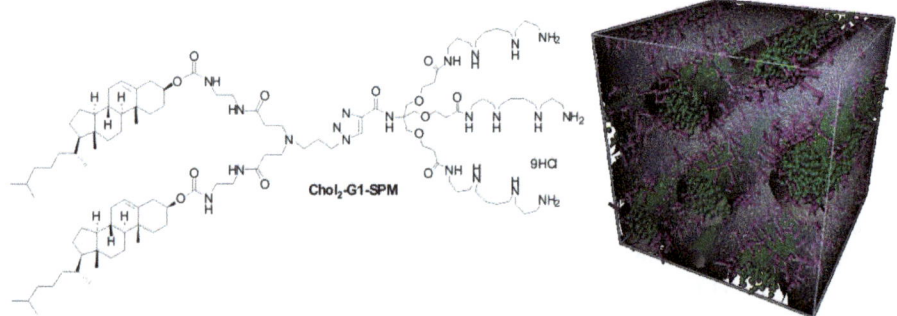

Figure 11 *Dendron **Chol₂-G1-SPM** and mesoscale model of cylindrical assembly mode*

In order to try and change the morphology of one of our self-assembled systems, we therefore synthesised **Chol₂-G1-SPM** (Fig. 11) which has a relatively small hydrophilic head group and a very large double-tailed hydrophobic unit.[41,43] Intriguingly, we found that not only was this dendron an effective DNA binder, but it was the most effective gene delivery system we have studied to date – much better than **Chol-G1-SPM** even though it bound DNA with a similar affinity. Mesoscale modelling of **Chol₂-G1-SPM** found that on increasing the volume fraction, the mode of assembly changed to give a cylindrical micellar hexagonal phase morphology (Fig. 11). Analogue **Chol-G1-SPM** did not exhibit this type of behaviour, with spherical micelles being the dominant and stable form. In consideration of Israeachvili's 'rules', packing parameters, P, of 0.24 and 0.47 for **Chol-G1-SPM** and **Chol₂-G1-SPM** respectively, supported the simulated morphologies. It is known that cylindrical morphologies can give rise to optimal gene delivery.[44]

Interestingly, we found the combination of **Chol₂-G1-SPM** and **Chol-G2-SPM** to be an even more effective vector – better than our positive control (poly(ethyleneimine)).[43] We proposed that co-assembly was enhancing gene delivery. The synthesis of **Chol₂-G1-SPM** however, is somewhat onerous, and we are therefore now using multiscale modelling to help us design modified self-assembling dendrons which assemble in similar ways, but are synthetically simpler and more accessible. We suggest that future experimental work in will be increasingly informed by the results of predictive multiscale molecular modelling in order to yield biological constructs for gene delivery with enhanced activity.

4.4 Self-Assembled Multivalency – Degradable Systems

We then applied our self-assembly approach to the degradable dendrons discussed in Section 2.3. To conjugate a hydrophobic group at the focal point of these ester/carbamate derived dendrons, we used the alkyne-modified dendron previously reported by Hawker and co-workers.[45] This dendron can be easily be conjugated using the dipolar cyclo-addition 'click' reaction.[46] In this way, we generated a library of hydrophobically-modified dendrons (Fig. 12).[47] We used DAPMA surface ligands, as they were synthetically easy to work with and more effective in gene delivery applications.[18]

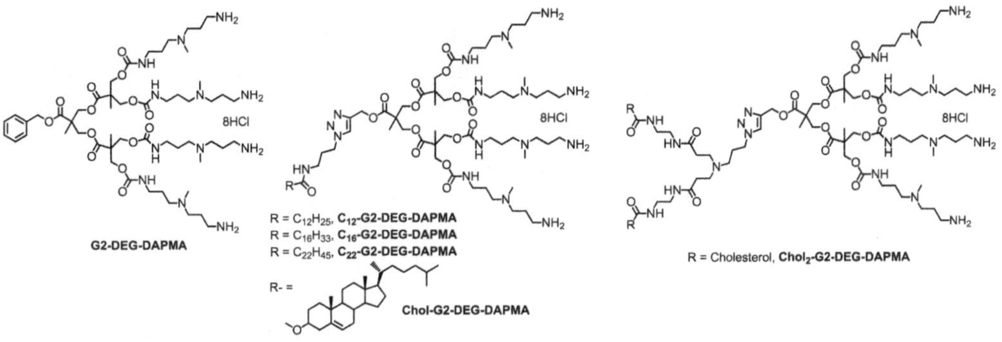

Figure 12 *Degradable hydrophobically modified systems*

Table 4 *Experimental and Theoretical Data for self-assembly and DNA binding of second generation **HYD-G2-DEG-DAPMA** demonstrating the impact of the hydrophobic unit on self-assembly parameters.*

Hydrophobic unit	Experimental				Theoretical			
	CMC^a	D_m^b	$Zeta^b$	CE_{50}^c	D_m^d	ΔG_{mic}^e	σ_m^f	ΔG_{bind}^g
None	n/a	n/a	+34.1	>10	n/a	n/a	n/a	n/a
C12	208	n/a	+42.6	>10	2.9	-63.6	1.77	-16.8
C16	37	5.93	+45.0	1.42	3.1	-75.7	1.89	-22.4
C22	2.0	6.96	+56.1	0.84	3.3	-92.3	2.09	-33.8
Chol	4.9	7.55	+56.3	0.66	3.9	-96.4	2.68	-71.2
Chol$_2$	4.9	15.04	+55.4	0.57	5.1	-99.6	2.15	-119.2

[a] CMC (μM) as measured using Nile Red assay. [b] D_m (nm) and Zeta potential (mV) determined by zeta-sizer. [c] CE_{50} represents the charge excess (ratio of protonatable nitrogen atoms on the dendron to deprotonatable phosphate groups on the DNA) at which 50% of EthBr is displaced. [d] D_m (nm) represents the micellar diameter. [d] N_{agg} represents the number of dendrons per self-assembled nanostructure. [e] ΔG_{mic} (kcal/mol) represents the energy of micellisation. [f] σ_m (e/nm^2) is the surface charge density of the self-assemblies. [g] ΔG_{bind} (kcal/mol) is determined by combined molecular dynamics and mesoscale modelling for the binding of dendrons to DNA.

We monitored the self-assembly of these dendrons using a Nile Red assay,[48] in which the hydrophobic dye is solubilised at concentrations above the critical micelle concentration (CMC, Table 4). As might be expected, the systems with more hydrophobic functionalisation assemble at lower concentrations, as the larger hydrophobic surface provides a greater driving force. Control **G2-DEG-DAPMA** did not aggregate <1 mM. For alkyl chain modified dendrons, as the hydrophobic chain at the focal point increases in length from C$_{12}$ to C$_{22}$, the CMC value drops from 208 μM to 2 μM, presumably a consequence of more effective packing of the longer hydrophobic chain. Cholesterol-functionalized dendrons exhibited low CMCs. Zeta sizing indicated that unfunctionalised **G2** and **C$_{12}$** systems assembled poorly. Conversely, **Chol**, **Chol$_2$**, and **C$_{22}$** functionalised systems formed well-defined aggregates with high zeta potentials. As the size of the hydrophobic unit increases, so did the diameter of the nanoscale assembly, from ca. 5.9 nm for C_{16} to 7.0 nm for C_{22} and 7.5 nm for **Chol**. Intriguingly, the assemblies formed by **Chol-G2-DEG-DAPMA** were significantly smaller than those formed by **Chol$_2$-G2-DEG-DAPMA**, although they exhibited roughly the same zeta potentials.

Multiscale modeling (Table 4) agreed with the experimental study in suggesting that, with the exception of **G2-DEG-DAPMA**, all dendrons self-assembled. It is possible to simulate the Gibbs free energy of transfer of a single amphiphilic molecule from the monomeric state to a micelle of aggregation number N_{agg}, commonly called the free energy of micellisation ΔG_{mic}. Pleasingly these values were in general agreement with the experimentally observed CMC values – as self-assembly becomes thermodynamically more favourable, the experimentally-observed CMC drops. Furthermore the trend in sizes of nanostructures was predicted by the modelling. There were some differences between theoretical and experimental D_m values – however, the general trends were reproduced. It must be remembered that these structures are solvated, and even though the modelling is performed in the presence of solvent, the hydrodynamic diameter determined experimentally will include solvent molecules, while these are not explicitly included in the diameters extracted from modelling – furthermore, the mesoscale methods applied somewhat under-estimate the dimensions of self-assemblies.

We then monitored the ability of the self-assemblies to bind DNA. Once again, the hydrophobic units induced large changes in DNA-binding ability (Table 4). The compounds which did not self-assemble well, were unable to bind DNA effectively. Conversely, the dendrons which self-assemble more effectively were much better DNA binders. Modelling suggested that increasing the alkyl chain length led to an increase in micellar surface charge density (σ_m) and improved DNA binding ability. We then performed a more detailed inspection by theoretical methods to try and unpick the subtle differences in binding. Quantitative modeling of micelle/DNA interactions at a fully atomistic level was used to rank the affinity of each type of modified dendron micelle towards DNA, ΔG_{bind}. This demonstrated that **Chol$_2$-G2-DEG-DAPMA** is a more effective binder than **Chol-G2-DEG-DAPMA**, in agreement with the experimental evidence, even though it has similar charge density. We suggest that the larger micelle size of **Chol$_2$-G2-DAPMA** plays a crucial role in allowing the charges to bind to the DNA double helix without overcrowding – as such, the ligands can be considered to be in a less overcrowded self-assembled nanoscale environment, making them more available for DNA binding. This is clearly related to the morphological effects described in Section 4.3.

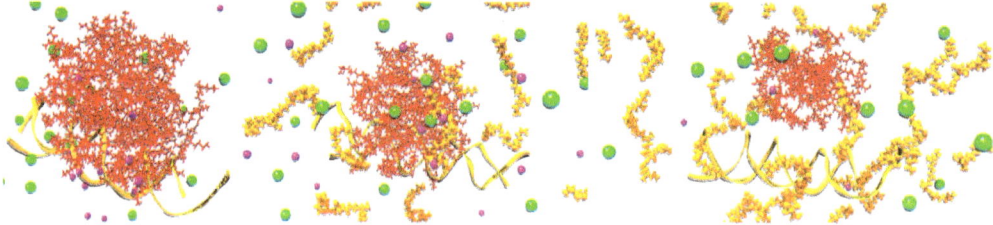

Figure 13 *Modelling the degradation and DNA binding ability of **Chol-G2-DEG-DAPMA***

A key feature of these dendrons was their potential to degrade under biologically relevant conditions, hence leading to self-assembled temporary multivalency. We used multiscale modelling to confirm that dendron degradation should lead to DNA release (Fig. 13). We detached surface ligands from the dendron by *in silico* degradation, and monitored the binding thermodynamics by MM/PBSA calculations. As the ligands were detached, DNA binding affinity decreased. Interestingly, the loss of DNA affinity was more marked for **Chol-G2-DEG-DAPMA** than the **Chol$_2$** analogue. We suggest this is a consequence of the two hydrophobic cholesterol units in **Chol₂-G2-DEG-DAPMA** being better able to maintain the self-assembled multivalent nanostructure during degradation, retaining a higher surface charge density, and allowing the nanostructure to bind DNA. These modeling observations agreed with our experimental results for gene delivery, in which **Chol-G2-DEG-DAPMA** was the better vector in transfection experiments.

An electrospray mass spectrometric assay was then used to probe dendron degradation experimentally at pH 7.4. We could determine the rate of loss of peaks associated with the dendron, and identify degradation products. Initially one of the branches is disconnected by ester bond hydrolysis. After this initial hydrolysis, the carboxylic acid undergoes decarboxylation. Subsequently, the second branch disconnects via ester hydrolysis. All dendrons degraded via the same pathway. The non-self-assembling dendron **G2-DEG-DAPMA** has an initial degradation rate of ca. 10.1 mmoldm^{-3h-1} at pH 7.4 – much faster than observed by Fréchet and co-workers for the same type of framework.[23] We suggested that the amine groups on our dendron periphery play an intramolecular role in catalyzing degradation. Interestingly, self-assembly appeared to have some impact on the rate of degradation, but these effects could not fully be rationalised.

Unfortunately, even though these dendrons have well-defined modes of degradation, which should diminish their affinity for DNA and enable DNA release, they did not appear to degrade within the cell and gave poor levels of transfection. We found that when complexed to DNA, the degradation of the dendron was prevented. We reasoned that the presence of DNA inhibits amine-catalysed intramolecular breakdown of the dendron framework. We are now developing systems which degrade via a different mechanism.

4.5 Self-Assembled Multivalency and Other Nanoscale Biological Targets – Heparin

Given we had developed a series of polycationic multivalent self-assembling dendrons which could bind polyanionic DNA with high-affinity as described above, we became interested in whether this type of system was also capable of binding to heparin. Heparin binding is a key medical target because this important anti-coagulant plays a key role *in vivo* during surgery.[49] When surgery is complete, a heparin reversal agent, protamine (a cationic protein), has to be employed, but unfortunately causes a significant number of negative side-effects.[50] There is therefore considerable interest in developing novel heparin reversal agents as protamine replacements.[51] We reasoned that self-assembled nanostructures might mimic protamine in terms of size and surface charge, but could potentially have better clinical outcomes as a consequence of the synthetic versatility and the potential of these nanostructures to degrade and/or disassemble.

We developed a self-assembling system, **C22-G1-DEG-DAPMA** using a combination of Fréchet dendron and click chemistry methodology (Fig. 14).[52] A Nile Red assay was used to demonstrate that the CMC of the dendron was 3.9±0.25 μM. We then employed a methylene blue displacement assay to determine the affinity of our self-assembled system for heparin (M_r 15,000 ± 2,000 Da).[53] In particular, in 1 mM tris buffer and 5 mM NaCl, the CE$_{50}$ (required to dsiplae 50% of methylene blue from its complex with heparin) was 0.74±0.10 for the dendron and 1.16±0.15 for protamine, i.e., the self-assembled system bound heparin with an affinity better than that of multivalent protamine. We used transmission electron microscopy (TEM) to visualise the self-assembling nanostructures. Nanospherical aggregates could be observed (diameter 8.5±1.5 nm), which in the absence of heparin were spread evenly across the TEM image. However, in the presence of heparin, the self-assembled micelles (diameter 6.5±1.0 nm) were preferentially located on the surface of heparin crystals and there was some evidence they were aligned along it in an ordered, nano-structured way. Importantly, heparin binding did not appear to induce loss in stability, morphological change or rearrangement of the nanoscale assemblies.

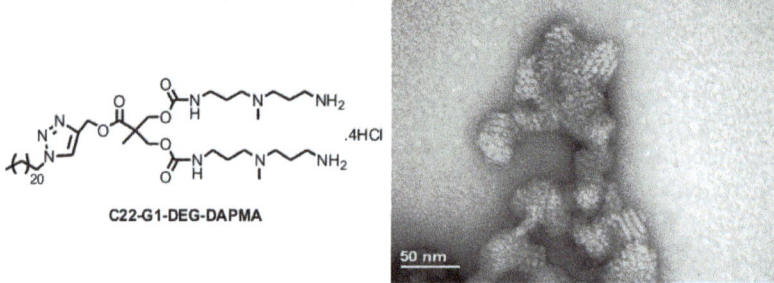

Figure 14 *Compound **C22-G1-DEG-DAPMA** and TEM image of the self-assembled spherical nanostructures in the presence of heparin*

We have recently started collaborative theoretical multiscale modelling of these heparin-binding nanostructures, and in this way, are gaining fundamental insight into differences between heparin binding and DNA binding. Furthermore, we intend to use the resulting insight to develop self-assembling systems which have high heparin affinity, low toxicity, stability in serum, and as a consequence, potential biomedical application.

4.6 Self-Assembled Multivalency and Other Nanoscale Biological Targets – Integrin

In addition to binding polyanions, we have been interested in multivalency effects in binding integrins – heterodimeric, transmembrane proteins with biological roles in cell signalling and adhesion, making them of interest in tissue engineering.[54] Some integrins are also over expressed on the surface of cancer cells making them an interesting target for anti-cancer treatments.[55] Arg-Gly-Asp (RGD) peptides have been shown to bind to integrins.[56] Integrin itself only has a single RGD binding site, and as such, the only benefits of multivalent binding to free integrin would appear to be limited to an effective ligand concentration effect. However, in biological systems, integrins are found in cell membranes and cluster in order to achieve focal adhesion – as such multivalency can offer additional benefits to binding. A number of reports of RGD-functionalised dendrimers binding integrin, with some increase in binding affinity have been published.[57]

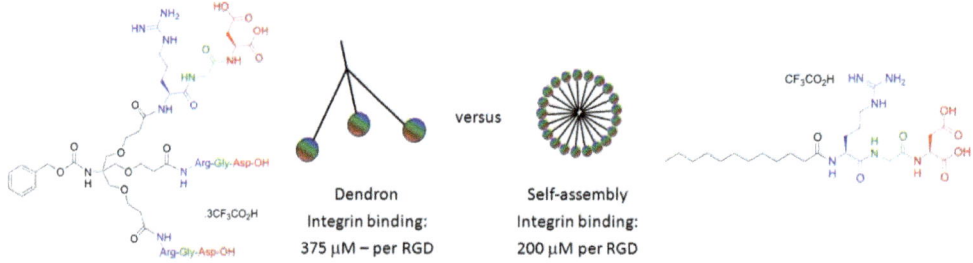

Figure 15 *Dendritic (left) versus self-assembled (right) multivalency in integrin binding*

We therefore wanted to quantify the difference between dendritic multivalency and self-assembled multivalency to determine whether there were fundamental differences between these approaches.[58] We synthesised **G1-RGD** (Fig. 15) and **G2-RGD** based on Newkome-type dendron scaffolds and assayed the ability of these compounds to bind integrin $\alpha_v\beta_3$, suspended in Triton X-100 surfactant using the displacement of a fluorescent probe from the integrin binding site, and monitoring the process by fluorescence polarisation.[59] The use of integrin in Triton X-100 mimics integrin proteins supported in a cell membrane. This assay gave us EC_{50} values for the binding of the RGD ligand to the protein – the effective concentration required to displace 50% of the fluorescent probe from the integrin binding site. We initially compared the performance of pure dendrons with a monovalent analogue. First generation **G1-RGD** was the most effective binding agent. The monovalent analogue was ineffective in the assay. Furthermore, more highly branched **G2-RGD** was not as good as **G1-RGD**, due to non-specific electrostatic binding effects and possibile crowding of the RGD ligands. We then tested a self-assembling monovalent RGD derivative, **C12-RGD** to compare it with the dendritic systems (Fig. 15). **C12-RGD** assembled into a spherical nanoscale architecture, and bound integrin much more effectively (EC_{50} = 200 μM) than the non-assembling monovalent analogue (EC_{50} > 1 mM). Notably, the self-assembly strategy was comparable to, if not more effective than, **G1-RGD** (EC_{50} = 125 μM, per RGD unit = 375 μM). This demonstrated that self-assembly is an effective strategy for ligand organisation and can compete, or be combined, with a dendritic approach. Self-assembly may even generate higher ligand densities, or systems which are more responsive and able to satisfy their biological binding partners.

5 SUMMARY AND PERSPECTIVES

In summary, dendrimers are fascinating multivalent systems which can bind nanoscale biological targets with enhanced affinity. By using a combined experimental and theoretical approach, we have been able to gain new insights into multivalent binding effects in dendrons. We have elucidated a novel 'sacrifice and screening' effect in which flexible multivalent arrays are able to optimise their interactions with a biological target.[9,15] Furthermore, we were able to dissect the thermodynamic parameters which underpin binding, leading us to conclude that not every charge is the same, and the charge-display on the multivalent array is crucial in optimising the entropic cost of binding.[18]

We then harnessed one of the real advantages of working with dendrons, modifying the focal point to enable the self-assembly of supramolecular dendrimers in which the multivalency gets multiplied up.[39] Once again, combining experimental and theoretical methods allowed us to understand how the self-organising hydrophobic units in the core of the supramolecular dendrimer tune the overall surface charge of the assembly, and hence the multivalent interactions with the binding partner. In this way, a lower generation dendron can even perform better than a higher generation analogue as a consequence of self-assembly.[41] We have also shown how degradability can be modelled, and elucidated the way in which as systems degrade, self-assembly can modify the affinity with which they continue to bind to their biological partners.[47] Furthermore, we have learned that dendron degradation is highly dependent on pH, nanostructure and the presence of the biological binding partner.

Finally, we have begun to explore multivalency effects in binding different biological targets. This has allowed us to generate self-assembling systems with high affinity for heparin,[52] and our work with RGD peptides has demonstrated that the self-assembly approach to multivalency can be competitive, in terms of binding affinity with a full dendritic approach.[58]

We believe that the combination of experiment and theory which we have been applying in this area is a powerful one, both in terms of providing fundamental insight into nanoscale recognition processes and enabling potential future applications in nanomedicine. In due course, we hope that this strategy will lead to novel nanoscale therapies for direct intervention *in vivo*.

6 REFERENCES

1 (*a*) F. Vögtle, G. Reichardt, N. Werner and A. J. Rackstraw, *Dendrimer Chemistry – Concepts, Syntheses, Properties, Applications*, Wiley-VCH, Weinheim, 2009. (*b*) G. R. Newkome and C. N. Moorefield, *Handbook of Dendrimers: Synthesis, Nanoscience and Applications*, Wiley-VCH, Weinheim, 2009.

2 (*a*) O. Rolland, C.-O. Turrin, A.-M. Caminade and J.-P. Marjoral, *New J. Chem.* 2009, **33**, 1809. (*b*) U. Boas, J.B. Christensen and P.M.H. Heegaard, *Dendrimers in Medicine and Biotechnology*, Royal Society of Chemistry, Cambridge, 2006. (*c*) B. Klajnert and M. Bryszewska, *Dendrimers in Medicine*, Nova Science, UK, 2007.

3 (*a*) M. Mammen, S.K. Choi and G.M. Whitesides, *Angew. Chem. Int. Ed.* 1998, **37**, 2755. (*b*) A. Mulder, J. Huskens and D.N. Reinhoudt, *Org. Biomol. Chem.* 2004, **2**, 3409. (*c*) J.D. Badjic, A. Nelson, S.J. Cantrill, W.B. Turnbull and J.F. Stoddart, *Acc. Chem. Res.* 2005, **38**, 723. (*d*) V. Martos, P. Castreño, J. Valero and J. de Mendoza, *Curr. Opin. Chem. Biol.* 2008, **12**, 698. (*e*) C. Fasting, C.A. Schalley, M. Weber, O. Seitz, S. Hecht, B. Koksch, J. Dernedde, C. Graf, E.W. Knapp and R. Haag, *Angew. Chem. Int. Ed.* 2012, **51**, 10472.

4 L. Mandolini, *Adv. Phys. Org. Chem.* 1986, **22**, 1.

5 J. Huskens, A. Mulder, T. Auletta, C. A. Nijhuis, M.J.W. Ludden and D.N. Reinhoudt, *J. Am. Chem. Soc.* 2004, **126**, 6784.

6 A. Barnard and D.K. Smith, *Angew. Chem. Int. Ed.* 2012, **51**, 6572.

7 For classic examples of dendrimers which bind and deliver DNA see: (*a*) J.-F. Kukowska-Latallo, A.U. Bielinska, J. Johnson, R. Spindler, D.A. Tomalia and J.R. Baker, *Proc. Natl. Acad. Sci. USA* 1996, **93**, 4897. (*b*) J. Haensler and F.C. Szoka, *Bioconjugate Chem.* 1993, **4**, 372. (*c*) J.S. Choi, E. J. Lee, Y.H. Choi, Y.J. Jeong and J.S. Park, *Bioconjugate Chem.* 1999, **10**, 62.

8 (*a*) M.L. Edelstein, M.R. Abedi and J. Wixon, *J. Gene Med.* 2007, **9**, 833. (*b*) M.A. Mintzer and E.E. Simanek, *Chem. Rev.* 2009, **109**, 259.

9 M.A. Kostiainen, J.G. Hardy and D.K. Smith, *Angew. Chem. Int. Ed.* 2005, **44**, 2556.

10 (*a*) G.R. Newkome and X. Lin, *Macromolecules* 1991, **24**, 1443. (*b*) J. K. Young, G. R. Baker, G.R. Newkome, K.F. Morris and C.S. Johnson Jr., *Macromolecules* 1994, **27**, 3464. (*c*) C.M. Cordona, R.E. Gawley and C. Gawley, *J. Org. Chem.* 2002, **67**, 1411.

11 (*a*) S.S. Cohen, *A Guide to Polyamines*, Oxford University Press, Oxford, 1998. (*b*) K. Igarashi and K. Kashiwagi, *Biochem. Biophys. Res. Commun.* 2000, **271**, 559.

12 (*a*) D. Bancroft, I.D. Williams, A. Rich and M. Egli, *Biochemistry* 1994, **33**, 1073. (*b*) V.A. Bloomfield, *Biopolymers* 1997, **44**, 269. (*c*) M. Saminathan, T. Anthony, A. Shirahata, L.H. Sigal, T. Thomas and T.J. Thomas, *Biochemistry* 1999, **38**, 3821. (*d*) Y. Burak, G. Ariel and D. Andelman, *Biophys. J.* 2003, **85**, 2100. (*e*) L. D'Agostino, M. di Pietro and A. Di Luccia, *FEBS J.* 2005, **272**, 3777.

13 (*a*) N. Korolev, A.P. Lyubartsev, A. Laaksonen and L. Nordenskiöld, *Biophys. J.* 2002, **82**, 2860. (b) N. Korolev, A.P. Lyubartsev, A. Laaksonen and L. Nordenskiöld, *Nucleic Acids Res.* 2003, **30**, 5971. (c) N. Korolev, A.P. Lyubartsev, A. Laaksonen and L. Nordenskiöld, *Eur. Biophys. J.* 2004, **33**, 671.

14 (*a*) B.F. Cain, B.C. Baguley and W.A. Denny, *J. Med. Chem.* 1978, **21**, 658. (*b*) H. Gershon, R. Ghirlando, S.B. Guttman and A. Minsky, *Biochemistry* 1993, **32**, 7143.

15 G.M. Pavan, A. Danani, S. Pricl and D.K. Smith, *J. Am. Chem. Soc.* 2009, **131**, 9686.

16 D.A. Case, T.A. Darden, T.E. Cheatham *et al. AMBER 9*, University of California, San Francisco, CA USA, 2006.

17 W.L. Jorgensen J. Chandrasekhar, J.D. Madura, R.W. Impey and M.L. Klein, *J. Chem. Phys.* 1983, **79**, 926.

18 S.P. Jones, G.M. Pavan, A. Danani, S. Pricl and D.K. Smith, *Chem. Eur. J.* 2010, **16**, 4519.

19 (*a*) J.-h.S. Kuo and Y.L. Lin, *J. Biotechnol.* 2007, **129**, 383. (*b*) J.-h.S. Kuo, M.-j. Liou and H.-c. Chiu, *Mol. Pharm.* 2010, **7**, 805.

20 J. Luten, C.F. van Nostruin, S.C. De Smedt, W.E. Hennink, *J. Controlled Rel.* 2008, **126**, 97.

21 M.A. Kostiainen, D.K. Smith and O. Ikkala, *Angew. Chem. Int. Ed.* **2007**, *46*, 7600.

22 (*a*) M.A. Kostiainen and H. Rosilo, H. *Chem. Eur. J.* 2009, **15**, 5656. (*b*) G.M. Pavan, M.A. Kostiainen and A. Danani, *J. Phys. Chem. B* 2010, **114**, 5686. (*c*) M.A. Kostiainen, J. Kotimaa, M.L. Laukkanen and G.M. Pavan, *Chem. Eur. J.* 2010, **16**, 6912. (*d*) M.A. Kostiainen, O. Kasyutich, J.J.L.M. Cornelissen and R.J.M. Nolte, *Nature Chem.* 2010, **2**, 394.

23 (*a*) E.R. Gillies and J.M.J. Fréchet, *J. Am. Chem. Soc.* 2002, **124**, 14137. (*b*) E.R. Gillies, E. Dy, J.M.J. Fréchet and F.C. Szoka, *Mol. Pharm.* 2005, **2**, 129. (*c*) C.C. Lee, E.R. Gillies, M.E. Fox, S.J. Guillaudeu, J.M.J. Fréchet, E.E. Dy and F.C. Szoka, *Proc. Natl. Acad. Sci. USA* 2006, **103**, 16649.

24 (*a*) H. Ihre, A. Hult and E. Soederlind, *J. Am. Chem. Soc.* 1996, **118**, 6388. (*b*) H. Ihre, A. Hult, J.M.J. Fréchet and I. Gitsov, *Macromolecules* 1998, **31**, 4061.

25 D.J. Welsh, S.P. Jones and D.K. Smith, *Angew. Chem. Int. Ed.* 2009, **48**, 4047.

26 J.G. Hardy, M.A. Kostiainen, D.K. Smith, N.P. Gabrielson and D.W. Pack, *Bioconjugate Chem.* 2006, **17**, 172.

27 (*a*) C. Dufes, I.F. Uchegbu and A. G. Schatzlein, *Adv. Drug Deliv. Rev.* 2005, **57**, 2177. (*b*) M. Guillot-Nieckowski, S. Eisler and F. Diederich, *New J. Chem.* 2007, **31**, 1111. (*c*) D.K. Smith, *Curr. Top. Med. Chem.* 2008, **8**, 1187.

28 (*a*) D.K. Smith, A.R. Hirst, C.S. Love, J.G. Hardy, S.V. Brignell and B. Huang, *Prog. Polym. Sci.* 2005, **30**, 220. (*b*) B.M. Rosen, C.J. Wilson, D.A. Wilson, M. Peterca, M.R. Imam and V. Percec, *Chem. Rev.* 2009, **109**, 6275.

29 (*a*) S.C. Zimmerman, F. Zeng, D.E.C. Reichert and S.V. Kolotuchin, *Science* 1996, **271**, 1095. (*b*) F. Zeng, S.C. Zimmerman, S.V. Kolotuchin, D.E.C. Reichert, Y.G. Ma, *Tetrahedron* 2002, **58**, 825. (*c*) P.S. Corbin, L.J. Lawless, Z.T. Li, Y.G. Ma, M.J. Witmer, S.C. Zimmerman, *Proc. Natl. Acad. Sci. USA* 2002, **99**, 5099. (d) Y. Ma, S.V. Kolotuchin, S.C. Zimmerman, *J. Am. Chem. Soc.* 2002, **124**, 13757.

30 (*a*) E.R. Gillies, J.M.J. Fréchet, *J. Org. Chem.* 2004, **69**, 46. (*b*) G.M. Dykes, L.J. Brierley, D.K. Smith, P.T. McGrail and G.J. Seeley, *Chem. Eur. J.* 2001, **7**, 4730. (*c*) G.M. Dykes, D.K. Smith, and G.J. Seeley, *Angew. Chem. Int. Ed.* 2002, **41**, 3254. (*d*) N. Yamaguchi, L.M. Hamilton and H.W. Gibson, *Angew. Chem. Int. Ed.* 1998, **37**, 3275. (*e*) H.W. Gibson, N. Yamaguchi, L. Hamilton and J.W. Jones, *J. Am. Chem. Soc.* 2002, **124**, 4653. (*f*) A.M. Elizarov, S.-H. Chiu, P.T. Glink, J.F. Stoddart, *Org. Lett.* 2002, **4**, 679. (*g*) H.-F. Chow, I.Y.-K. Chan, P.-S. Fung, T.K.-K. Mong and M.F. Nongrum, *Tetrahedron* 2001, **57**, 1565. (*h*) M. Kawa and J.M.J. Fréchet, *Chem. Mater.* 1998, **10**, 286. (*i*) D.L. Stone, G.M. Dykes and D.K. Smith *Dalton Trans.* 2003, 3902.

31 (*a*) J.C.M. van Hest, D.A.P. Delnoye, M.W.P.L. Baars, M.H.P. van Genderen and E.W. Meijer, *Science* 1995, **268**, 1592. (*b*) J.C.M. van Hest, D.A.P. Delnoye, M.W.P.L. Baars, C. Elissen-Román, M.H.P. van Genderen and E.W. Meijer, *Chem. Eur. J.* 1996, **2**, 1616.

32 J.E. Kingerywood, K.W. Williams, G.B. Sigal and G.M. Whitesides, *J. Am. Chem. Soc.* 1992, **114**, 7303.

33 (*a*) J.A. Zupancich, F.S. Bates and M.A. Hillmyer, *Biomacromolecules* 2009, **10**, 1554. (*b*) Y.-B. Lim, E. Lee and M. Lee, *Angew. Chem. Int. Ed.* 2007, **46**, 3475. (*c*) Y.-B. Lim, O.-J. Kwon, E. Lee, P.-H. Kim, C.-O. Yun and M. Lee, *Org. Biomol. Chem.*, 2008, **6**, 1944. (*d*) M.O. Guler, L. Hsu, S. Soukasene, D.A. Harrington, J.F. Hulvat and S.I. Stupp, *Biomacromolecules* 2006, **7**, 1855. (*e*) Z. Huang, T.D. Sargeant, J.F. Hulvat, A. Mata, P. Bringas, C.-Y. Koh, S.I. Stupp and M.L. Snead, *J. Bone and Mineral Res.* 2008, **23**, 1995. (*f*) M. Zhou, A.M. Smith, A.K. Das, N.W. Hodgson, R.F. Collins, R.V. Ulijn and J.E. Gough, *Biomaterials* 2009, **30**, 2523.

34 (*a*) I. Toth, T. Sakthivel, A.F. Wilderspin, H. Bayele, M. O'Donnell, D.J. Perry, K.J. Pasi, C.A. Lee and A.T. Florence, *STP Pharm. Sci.* 1999, **9**, 93. (*b*) D.S. Shah, T. Sakthivel, I. Toth, A.T. Florence and A.F. Wilderspin, *Int. J. Pharm.* 2000, **208**, 41. (*c*) K.T. Al-Jamal, C. Ramaswamy, B. Singh and A.T. Florence, *J. Drug Deliv. Sci. Technol.* 2005, **15**, 11. (*d*) H.K. Bayele, T. Sakthivel, M. O'Donell, K.J. Pasi, A.F. Wilderspin, C.A. Lee, I. Toth and A.T. Florence, *J. Pharm. Sci.* 2005, **94**, 446. (*e*) H.K. Bayele, C. Ramaswamy, A.F. Wilderspin, K.S. Srai, I. Toth and A.T. Florence, *J. Pharm. Sci.* 2006, **95**, 1227.

35 (*a*) K.C. Wood, S.R. Little, R. Langer and P.T. Hammond, *Angew. Chem. Int. Ed.* 2005, **44**, 6704. (*b*) K.C. Wood, S.M. Azarin, W. Arap, R. Pasqualini, R. Langer, P.T. Hammond, *Bioconjugate Chem.* 2008, **19**, 403. (*c*) Z. Poon, J.A. Lee, S. Huang, R. J. Prevost and P.T. Hammond, *Nanomedicine* 2011, **7**, 201

36 (*a*) D. Joester, M. Losson, R. Pugin, H. Heinzelmann, E. Walter, H.P. Merkle and F. Diederich, *Angew. Chem. Int. Ed.* 2003, **42**, 1486. (*b*) M. Guillot, S. Eisler, K. Weller, H.P. Merkle, J.L. Gallani and F. Diederich, *Org. Biomol. Chem.* 2006, **4**, 766.

37 S. Malhotra, H. Bauer, A. Tschiche, A. M. Staedtler, A. Mohr, M. Calderon, V.S. Parmar, L. Hoeke, S. Sharbati, R. Einspanier and R. Haag, *Biomacromolecules* 2012, **13**, 3087.

38 T. Yu, X. Liu, A.L. Bolcato-Bellemin, Y. Wang, C. Liu, P. Erbacher, F. Qu, P. Rocchi, J.-P. Behr and L. Peng, *Angew, Chem. Int. Ed.* 2012, **51**, 8478.

39 S.P. Jones, N.P. Gabrielson, C.-H. Wong, H.-F. Chow, D.W. Pack, P. Posocco, M. Fermeglia, S. Pricl and D.K. Smith, *Mol Pharm*, 2011, **8**, 416.

40 (*a*) P.J. Hoogerbrugge, J. Koelman, *Europhys. Lett.* 1992, **19**, 155. (*b*) P. Español and P. Warren, *Europhys. Lett.* 1995, **30**, 191. (*c*) R.D. Groot and P.B. Warren, *J. Chem. Phys.* 1997, **107**, 4423. (*d*) R.D. Groot and K.L. Rabone, *Biophys. J.* 2001, **81**, 725.

41 P. Posocco, S. Pricl, S. Jones, A. Barnard and D.K. Smith, *Chem. Sci.* 2010, **1**, 393

42 (*a*) J.N. Israelachvili, D.J. Mitchell and B.W. Ninham, *J. Chem. Soc. Faraday Trans.II* 1976, **72**, 1525. (*b*) J.N. Israelachvili, D.J. Mitchell and B.W. Ninham, *Biochim. Biophys. Acta* 1977, **470**, 185.

43 S.P. Jones, N.P. Gabrielson, D.W. Pack and D.K. Smith, *Chem Commun*, **2008**, 4700.

44 (*a*) I. S. Zuhorn, J. B. F. N. Engberts and D. Hoekstra, *Eur. Biophys. J. Biophys. Lett.* 2007, **36**, 349. (*b*) J. O. Radler, I. Koltover, T. Salditt and C. R. Safinya, *Science* 1996, **275**, 810. (*c*) A. El Oahabi, M. Thiry, V. Pector, R. Fuks, J. M. Ruysschaert and M. van den Branden, *FEBS Lett.* 1997, **414**, 187.

45 P. Wu, M. Malkoch, J.N. Hunt, R. Vestberg, E. Kaltgrad, M.J. Finn, V.V. Fokin, K.B. Sharpless, C.J. Hawker, *Chem. Commun.* 2005, 5775.

46 H.C. Kolb, M.G. Finn and K.B. Sharpless, *Angew. Chem. Int. Ed.* **2001**, *40*, 2004.

47 A. Barnard, P. Posocco, S. Pricl, M. Calderon, R. Haag, M.E. Hwang, V.T. Shum, D.W. Pack and D.K. Smith, *J. Am. Chem. Soc.* 2011, **133**, 20288.

48 M.C.A. Stuart, J.C. van de Pas and J.B.F.N. Engberts, *J. Phys. Org. Chem.* 2005, **18**, 929.

49 (*a*) D.L. Rabenstein, *Nat. Prod. Rep.* 2002, **19**, 312. (*b*) S. Middeldorp, *Thrombosis Res.* 2008, **122**, 753. (*c*) N.S. Gandhi and R.L. Mancera, *Drug Disc. Today* 2010, **15**, 1058.

50 (*a*) J.C. Horrow, *Anesthesia and Analgesia* 1985, **64**, 348. (*b*) S.E. Kimmel, M.A. Sekeres, J.A. Berlin, L.R. Goldberg and B.L. Strom, *J. Clin. Epidemiol.* 1998, **51**, 1. (*c*) R. Porsche and Z.R. Brenner, *Heart Lung* 1999, **28**, 418. (*d*) M. Nybo and J.S. Madsen, *Basic Clin. Pharmacol.* 2008, **103**, 192. (*e*) Y.-Q. Chu, J.-J. Cai, D.-C. Jiang, D. Jia, S.-Y. Yan and Y.-Q. Wang, *Clin. Ther.* 2010, **32**, 1729. (*f*) J.J. van Veen, R.M. Maclean, K.K. Hampton, S. Laidlaw, S. Kitchen, P. Toth and M. Makris, *Blood Coagulation and Fibrinolysis* 2011, **22**, 565.

51 (*a*) T.W. Wakefield, P.C. Andrews, S.K. Wrobleski, A.M. Kadell, A. Fazzalari, B.J. Nichol, T. Van der Kooi and J.C. Stanley, *J. Surgical Res.* 1993, **56**, 586. (*b*) M. Kikura, M.K. Lee and J.H. Levy, *Anesthesia & Analgesia* 1996, **83**, 223. (*c*) M. Schuksz, M.M. Fuster, J.R. Brown, B.E. Crawford, D.P. Ditto, R. Lawrence, C.A. Glass, L. Wang, Y. Tor and J.D. Esko, *Proc. Natl. Acad. Sci. USA* 2008, **105**, 13075. (*d*) B. Kalaska, E. Sokolowska, K. Kaminski, K. Szczubialka, K. Kramkowski, A. Mogielnicki, M. Nowakowska and W. Buczko, *Eur. J. Pharm.* 2012, **686**, 81.

52 A.C. Rodrigo, A. Barnard, J. Cooper and D.K. Smith, *Angew. Chem. Int. Ed.* **2011**, *50*, 4675.

53 Q.C. Jiao, Q. Liu, C. Sun and H. He, *Talanta* 1999, **48**, 1095.

54 (*a*) R.O. Hynes, *Cell* 1992, **69**, 11. (*b*) L. Perlin, S. MacNeil and S. Rimmer, *Soft Matter* 2008, **4**, 2331.

55 (*a*) P.C. Brooks, A.M.P. Montgomery, M. Rosenfeld, R.A. Reisfeld, T.H. Hu, G. Klier and D.A. Cheresh, *Cell* 1994, **79**, 1157. (*b*) P.C. Brooks, R.A.F. Clark and D.A. Cheresh, *Science* 1994, **264**, 569.

56 M.D. Pierschbacher and E. Ruoslahti, *Nature* 1984, **309**, 30.

57 (*a*) D.T.S. Rijkers, G.W. van Esse, R. Merkx, A.J. Brouwer, H.J.F. Jacobs, R.J. Pieters and R.M.J. Liskamp, *Chem. Commun.* 2005, 4581. (*b*) I. Dijkgraaf, A.Y. Rijnders, A. Soede, A.C. Dechesne, G.W. van Esse, A.J. Brouwer, F.H.M. Corstens, O.C. Boerman, D.T.S. Rijkers and R.M.J. Liskamp, *Org. Biomol. Chem.* 2007, **5**, 935. (*c*) E. Garanger, D. Boturyn, Z.H. Jin, P. Dumy, M.C. Favrot and J.L. Coll, *Mol. Ther.* 2005, **12**, 1168. (*d*) E. Garanger, D. Boturyn, J.L. Coll, M.C. Favrot and P. Dumy, *Org. Biomol. Chem.* 2006, **4**, 1958.

58 D.J. Welsh and D.K. Smith, *Org. Biomol. Chem.* 2011, **9**, 4795.

59 W. Wang, Q. Wu, M. Pasuelo, J.S. McMurray and C. Li, *Bioconjugate Chem.* 2005, **16**, 729.

Subject index